UNDERSTANDING AND CARING FOR HUMAN DISEASES

Understanding and Caring for Human Diseases

Marcia Borgstadt, RN

Delmar Publishers

I ⓣ P™ An International Thomson Publishing Company

Albany • Bonn • Boston • Cincinnati • Detroit • London • Madrid
Melbourne • Mexico City • New York • Pacific Grove • Paris • San Francisco
Singapore • Tokyo • Toronto • Washington

NOTICE TO THE READER

f the products described herein or perform any independent analysis in connection with any of
sher does not assume, and expressly disclaims, any obligation to obtain and include information
rer.

nd adopt all safety precautions that might be indicated by the activities described herein and to avoid all potential hazards. By following the instructions contained herein, the reader willingly assumes all risks in connection with such instructions.

The publisher makes no representations or warranties of any kind, including but not limited to, the warranties of fitness for particular purpose or merchantability, nor are any such representations implied with respect to the material set forth herein, and the publisher takes no responsibility with respect to such material. The publisher shall not be liable for any special, consequential, or exemplary damages resulting, in whole or in part, from the readers' use of, or reliance upon, this material.

Cover photos: (right) From Hegner, *Nursing Assistant: A Nursing Process Approach, 7th edition,* copyright © 1995, Delmar Publishers; (left) From Keir, et al., *Medical Assisting: Administrative and Clinical Competencies, 3rd edition,* copyright © 1993, Delmar Publishers

Cover design courtesy John DiSieno

Delmar Staff:
Publisher: Tim O'Leary
Acquisitions Editor: Sandy Clark
Senior Project Editor: Andrea Edwards Myers
Production Editor: Carolyn Miller
Marketing Manager: Maura Theriault

COPYRIGHT © 1997
By Delmar Publishers
a division of International Thomson Publishing Inc.

The ITP logo is a trademark under license

Printed in the United States of America

For more information, contact:

Delmar Publishers
3 Columbia Circle, Box 15015
Albany, New York 12212-5015

International Thomson Publishing Europe
Berkshire House 168–173
High Holborn
London, WC1V 7AA
England

Thomas Nelson Australia
102 Dodds Street
South Melbourne, 3205
Victoria, Australia

Nelson Canada
1120 Birchmount Road
Scarborough, Ontario
Canada M1K 5G4

International Thomson Editores
Campos Eliseos 385, Piso 7
Col Polanco
11560 Mexico D F Mexico

International Thomson Publishing Gmbh
Königswinterer Strasse 418
53227 Bonn
Germany

International Thomson Publishing Asia
221 Henderson Road #05–10
Henderson Building
Singapore 0315

International Thomson Publishing – Japan
Hirakawacho Kyowa Building, 3F
2-2-1 Hirakawacho
Chiyoda-ku, 102 Tokyo
Japan

1 2 3 4 5 6 7 8 9 10 XXX 02 01 00 99 98 97 96

Library of Congress Cataloging-in-Publication Data

Borgstadt, Marcia.
    Understanding and caring for human diseases / Marcia Borgstadt.
       p.   cm.
    Includes bibliographical references and index.
    ISBN 0-8273-6605-1
    1. Medicine—Vocational guidance—Juvenile literature.
    [1. Medicine—Vocational guidance. 2. Health occupations.
    3. Vocational guidance.] I. Title.
    R690.B646 1996   95-13518
    616—dc20   CIP
                                             AC

Contents

Preface

Understanding and Caring for Human Diseases is based on course materials successfully used in practice for several years. Targeted for advanced health occupations course work, this textbook provides an understanding of basic human diseases to students who may branch off into the many diversified health occupations fields. All health care professionals must have a basic understanding of diseases and their attendant care. With this understanding, they are able to provide comfort and basic care tailored to the specific needs of their patients as determined by their conditions. In addition, with knowledge of diseases and their care, health care providers at any level are better able to note and report any situations that require immediate intervention.

This comprehensive text on understanding human diseases makes the subject matter interesting and easy to follow. The text is divided into units according to body systems and major disease categories. Chapters include the following components as appropriate to the particular disease being discussed:

- Objectives
- Introduction
- Physiology
- Statistics
- Risk Factors or Causes
- Signs, Symptoms, and Associated Care

- Diagnosis
- Treatment
- Considerations for Care
- For More Information
- Assignment Sheet

Key supplemental information may be included as sections within the appropriate chapters.

The scope of this text is based on the incidence rates of common diseases of interest to the typical health occupations student. Diseases of lower incidence are left for the student to investigate in references listed in the bibliography.

Other features of the text include:
- Practical interventions for signs and symptoms
- Learning objectives and key terms highlighted throughout the text
- Key terms defined on the text page on which they first appear
- *Italic* terms referring to laboratory tests, found in Appendix A, or procedures used for diagnosis or treatment, found in Appendix B
- Chapter assignment sheets at the end of each chapter
- Comprehensive glossary of terms
- Valuable appendices containing information on:
  - —Laboratory Values
  - —Procedures for Diagnosis and Treatment
  - —Universal Precautions
  - —Vital Signs

The associated care is described for a majority of the listed symptoms. The associated care has been listed in its entirety for each chapter rather than having the student refer to an appendix of the book.

The assignment sheets located at the end of the chapter are designed to help the student remember the information in a logical sequence. Students need to have mastered the information prior to being able to answer questions about the material. Once the student has mastered the basics, he or she is ready to apply that knowledge and some higher-order thinking skills to the Knowledge Into Action questions. These questions are case studies/situational analyses that pose medical and ethical dilemmas requiring knowledge and reflection, provoking thoughtful and creative answers from the student.

The *Instructor's Guide*, as a supplement to the text, provides activities that will stimulate the student's insight. When the text and *Instructor's Guide* are used in tandem, the learning needs of students are well covered. Students' complete grasp of the subject matter is enhanced when the hands-on activities included in the *Instructor's Guide* are presented. Hands-on activities not only enhance the learning process for students but make the subject matter fun and exciting for both teacher and students.

Author's Note

Since regulations vary from state to state regarding procedures that can be performed by a student in health occupations, it will be important to check specific regulations in each state. A health occupation worker should never perform any procedure without checking legal responsibilities. In addition, no procedure should be performed by the student unless the student has been taught and has been authorized to do so. Though not always specifically stated, the care and treatment procedures in this text often require a physician prescription and cannot be administered without authorization. The author bears no liability for the actions of students applying the principles and procedures described in this text.

Acknowledgments

The author and Delmar Publishers would like to thank those individuals who reviewed the manuscript and offered suggestions, feedback, and assistance. Their work is greatly appreciated.

Virginia Burke
Ogeechee Technical Institute

Tom Chartier
Woodbury Central High School

Sue A. Hunt
Middlesex Community College

Deborah Iles
Central Ohio J.V.S.D.

Doris Jones
Metropolitan Vocational Center

Burnie Kelley
Ozark Vocational School

Jacquelyn King
Southern Illinois University

Kathy Neeb
Minneapolis Technical College

Barbara Wortman
Fair Park Medical Careers Magnet

ABOUT THE AUTHOR

Marcia Borgstadt, RN, teaches Health Occupations and ProMed courses at East Central MultiDistrict Vocational-Technical School in Brookings, South Dakota. Juniors and seniors in high school take these nonsequential courses to experience the exciting field of health care.

Over a decade of Ms. Borgstadt's hospital and clinical nursing has formed a foundation for teaching others about medical terminology, understanding diseases, and patient care. She has been recognized as a state and regional Outstanding New Vocational Teacher by her American Vocational Association colleagues. Her health occupations program has been recognized as the state's best and is the basis for this textbook and related *Instructor's Guide*.

DEDICATION

I would like to thank Gary, Jenny, and Angie for their support and encouragement during the development of this textbook. Their love made the resulting textbook possible.

UNIT 1

CANCERS

Breast Cancer

OBJECTIVES

Upon completion of this chapter, the student should be able to:

- Define the key terms listed throughout the chapter
- State a specific definition for breast cancer
- Describe the incidence of breast cancer
- Describe the survival rates of breast cancer
- List specific sites of metastasis for breast cancer
- List the risk factors and contributing factors for breast cancer
- List specific interventions to decrease the risk of breast cancer
- Describe specific signs and symptoms associated with breast cancer
- Identify specific methods of diagnosis for breast cancer
- Identify specific methods of treatment for breast cancer
- Describe post-operative care associated with lumpectomies and mastectomies
- Describe specific considerations for care to keep in mind when caring for a patient with breast cancer

KEY TERMS

Malignancy – cancerous

Pectoral – chest

Adipose – fat tissue

Areola – colored area of tissue around the nipple of the breast

INTRODUCTION AND PHYSIOLOGY

Breast cancer is defined simply as a **malignancy** of the breast tissue. The breasts are located on the chest directly over the **pectoral** muscles. The size of the breasts is determined by the amount of **adipose** (fat) tissue contained in the breast. The ducts located within the breast are used to carry milk, which is secreted by the breast, toward the nipple. The nipple, which is located in the center of the breast, is surrounded by a dark-colored pink tissue called the **areola**. (See Figure 1-1.)

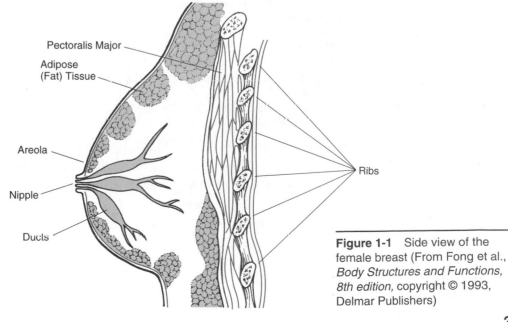

Pectoralis Major

Adipose (Fat) Tissue

Areola

Nipple

Ducts

Ribs

Figure 1-1 Side view of the female breast (From Fong et al., *Body Structures and Functions, 8th edition,* copyright © 1993, Delmar Publishers)

Quadrant – a specific region of the abdomen that has been divided into four separate portions by one horizontal and one vertical line through the umbilicus

Metastasized – spread from one point to another point within the body; generally refers to the spread of cancer within the body

Lymph nodes – tissue located along the lymph vessels that is an important part of the lymph system (immune system); lymph nodes filter pathogens from the bloodstream and produce monocytes and lymphocytes

Axillary – armpit

Adrenal glands – small endocrine glands located on the top portion of each individual kidney; responsible for manufacturing and storing the hormones epinephrine, norepinephrine, sex hormones, aldosterone, and cortisol

Lymph system – system of the body that has the primary function of detecting pathogens in the body and removing or destroying the foreign pathogen; also known as the immune system

Adjacent – situated next to

Alleviating – lessening the severity of symptoms or a disease

Nulliparity – condition referring to a female who has not produced a viable (living or capable of living) offspring

Menopause – cessation of the menstrual cycle in the female; generally occurring between the ages of 45 and 55

Menstruation – monthly discharge of blood and tissues from the lining of the uterus in a female who is not pregnant; generally a cycle of 28 days

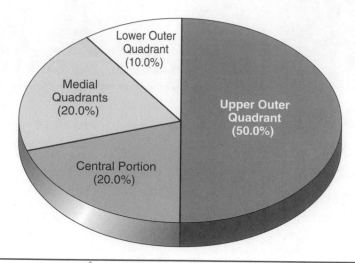

Figure 1-2   Breast cancer incidence by quadrant

STATISTICS

Breast cancer is the predominant form of cancer affecting females in the United States. Nearly 150,000 new cases of breast cancer are reported annually in the United States. Breast cancer is the second leading cause of female cancer deaths in the United States claiming 38,000 lives annually. Although breast cancer has been reported primarily in women, it has been reported in men. It is also rare in women under the age of 35 with more than two-thirds of all breast cancers occurring in females over the age of 50. Breast cancer affects one out of every nine women in the United States and occurs most frequently in the upper outer **quadrant** of the left breast. (See Figure 1-2.)

SURVIVAL RATES

The overall survival rate for breast cancer is approximately 50% for 10 years post-diagnosis. The five-year survival rate depends on whether the cancer is localized to the breast (85% survival rate) or if the cancer has **metastasized** to **lymph nodes** (55% survival rate).

SITES OF METASTASIS

Common sites of metastasis for breast cancer include **axillary** lymph nodes, **adrenal glands**, bones, liver, and lungs. Breast cancer has the capability of metastasizing via the bloodstream, **lymph system**, and also to **adjacent** tissues and organs.

RISK FACTORS

Approximately 80 to 90% of all cancers in the United States are caused by risk factors that would be totally preventable by **alleviating** the risk factors themselves. Predisposing risk factors for breast cancer include the following:

1. Females over the age of 45
2. Family history of breast cancer
3. Prior history of breast cancer
4. First pregnancy after age 35
5. **Nulliparity**
6. Late **menopause**
7. Early age at onset of **menstruation**

Endometrial – of the mucous membrane that lines the interior of the uterus

Cervical – the neck or cervix of the female reproductive organs

Fibrocystic – abnormal growth of fibrous tissue

Contraceptives – methods used to prevent a pregnancy from occurring

Obesity – the state of being overweight; generally refers to those people who are a minimum of 20 to 30% over their recommended weight

Diabetes – a condition in which there is either a complete lack of insulin, inadequate amounts of insulin, or the body's cells are not able to use the insulin efficiently

Hypertension – high blood pressure

Mammography – x-ray of the breast tissue; used in the diagnosis of breast cancer and other diseases affecting the breast

Asymmetry – unequal in size or shape compared to the corresponding body part on the opposite side of the body; also refers to irregular edges of a mole or rash

Retraction – pulling back

Edema – accumulation of fluid in the tissues that results in swelling and weight gain

8. History of **endometrial** or **cervical** cancer
9. History of **fibrocystic** breast disease
10. Use of oral **contraceptives**
11. Use of alcohol and tobacco
12. Exposure to radiation
13. Caucasians in the middle to upper socioeconomic class
14. **Obesity**
15. High intake of dietary fat
16. **Diabetes**
17. **Hypertension**

INTERVENTIONS FOR RISK FACTORS

1. Monthly *breast self-examination*
2. Annual physical examination by physician (every 3 years prior to age 40 and annually after age 40)
3. Annual *mammography* for women over the age of 50, with baseline mammogram at age 35
4. Report unusual findings on breast self-examination promptly to physician
5. Use alternative forms of birth control (See Figure 1-3)
6. Decrease or cease use of alcohol and tobacco. Daily consumption of alcohol increases the risk of breast cancer by 50% over women who don't consume alcoholic beverages.
7. Minimize exposure to radiation
8. Weight loss program
9. Reduce intake of dietary fat
10. Selenium has been shown to reduce breast cancers in areas in which large amounts of selenium are found in the soil. Selenium is found in water-packed tuna, shellfish, organ meats, muscle meats, whole grain cereals, and brazil nuts.
11. Exercise regularly. Lack of exercise doubles the risk of breast cancer over women who participate in an exercise program.

SIGNS, SYMPTOMS, AND ASSOCIATED CARE

1. Nontender lump, which may be movable and does not change in size with menstrual cycle. Note that approximately 25% of breast lumps prove to be cancerous.
2. **Asymmetry** of breasts
3. Bleeding or discharge from the nipple
4. Change in skin temperature of the breast
5. Pain to breast or surrounding area
6. **Retraction** of the nipple
7. Orange-peel effect to the skin of the breast
8. **Edema** to arm on the affected side

The signs and symptoms of this disease are signals that breast cancer should be considered as a diagnosis. Associated care for these signs and symptoms is aimed at patient comfort measures and staff protection measures.

Methods of Contraception			
Method	Percentage of Couples Using Method	Percentage of Women Who Avoid Pregnancy in a Given Year	Percentage of Women Experiencing Accidental Pregnancy during 1st Year of Use
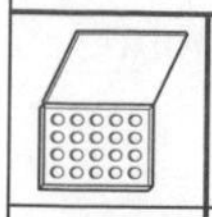 Oral Contraceptive	18.5	97	3
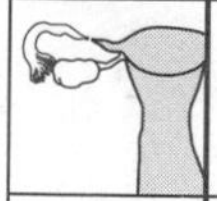 Female Sterilization	16.6	99.6	0.4
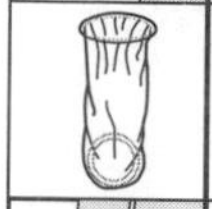 Male Condom	8.8	86	12
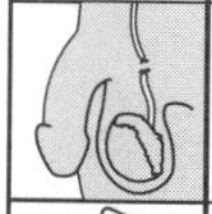 Male Sterilization	7	99.8	0.15
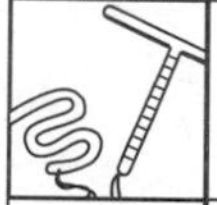 IUD	1.2	94	3
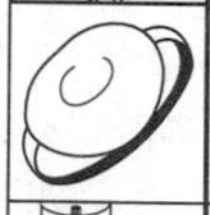 Sponge	0.7	72 – 82	18 – 28
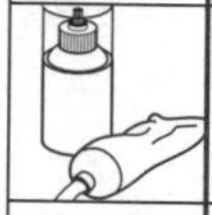 Spermicide	0.6	79	21
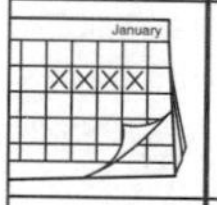 Rhythm/Chance	1.8	80	85
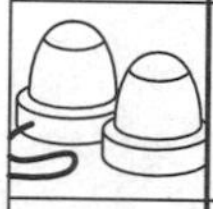 Cervical Cap	1	73 – 92	18
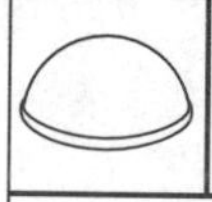 Diaphragm	1	84	18
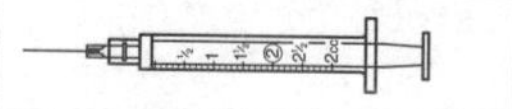 Depro-Provera (injectable progestogen)	Statistics Unavailable		0.3
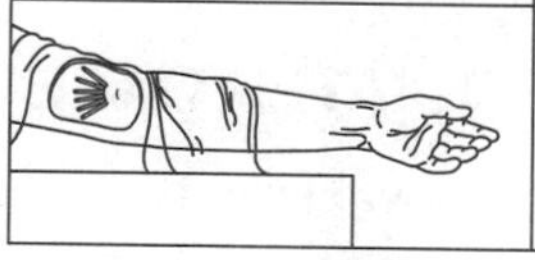 Implants Norplant Capsules	Statistics Unavailable		0.04

Figure 1-3   Alternate forms of birth control (From Anderson, *Basic Maternal/Newborn Nursing, 6th edition,* copyright © 1994, Delmar Publishers)

DIAGNOSIS

1. *Breast self-examination*
   - Learn proper procedure
   - Perform monthly
   - Best time to perform is immediately following menstrual cycle monthly
   - Must be continued for a lifetime
   - Between the ages of 20 to 40, a physician should perform breast exam every 3 years

Biopsy – removal of a small piece of tissue for examination under a microscope; procedure used to diagnose specific diseases, especially cancer

Hormonal receptor assay – test that helps in the determination of an estrogen- versus a progesterone-dependent tumor

Estrogen – female sex hormone produced by the ovary

Progesterone – hormone secreted by the ovary

Lumpectomy – surgical removal of a lump

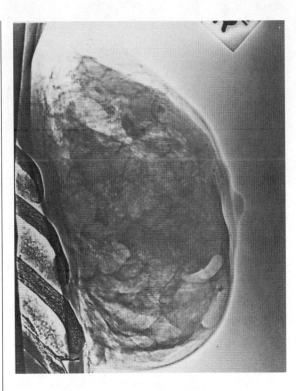

Figure 1-4   A mammogram is routinely done to detect the presence of tumors in the breast. (From Carlton, *Principles of Radiographic Imaging: An Art and a Science*, copyright © 1992, Delmar Publishers)

- Between the ages of 40 to 50, a physician should perform breast exam every 2 years
- Over age 50, a physician should perform breast exam annually

2. *Mammography* (See Figure 1-4)

- Between the ages of 35 and 40, all women should have a baseline mammogram
- Between the ages of 40 and 50, women should have a mammogram every 2 years
- Over age 50, women should have a mammogram annually

3. *Ultrasound*

4. *X-ray*

5. *Biopsy* of the tumor

6. Physical examination

7. Methods to check for metastasis

- Laboratory work, e.g. *SGOT, SGPT, bilirubin, albumin, alkaline phosphatase,* and *prothrombin time*
- *Bone scan*
- *Liver scan*
- *Brain scan*
- *Chest x-ray*

8. **Hormonal receptor assay** helps in the determination of an **estrogen-** versus a **progesterone**-dependent tumor

TREATMENT

1. Surgery

   a. *Lumpectomy*—surgical removal of the breast lump; frequently followed by radiation therapy

Mastectomy – surgical removal of the breast

Palliative – treatment offered for purposes of comfort rather than purposes of cure

Androgens – hormones that are important in the development of secondary sex characteristics in males

Progestin – class of hormones that includes the hormone progesterone

Phlegm – mucous from the respiratory tract

Dyspnea – difficulty with breathing

Diaphoresis – extreme perspiration or sweating

b. *Mastectomy*
- Simple mastectomy—surgical removal of the breast and several of the axillary lymph nodes (optional)
- Modified radical mastectomy—surgical removal of the breast and axillary lymph nodes
- Radical mastectomy—surgical removal of the breast, axillary lymph nodes, and chest muscles

2. *Chemotherapy*
- Often used in conjunction with surgery or radiation
- Examples include methotrexate, 5-FU, doxorubicin, and cyclophosphamide
- May be used as a curative measure or for **palliative** treatment

3. Hormonal therapy
- Commonly used for breast cancer that has metastasized or in cases of recurrence
- Examples of hormonal therapy include **androgens**, estrogen, **progestin**, and tamoxifen

4. *Radiation therapy*
- Often used in conjunction with surgery and chemotherapy
- May be used to shrink a tumor to make it more accessible by surgery
- May be used as palliative treatment to shrink the tumor

5. *Bone marrow transplant*
- May be indicated when high doses of chemotherapy are used

POST-OPERATIVE CARE

1. Assessment of pain after surgery and offer pain relief methods as directed by physician
2. Instruct patient regarding need for coughing and deep-breathing exercises to reduce the risk of respiratory complications. Symptoms of respiratory complications include:
   - Cough
   - Green or blood-tinged **phlegm**
   - Chest pain
   - **Dyspnea**
   - Fever
   - Weakness, fatigue
   - **Diaphoresis**
3. Instruct patient regarding exercising the affected arm(s) to avoid complications
4. Instruct patient regarding special care precautions of the affected arm(s) after surgery
   - Avoid injury to the affected arm
   - Do not lift or carry heavy items with the affected arm
   - Avoid long-term or repetitive activities with the affected arm
   - Instruct medical personnel regarding history of breast cancer and refrain from blood pressures in the affected arm, as well as intravenous (IV) lines and blood being drawn in the affected arm

Activities of daily living (ADLs) – personal care activities such as eating, bathing, elimination, ambulation, and dressing

Vital signs – the measurements of temperature, pulse, respirations, and blood pressure; *see* Appendix D

Phlebotomy – withdrawal of blood from a vein

Intravenous (IV) – the area within the veins of the body or the introduction of fluids into the veins of the body

Lymphedema – swelling of an extremity due to obstruction of the lymph vessels

Unilateral – one side of the body

Prosthesis – artificial limb or body part; frequently refers to breast prosthesis or artificial limb

Imaging – imaging oneself in a different setting, often used as a method of pain relief

5. Encourage activity after surgery as well as participation in **activities of daily living (ADLs)**

6. Discussion of body image and sexual activity related to mastectomy

7. Include spouse/significant other in the instructions and education

8. Change dressings to wound as needed and assess for signs of infection:
   - Redness
   - Swelling
   - Discharge
   - Odor
   - Increased pain
   - Area hot to touch
   - Fever

9. Monitor **vital signs** (See Appendix D)

10. Avoid use of affected arm for **phlebotomy**, blood pressures, **intravenous (IV)** lines, or injections due to chance of **lymphedema** due to obstructed lymph flow following surgery

11. Monitor care of wound drains if present after surgery

CONSIDERATIONS FOR CARE

1. Education
   - Nutrition guidelines
   - Need to continue breast self-examination, physical examinations, and mammography if **unilateral** mastectomy or lumpectomy
   - Instruct regarding informing female relatives of diagnosis of breast cancer due to the increased incidence among relatives

2. Inform regarding support groups such as American Cancer Society and Reach to Recovery (a group of volunteers who have had mastectomies and will offer advice, encouragement, and assistance with **prosthesis** after surgery)

3. Encourage patient and family to verbalize feelings and concerns

4. Discuss body image and sexual activity

5. Assist and encourage patient in obtaining a prosthesis

6. Comfort measures such as relaxation techniques, **imaging**, massage, and pain medications as directed by physician

7. Wear a brassiere prior to surgery and post-operatively to maintain breast support

FOR MORE INFORMATION

American Cancer Society
1599 Clifton Road, NE
Atlanta, GA 30329

ASSIGNMENT SHEET: BREAST CANCER

Short Answer

1. Write a brief definition for the terms listed throughout the chapter.

2. Write a brief definition for breast cancer.

3. Describe the incidence of breast cancer.

4. Describe the survival rate of breast cancer.

5. List five (5) possible sites for metastasis of breast cancer and describe how each of the sites could be diagnosed.

6. Describe three (3) methods of how breast cancer could metastasize to other areas of the body.

7. List seventeen (17) risk factors for breast cancer.

8. Describe eleven (11) specific interventions to reduce the risk of breast cancer.

9. Describe eight (8) signs and symptoms of breast cancer.

10. List and describe eight (8) specific methods used to diagnose breast cancer.

11. List and describe five (5) specific methods used to treat breast cancer.

12. List eleven (11) specific post-operative interventions for the patient who has had a lumpectomy or mastectomy.

13. List seven (7) specific signs and symptoms of a wound infection.

14. List seven (7) specific considerations for care to keep in mind when caring for a patient who has breast cancer.

15. List four (4) specific post-operative special care precautions to give the patient regarding care of the affected arm.

16. Describe each of the following procedures used in the diagnosis or treatment of breast cancer.
    a. Breast self-examination
    b. Mammogram
    c. Ultrasound
    d. X-ray
    e. Biopsy
    f. Bone scan
    g. Liver scan
    h. Brain scan
    i. Lumpectomy
    j. Mastectomy
    k. Chemotherapy
    l. Radiation therapy
    m. Bone marrow transplant

17. Write the normal ranges for each of the following laboratory tests.
    a. SGOT
    b. SGPT
    c. Bilirubin
    d. Albumin
    e. Alkaline phosphatase
    f. Prothrombin time

KNOWLEDGE INTO ACTION

1. Mr. Darien Jones, whose wife just underwent a double mastectomy, is crying in the visitor's lounge as you are walking by. He says to you, "I'm afraid my wife won't take this all very well. She said she won't feel very feminine any more. I'm also scared I won't know how to respond to her or how to comfort her." What will your response be regarding Mrs. Jones' feelings as well as those of her husband?

2. Your neighbor has recently read an article about breast cancer and breast self-examination. She asks you, "What exactly should I be looking for that might indicate I might have breast cancer?" What will your response be?

3. Cora Green, an 82-year-old widow who lives next to you, recently had a left mastectomy. She is concerned about her limitations concerning her left arm and is afraid she will cause injury to the left arm. What will your response be regarding her limitations regarding her left arm as well as methods to prevent injury to the left arm?

Bladder Cancer

OBJECTIVES

Upon completion of this chapter, the student should be able to:

- Define the key terms listed throughout the chapter
- State a specific definition for bladder cancer
- Describe the physiology of the bladder
- Describe the incidence of bladder cancer
- List the contributing risk factors for bladder cancer
- Describe the signs and symptoms associated with bladder cancer
- Identify specific methods for diagnosis of bladder cancer
- Identify specific methods for treatment of bladder cancer
- Describe considerations for caring for a patient with bladder cancer

KEY TERMS

Papillary – nipple of the breast

Ulceration – lesion on the skin or mucous membrane

Pelvis – region located below the abdomen

Urethra – tube from which urine passes from the bladder to the outside of the body

Mucous membrane – membrane that lines organs or systems that are open to the air and secrete mucous

Milliliter (ml) – unit of liquid measurement; 1/1000 of a liter

Sphincter – muscular opening between two parts of the body that, when contracted, prevents passage of material from one part to the next and also prevents reflux back into the original part of the body

INTRODUCTION

Bladder cancer is a malignant growth found either within the bladder wall or on the surface of the bladder. Approximately 88% of all bladder cancers result from two main types of bladder cancers:

1. **Papillary** is the most common type of bladder cancer and is also the most easily cured. With papillary cancer, the malignant cells grow from the bladder wall to the inside of the bladder.
2. Transitional cell cancer is the second most common type of bladder cancer. This type of cancer penetrates the bladder wall resulting in a high risk of infection and **ulceration** in the bladder wall and surrounding tissues. Infection resulting from this form of bladder cancer may lead to death.

PHYSIOLOGY OF THE BLADDER

The bladder is a hollow organ located in the **pelvis**. The function of the bladder is to collect and store urine from the kidneys until it is ready to leave the body through the **urethra**. The bladder itself is a muscular organ that is lined with a **mucous membrane**. The bladder, when empty, is approximately 2 inches (5 cm) in length. The normal capacity of the bladder is 450 **milliliters** (approximately 1 pint) of urine and will then extend to 5 inches (12.5 cm) in length. A **sphincter** located at the urethral outlet of the bladder, prevents urine from leaking from the bladder until the time of voluntary urination. (See Figure 2-1.)

STATISTICS

Bladder cancer is responsible for 2 to 4% of all cancers in the United States. Almost 52,000 new cases of bladder cancer are reported annually. Approximately 75% of bladder cancers occur in males and occur most often in the 50 to 70 year age group. There has been a documented increase in bladder cancer in the United States due to

Carcinogens – substances that cause cancer or have the ability to cause or increase the risk of developing cancer

Chronic – long-term

Hematuria – presence of blood in the urine

Anemia – decrease in red blood cells (RBCs), hemoglobin, or blood loss

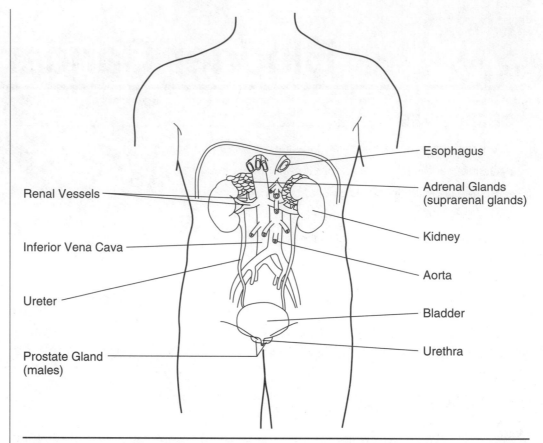

Renal Vessels

Inferior Vena Cava

Ureter

Prostate Gland
(males)

Esophagus

Adrenal Glands
(suprarenal glands)

Kidney

Aorta

Bladder

Urethra

Figure 2-1   The urinary system (From Shapiro, *Basic Maternal/Pediatric Nursing,* copyright © 1994, Delmar Publishers)

increased longevity of Americans as well as an increase in environmental **carcinogens**. Localized tumors of the bladder allow a 70% five-year survival rate in males and 76% survival rate for females.

RISK FACTORS

1. Tobacco use has been shown to increase the incidence of bladder cancer by two to four times and has been shown to cause 35% of all types of cancers.

2. People with **chronic** bacterial infections have an increased incidence of bladder cancer.

3. People who live in highly populated areas where there is an increased amount of industry, especially chemical dyes used by industry, have an increased incidence of bladder cancer.

SIGNS, SYMPTOMS, AND ASSOCIATED CARE

Early bladder cancer may exhibit no symptoms. A person may have bladder cancer for 15 to 20 years prior to the onset of symptoms.

1. Painless **hematuria** is present in 85% of cases

   • Save 3 consecutive urine samples to monitor for improving or worsening hematuria

   • Monitor for **anemia**

   • Avoid blood thinners

   • Provide reassurance for patient

Urinal – container males use to urinate into

Commode – portable toilet frequently seen in a hospital or long-term care facility; used for a patient who has difficulty ambulating to the bathroom

Incontinent – inability to control urination or defecation; may be due to muscle damage, neurological damage, or confusion

Dysuria – painful urination

Flank – area of the back and side between the lower edge of the ribs to the upper area of the ilium

- Monitor for hematuria
- Avoid use of aspirin and aspirin-containing products as they interfere with normal *platelet* function

2. Increased frequency of urination
   - Provide patient opportunity to use the restroom, **urinal**, or **commode** frequently (See Figure 2-2)
   - Provide night light for patient who needs to urinate during the night
   - Watch for signals that the patient needs to urinate if the patient seems confused
   - Change bedding or briefs frequently and provide meticulous skin care for the patient who may be **incontinent**
   - Assist patient to bathroom as needed
   - Be aware of frequency when planning treatments or when traveling
   - Provide a method for patient to contact staff if assistance is needed
   - Respond promptly to patient request for assistance

3. **Dysuria**
   - Offer comfort to the patient experiencing pain
   - Increase fluid intake up to 3000 milliliters (ml) per day

4. Urgency
   - Be aware of a place where the patient can urinate when out of her own environment
   - Respond to the patient's request immediately when she signals the need to go to the bathroom
   - Have equipment on hand and ready for the patient when she signals the need to go to the bathroom
   - Provide a method for patient to contact staff if assistance is needed
   - Encourage frequent urination schedule to avoid problems associated with urgency and possible incontinence

5. **Flank**, pelvic, or back pain
   - Administer pain medications as directed by physician
   - Position patient to relieve or reduce pain
   - Avoid constrictive garments or undergarments
   - Offer comfort measures such as heat, massage, relaxation techniques, and imaging techniques to relieve pain
   - Encourage patient to report pain before it becomes too severe

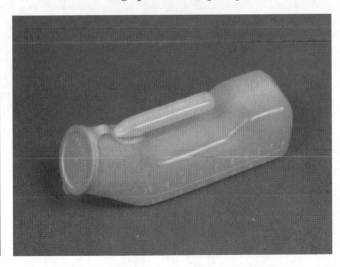

Figure 2-2   Male urinal (From Hegner, *Nursing Assistant: A Nursing Process Approach, 7th edition,* copyright © 1995, Delmar Publishers)

Jobst stockings – highly elasticized stocking that is worn to increase venous blood return and lymphatic vessel return from the extremities

Extremity – refers to the arms or legs of the body; limb

Cyanosis – blue discoloration of the skin due to decreased hemoglobin and oxygenation of the blood

Intake and output (I and O) – record that is kept of all fluids taken into the body and all the fluids that leave the body

Nocturia – increased frequency of urination during the night

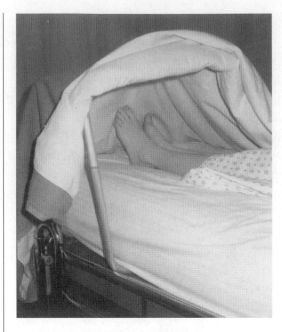

Figure 2-3   A bed cradle is used to reduce pressure to extremities from linens and blankets.

- Monitor appetite due to pain
- Encourage activity as able
- Assist with activities of daily living (ADLs) as needed due to pain

6. Leg edema due to lymph node involvement
   - Avoid constrictive clothing or undergarments
   - Restrict salt in diet as prescribed by physician
   - Provide elastic stockings or **Jobst stockings** as necessary to reduce swelling
   - Monitor edema on a routine basis
   - Encourage patient to elevate edematous **extremity** above the level of the heart to reduce swelling
   - Monitor for skin breakdown in edematous areas
   - Monitor for symptoms of decreased circulation in edematous areas such as cool to touch, **cyanosis**, and decreased sensation
   - Obtain baseline weight and monitor on a routine basis
   - Monitor **intake and output (I and O)**
   - Utilize a bed cradle to reduce pressure from linens and blankets (See Figure 2-3)

7. **Nocturia**
   - Assist patient to the bathroom as needed
   - Monitor patient during the night if going to bathroom
   - Use a night light, especially if in new surroundings or confused, for patient safety to get to the bathroom
   - Provide a urinal or commode for patient use (See Figure 2-4)
   - Provide a method for patient to call for help if needed during the night

DIAGNOSIS

1. *Cystoscopy* is used for visualization of the tumors, biopsy, and follow-up (See Figure 2-5)
2. *Biopsy* is used to determine type of growth present
3. *Intravenous pyelography* is used to determine condition of kidneys and ureters

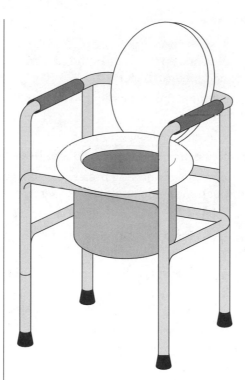

Figure 2-4   Bedside (portable) commode

4. *CT scan* can determine tumor position and size as well as metastasis
5. Symptoms stated by patient
6. Physical examination
7. *Urinalysis*
8. *Excretory urography*
9. *CBC*

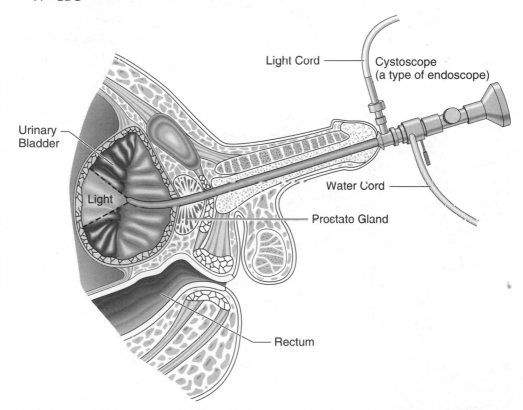

Figure 2-5   Cystoscopy (From Layman, *The Medical Language,* copyright © 1995, Delmar Publishers)

Cystectomy – surgical removal of a fluid-filled sac or the urinary bladder

Ureter – narrow tube that carries urine from the kidney to the bladder

Distal – farthest from the point of attachment

Ileum – distal portion of the small intestine; small intestine is divided into three parts: the duodenum, jejunum, and ileum; varies in total length from 8 to 15 feet

Stoma – artificial opening created between two cavities in the body or between a cavity and the outside (surface) of the body

Sigmoid colon – portion of the large intestine between the transverse colon and the rectum

Colon – the main portion of the large intestine extending from the ileum to the rectum

Rectum – distal five inches of the large intestine; responsible for storing feces until they are ready to be expelled from the body

Catheter – tube inserted into an opening in the body to drain or inject fluid

Posterior – back side or back part

Intravesical – inside the bladder

Chemotherapy – instillation of antineoplastic chemicals for the purpose of treating malignancies

Antineoplastic – substance used in the treatment of cancerous growths (neoplasm)

Systemic – refers to the entire body

Dehydration – reduced fluid level in the body resulting from extreme fluid loss from the body or severe reduction in the amount of fluid taken into the body

TREATMENT

Treatment of the cancer depends on the stage of the cancer, the degree of metastasis, as well as the patient's age and medical history.

1. Surgical removal of the tumor is possible when the tumor has not metastasized.
2. *Cystectomy* with diversion of the urine.
    *   *Ileal conduit*—connecting **ureters** to the **distal ileum** and creating a **stoma**
    *   *Ureterosigmoidostomy*—connecting ureters to the **sigmoid colon** routing urine flow through the **colon** and urine is excreted through the **rectum**
    *   *Ureterostomy*—attaching the ureter to a stoma in the skin of the abdomen
    *   *Nephrostomy*—placement of a **catheter** through the **posterior** flank directly into the kidney
3. **Intravesical** *chemotherapy*—instillation of **antineoplastic** agent directly into the bladder
4. **Systemic** chemotherapy, e.g. Thiotepa, Cyclophosphamide (Cytoxan), Doxorubicin (Adriamycin), Cisplatin
5. *Radiation therapy*—internal or external

CONSIDERATIONS FOR CARE

1. Educate patient and family regarding the disease process and forms of treatment.
2. Instruct patient and family regarding well-balanced meals and fluid intake requirements.
3. Encourage a form of contraception if the patient is of child-bearing age, as chemotherapy has been shown to increase the incidence of birth defects.
4. Encourage the patient and family to verbalize their feelings.
5. Make patient and family aware of support group options.
6. Monitor intake and output to observe for **dehydration** and other problems associated with urination and urinary diversion systems. Symptoms of dehydration include:
    *   Decreased urine output
    *   Dry skin
    *   Dry mouth and eyes
    *   **Constipation**
    *   **Tenting** of skin
    *   Concentrated urine
    *   Confusion
    *   **Hypotension**
7. If the patient has a stoma post-operatively:
    *   Observe the stoma for symptoms of infection, such as redness, swelling, discharge, and odor.
    *   Educate patient and family regarding the care of the stoma.
    *   Monitor skin integrity around the stoma and instruct the patient and family regarding skin care techniques.
8. Educate patient regarding what to expect in the event of chemotherapy and radiation.

Constipation – difficulty having a bowel movement due to the feces being hard, dry, or large in diameter

Tenting – loss of elasticity of the skin caused by dehydration; causes skin to return slowly to its normal position when pinched

Hypotension – low blood pressure

Perineal – external floor of the pelvis

9. Instruct patient and family regarding foods that may give urine a strong odor when wearing a urinary diversion device, e.g. cabbage and broccoli.

10. Educate patient and family regarding methods to avoid bladder infections.
    - Increase fluids to 3000 ml per day
    - Encourage intake of cranberry juice and other juices.
    - For females, wipe **perineal** area from front to back.
    - Wear cotton undergarments to absorb moisture.
    - Avoid bubble baths, strong soaps, scented powders, and sprays and lotions to perineal area.

11. Monitor laboratory values such as *hemoglobin*, *hematocrit*, *BUN*, and *creatinine*.

12. Monitor intake and output (I and O).

13. Monitor for abnormal function of the urinary system. Be aware of symptoms of complications:
    - Dysuria
    - Hematuria
    - Frequency of urination
    - Low back or pelvic pain
    - Presence of a pelvic mass

FOR MORE INFORMATION

American Cancer Society
1599 Clifton Road, NE
Atlanta, GA 30329
1-800-ACS-2345

ASSIGNMENT SHEET: BLADDER CANCER

Short Answer

1. Write a brief definition for bladder cancer.

2. Describe the incidence of bladder cancer.

3. Describe the function of the bladder.

4. List and describe three (3) contributing risk factors for bladder cancer.

5. List seven (7) signs and symptoms of bladder cancer and associated care for each of these symptoms.

6. List and describe nine (9) methods used to aid in the diagnosis of bladder cancer.

7. List and describe five (5) methods used to treat bladder cancer.

8. List thirteen (13) considerations for caring for a patient with bladder cancer.

9. List eight (8) specific symptoms of dehydration.

10. Describe why there could be an increased incidence of bladder cancer in densely populated industrial areas.

11. Write the normal ranges for each of the following laboratory tests and describe the purpose of each of the tests.
    a. Hemoglobin (Hg)
    b. Hematocrit (Hct)
    c. Blood urea nitrogen (BUN)
    d. Creatinine
    e. Platelet
    f. Red blood cell count (RBC)
    g. White blood cell count (WBC)

12. Describe each of the following procedures used in the diagnosis or treatment of bladder cancer.
    a. Cystoscopy
    b. Biopsy
    c. Intravenous pyelography
    d. CT scan
    e. Urinalysis
    f. Excretory urography
    g. Chemotherapy
    h. Radiation therapy

KNOWLEDGE INTO ACTION

1. Larry Peterson, a patient who has a high frequency of urination, is concerned that he might not be able to make it to the bathroom in time. List three methods that could be used to assist Mr. Peterson.

2. Cece Johnson is scheduled for a cystoscopy and intravenous pyelography (IVP) in the morning to rule out a diagnosis of bladder cancer. She says to you, "The doctor says I'm having those two tests in the morning, but he had to leave before he could explain them to me. Can you tell me what they are?" What will your response be?

3. Dale Jensen is being discharged from the hospital after having a ureterostomy because of bladder cancer. While you are helping him pack his belongings, he says to you, "I read in this booklet that I need to drink lots of fluid so I don't get dehydrated. How would I know if I was dehydrated?" What will your response be regarding the symptoms of dehydration?

Colorectal Cancer

OBJECTIVES

Upon completion of this chapter, the student should be able to:

- Define the key terms listed throughout the chapter
- Describe the physiology of the colon and rectum
- State a specific definition for colorectal cancer
- Describe the incidence of colorectal cancer
- List the risk factors for colorectal cancer
- Describe the signs and symptoms of colorectal cancer and give the rationale for each
- Identify specific methods for diagnosis of colorectal cancer
- Identify specific methods for treatment of colorectal cancer
- Describe specific methods of caring for a colostomy
- Describe considerations for caring for a patient with colorectal cancer

KEY TERMS

Neoplastic – refers to the tissue growth of a neoplasm

Epithelium – covering of internal and external organs

Adenocarcinomas – cancerous tumors of a gland

Cecum – first part of the large intestine; situated between the ileum of the small intestine and the ascending colon

Ascending colon – portion of the large intestine located between the distal ileum and the transverse colon

Transverse colon – portion of the large intestine located between the ascending and the descending colons

Descending colon – portion of the large intestine between the transverse colon and the sigmoid colon

Anus – external opening of the rectum

INTRODUCTION

Colorectal cancer is characterized by uncontrolled growth of **neoplastic** cells that often invade surrounding tissue with metastasis common to other sites. Colorectal cancers are cancers that originate in the cecum, colon, or rectum. The most-frequent sites for metastasis of colorectal cancers are to the liver and lungs. The majority of colorectal cancers begin in the lining, or **epithelium**, of the colon. These specific cancers are referred to as **adenocarcinomas**.

PHYSIOLOGY OF THE COLON AND RECTUM

The function of the colon and rectum is to absorb water from digested food and hold solid wastes until they are ready to be expelled and eliminated as solid wastes. The large intestine is approximately 5 feet in length and 2 inches in diameter. The first part of the large intestine is the **cecum**, which is separated from the ileum of the small intestine by a sphincter. The sphincter prevents digested food from backing up into the small intestine. The second portion of the large intestine is the **ascending colon** followed by the **transverse colon**. Finally, the **descending colon** is followed by the sigmoid colon, which empties into the rectum. The rectum is approximately 5 inches in length and stores solid wastes until they are ready to be expelled. The solid wastes are emptied out of the body through the **anus**. (See Figure 3-1.)

STATISTICS

More than 138,000 new cases of colorectal cancer are diagnosed annually in the United States with approximately 60,000 people dying annually from the disease. It accounts for 15% of all new cancers diagnosed. Colorectal cancer has the second highest death rate for any type of cancer in the United States. Men and women are affected equally by the disease with those over the age of 50 most affected. Less than 6% of all colorectal

Diarrhea – the passing of liquid or semisolid bowel movements (feces); diarrhea results due to the fact that the waste products pass through the intestinal tract so rapidly that fluid and nutrients are not reabsorbed into the body

Hemoccult® – test used to check for the presence of blood in feces

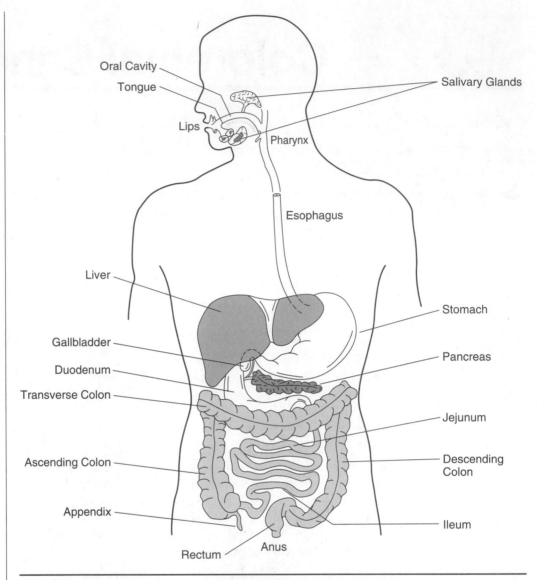

Oral Cavity

Tongue

Salivary Glands

Lips

Pharynx

Esophagus

Liver

Stomach

Gallbladder

Pancreas

Duodenum

Transverse Colon

Jejunum

Ascending Colon

Descending Colon

Appendix

Ileum

Rectum

Anus

Figure 3-1 The digestive tract. The small intestine is actually longer than shown.

cancers are diagnosed prior to the age of 50. Approximately 5 to 6% of all people in the United States will develop colorectal cancer in their lifetime with a five-year survival rate of 70 to 75%. The most frequent site of metastasis for colorectal cancer is to the liver and lungs. Approximately 50% of patients with colorectal cancer also have involvement of the local lymph nodes.

RISK FACTORS

1. Over 50 years of age
    - Annual physical examinations with *digital rectal examination*
    - Report symptoms of rectal bleeding, abdominal pain, extreme constipation, **diarrhea**, weight loss, and other symptoms of colorectal cancer
    - *Stools for occult blood (**Hemoccult**®)* checked annually or as directed by a physician
    - *Proctosigmoidoscopy* should be done annually after the age of 50. When the person has had two consecutive normal tests, they often can be done every 3 to 5 years thereafter.

Fiber – substances that remain after the digestion of foods in the digestive tract; bulk

Carbohydrate – important energy source found in many foods; substance made of hydrogen, oxygen, and carbon; primary food sources of carbohydrates are sugars (simple carbohydrates) and starches (complex carbohydrates)

Polyposis – condition of having many polyps

Polypectomy – surgical removal of a polyp

Ulcerative colitis – condition of inflammation of the colon resulting in formation of ulcers in the mucous membrane of the colon

Diverticulosis – presence of diverticulum (sacs or pouches) in the intestinal tract

2. High-fat, low-**fiber** diet; high refined **carbohydrates**
   - Education regarding the importance of a low-fat, high-fiber diet
   - Fat should make up less than 20 to 30% of the total daily calories (See Table 3-1)
   - Fiber intake should be 20 to 35 grams per day (See Table 3-2)
   - High fiber includes whole grain, fruits (especially prunes), and vegetables
3. Multiple **polyposis** (Gardner's syndrome)
   - Regular physical examinations for patients at risk
   - **Polypectomy** (surgical removal of polyps) should reduce the risk
4. Chronic **ulcerative colitis**
   - Monitor stools for presence of bleeding (*Hemoccult*®)
   - Regular physical examinations for patient
   - Administer diet as prescribed by physician
5. **Diverticulosis**
   - There is no evidence that diverticulosis increases the risk of colorectal cancer though the two are often present together and the symptoms may mimic each other
   - Symptoms of increased abdominal pain, weight loss, and presence of blood in stools should be reported to a physician promptly

Table 3-1   Fat Content of Foods

Food	Serving Size	Total Fat (grams)	Saturated Fat (grams)	Unsaturated Fat (grams)
Whole milk	1 cup	9	5	3
Skim milk	1 cup	trace	trace	trace
Cheddar cheese	1 oz	9	5	3
Cottage cheese	1 cup	1	trace	trace
Ice cream	1 cup	14	8	5
Eggs	1 each	6	2	3
Bacon	3 slices	8	3	4
Hamburger	3 oz (broiled)	17	8	8
Chicken	3 oz (breast)	3	1	1
Cashews	1 cup	64	11	45
Asparagus	1 cup	trace	0	0
Green beans	1 cup	trace	0	0
Corn	1 cup	2	trace	trace
French fries	10 each	7	2	5
Sweet potatoes	1 each	6	2	4
Avocado	1 each	37	7	22
Banana	1 each	trace	0	0
Apple	1 each	trace	0	0
Orange	1 each	trace	0	0
Choc. cake	1 slice	9	3	5
Choc. chip cookie	1 each	3	1	2
Doughnut	1 each	6	1	4
Butter	1 tbsp	12	6	4
Margarine	1 tbsp	12	2	9
Cr. mush. soup	1 cup	14	4	9

Hemorrhoids – enlargement of the vessels of the mucous membrane of the anus or rectum

Obstruction – blockage

Serum – portion of the blood remaining after the clotting factors have been removed or separated

Electrolytes – compounds capable of transmitting an electrical current, e.g. sodium, potassium, and chloride

Table 3-2   Fiber Content of Foods

Food	Serving Size	Fiber (grams)
Apple	1 each, medium	3.3
Banana	1 each	6.0
Orange	1 each, medium	4.6
Prunes	4 each, dried	5.3
Peanuts	½ cup	5.8
Baked beans	1 cup	18.7
Celery	1 stalk	0.8
Peas	1 cup	11.4
Potato	1 each, baked	1.5
White bread	1 slice	0.8
Wheat bread	1 slice	2.5
Bran cereal	½ cup	10.0
Rice Krispies	1 cup	1.5

6. Exposure to asbestos
    - Take necessary precautions to reduce exposure to asbestos

SIGNS, SYMPTOMS, AND ASSOCIATED CARE

1. Blood in stools due to irritation in the lining of the colon from the tumor, or bleeding from the tumor itself
    - Offer reassurance to patient
    - Monitor for anemia in the presence of bloody stools
    - Check for the presence of blood in stools (*Hemoccult*®)
    - Monitor amount, frequency, and consistency of stools
    - Provide meticulous skin care to the anal area

2. Rectal bleeding due to irritation in the lining of the colon from the tumor or bleeding from the tumor itself
    - Monitor for presence of rectal bleeding
    - Monitor for anemia in the presence of rectal bleeding
    - Offer reassurance to patient

    People with **hemorrhoids** have a tendency to overlook rectal bleeding and need to be educated regarding the fact that an examination needs to be done by a physician to determine the cause of the rectal bleeding.

3. Diarrhea due to partial **obstruction** and need for stool to pass by the partial obstruction
    - Monitor number, amount, and consistency of stools
    - Monitor intake and output (I and O) to avoid dehydration. Symptoms of dehydration include decreased urine output, constipation, dry skin, tenting of skin, dry mouth, dry eyes, concentrated urine, hypotension, and confusion.
    - Monitor **serum electrolytes** (*sodium*, *potassium*, and *chloride*)
    - Provide meticulous skin care, especially if incontinent
    - Monitor for presence of hemorrhoids

Sitz baths – baths that soak the buttocks and hips; frequently used after the vaginal delivery of an infant or after rectal surgery

Topical – a specific area of the body; often refers to medication or ointments applied to the skin

Suppositories – cone-shaped, semisolid substances that may be inserted into the rectum, vagina, or urethra for the purpose of administering treatment or medication

Peristalsis – muscular contractions of the gastrointestinal tract

Hemoglobin – protein found in the red blood cells that contains iron; function is to enable the red blood cells to transport oxygen and carbon dioxide in the bloodstream

Hematocrit – percentage by volume of the number of red blood cells in the blood

Pallor – pale; absence of color

Vertigo – dizziness

Emesis – vomiting

Fecal – refers to bowel movements or stools passed from the intestines

Antiemetics – substances that prevent or treat nausea and vomiting

Aspiration – inhalation or drawing in of a foreign body into the lungs; also refers to removal of fluid from a certain site in the body, e.g. knee or spine

Vomit – expulsion of material from the stomach to the mouth

Laxatives – medications or substances given to promote a bowel movement by increasing peristalsis or by absorbing fluid from the surrounding tissues to loosen the consistency of the feces

- Monitor for rectal discomfort and offer **sitz baths**, warm soaks, and **topical** ointments or *suppositories*
- Provide frequent skin care, especially to anal area to prevent skin breakdown
- Monitor for presence of blood in stools (*Hemoccult*®)
- Offer reassurance to patient
- Avoid foods that are too hot or too cold as they increase **peristalsis**

4. Anemia due to blood loss
   - Administer blood transfusions and iron supplements as necessary
   - Monitor *hemoglobin* and *hematocrit*
   - Monitor for weakness and assist with activities of daily living (ADLs) as necessary due to weakness. Protect from possible injury due to weakness.
   - Monitor physical symptoms of anemia, such as **pallor**, weakness, and **vertigo**

5. Vomiting due to obstruction or partial obstruction; **emesis** may contain **fecal** material
   - Administer **antiemetics** before meals as prescribed by physician
   - Offer food choices according to patient preference
   - Control odors and unpleasant sights in room
   - Offer fluids frequently to prevent dehydration
   - Monitor intake and output (I and O) to avoid dehydration
   - Monitor serum electrolytes
   - Encourage rest periods after meals
   - Avoid foods that are spicy, rich, or previously disagreeable to patient
   - Provide container for patient to vomit into as needed; this should be cleaned whenever used and changed on a frequent basis
   - Administer meticulous mouth care
   - Prevent **aspiration** of **vomit**
   - Employ universal precautions at all times when coming in contact with blood or body fluids (See Appendix C)
   - Avoid greasy foods as they tend to stay in the stomach a long period of time
   - Avoid cooking food if possible due to increased nausea with odors of foods
   - Avoid hot foods as necessary due to the increased odors of hot foods
   - Encourage to eat in well-ventilated area to decrease the accumulation of odors of foods while eating

6. Obstruction due to tumor growth
   - Monitor for symptoms of obstruction such as absence of stools, diarrhea, bloating, nausea, vomiting, abdominal pain, and fever
   - Avoid use of **laxatives** if obstruction is suspected
   - Refrain from giving patient foods or liquids by mouth in the event of suspected obstruction

7. Constipation regardless of increased fiber, fluids, and exercise due to mal-absorption of nutrients and fluids
   - Encourage fluids, fiber, fresh fruits, and fresh vegetables
   - Encourage a high-fiber diet
   - Increase exercise as tolerated

Flatus – gas in the intestinal tract

Girth – measurement of the circumference of the abdomen

Malabsorption – inadequate or altered absorption of vitamins, minerals, and other nutrients from the digestive tract

Parenteral – route for nourishment or medication that does not include the alimentary canal, e.g. intravenous, intramuscular, and subcutaneous

- Administer enemas, suppositories, stool softeners, and laxatives as prescribed by physician (See Figure 3-2)
- Monitor frequency, number, and consistency of stools
- Monitor for possible bowel obstruction
- Establish regular bowel routine
- Provide privacy for bowel routine as able

8. Lower abdominal pain due to abdominal distention and often from metastasis
   - Assist with position for patient comfort
   - Avoid constrictive garments and undergarments
   - Assist with methods to promote comfort, such as relaxation techniques, imaging, massage, and warm baths
   - Monitor for level of pain and offer comfort measures as necessary
   - Administer medications as necessary and as prescribed by physician for the control of pain
   - Encourage patient to request pain relief methods before pain becomes too severe

9. Abdominal distention, due to retention of stool, and **flatus**, due to retention of fluid high in protein and electrolytes
   - Assist with position for patient comfort
   - Measure abdominal **girth** on routine basis (Mark area so the same area is measured each time for accuracy.)
   - Encourage nonconstrictive clothing and undergarments
   - Avoid foods that increase formation of intestinal gas, such as onions, spicy foods, carbonated beverages (including beer), foods from the cabbage family, and beans
   - Monitor abdominal distention

10. Weight loss due to poor nutrition and **malabsorption** of minerals
    - Obtain baseline weight and monitor weight on a routine basis
    - Encourage patient to participate in dietary choices
    - Provide nutritional supplements and vitamins as necessary
    - Encourage family and friends to bring in food that is appealing to patient as his dietary restrictions allow
    - Administer **parenteral** fluids as necessary
    - Monitor intake and output (I and O)
    - Encourage rest periods before and after meals

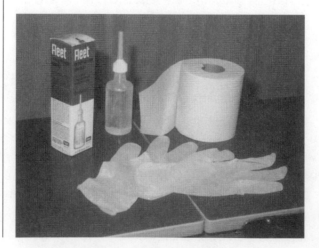

Figure 3-2 Equipment used for enema administration

Hepatomegaly – refers to enlargement of the liver

Tachycardia – rapid heart rate; generally refers to a pulse greater than 100 to 110 beats per minute

Metabolized – combined chemical and physical changes occur within the body

Jaundice – yellow discoloration of the skin, mucous membranes, and eyes due to an accumulation of bilirubin in the blood

Cachexia – general wasting away of weight and body tissue often seen in chronic and debilitating illness

- Avoid unpleasant sights and odors in room to make meals more appealing
- Provide meticulous mouth care
- Monitor for skin breakdown due to loss of body tissue
- Encourage clothing styles that do not draw attention to weight loss
- Monitor for symptoms of dehydration, such as decreased urine output, constipation, dry skin, tenting of skin, dry mouth, dry eyes, concentrated urine, hypotension, and confusion

11. Weakness due to anemia and poor absorption of minerals
    - Assist patient with ADLs as necessary
    - Schedule care, activities, and treatment around patient's rest schedule
    - Schedule phone calls and visitors around patient's energy level and rest schedule
    - Encourage frequent rest periods
    - Provide assistance as needed to prevent injury due to weakness
    - Provide a method for patient to call for assistance
    - Encourage patient to set realistic goals of activities
    - Allow adequate time to do activities and procedures to avoid frustration or possible injury
    - Encourage exercise to maintain/promote muscle strength
    - Provide cane or walker for additional assistance with ambulation and transfer
    - Provide private room as able for patient to promote rest periods

12. **Hepatomegaly** due to metastasis
    - Monitor for hepatomegaly
    - Avoid abdominal injury in the presence of hepatomegaly
    - Monitor for signs of internal bleeding in the presence of hepatomegaly, such as abdominal pain, **tachycardia**, hypotension, and abdominal distention
    - Monitor liver function with serum laboratory tests, e.g. *SGOT, SGPT, bilirubin, albumin, alkaline phosphatase*, and *prothrombin time*
    - Monitor for bleeding tendencies in the presence of hepatomegaly
    - Educate to avoid the use of alcohol and medications *metabolized* in the liver
    - Monitor for **jaundice**

13. **Cachexia** due to anemia, poor absorption of minerals, or loss of appetite

14. Metastasis to other organs, most frequently the liver

15. Pallor due to anemia and blood loss
    - Administer blood transfusion as necessary if pallor due to anemia
    - Encourage clothing and makeup to enhance skin coloring as patient desires

16. Dyspnea due to abdominal distention or metastasis
    - Assist with position for patient comfort
    - Administer oxygen as needed and as directed by physician
    - Encourage nonconstrictive garments and undergarments
    - Provide fan in room to circulate air and assist in making breathing easier
    - Encourage frequent rest periods to conserve energy
    - Arrange schedule of activities around patient rest periods
    - Assist with ADLs as necessary

Hypoxia – decreased oxygen intake

Syncope – fainting; loss of consciousness

Lymphadenopathy – refers to disease of the lymph nodes; generally accompanied by enlargement of the lymph nodes

- Assess breath sounds on routine basis
- Observe for signs of **hypoxia**, such as cyanosis, diaphoresis, decreased level of consciousness, and confusion
- Monitor ease of respirations and respiratory rate
- Encourage to do as many activities as possible in a sitting position, e.g. dressing, bathing, cooking, and cleaning
- Humidify air as needed
- Provide reassurance to patient
- Treat cause of dyspnea

17. Vertigo due to anemia and malabsorption of minerals
    - Monitor for vertigo
    - Monitor vital signs (See Appendix D)
    - Assist with ambulation and transfer to prevent injury in the presence of vertigo
    - Educate patient to ask for assistance when out of bed in presence of **syncope**
    - Provide method for patient to call for assistance

18. **Lymphadenopathy** due to metastasis
    - Monitor for lymphadenopathy
    - Assist with position for patient comfort
    - Provide comfort measures as necessary due to lymphadenopathy

19. "Ribbonlike" stools due to partial obstruction or colon spasms
    - Monitor color, number, consistency, and amount of stools

20. Black, tarry stools due to blood in the stools
    - Monitor stools for amount of bleeding
    - Offer reassurance to patient
    - Monitor for anemia in the presence of bloody stools
    - Monitor for the presence of blood (*Hemoccult®*)
    - Monitor amount, frequency, and consistency of stools

21. Increased intestinal gas due to inability to pass due to partial obstruction
    - Avoid foods that increase intestinal gas formation
    - Encourage fluids
    - Control odors in patient room with ventilation and room deodorizers
    - Provide private room if available
    - Prevent embarrassment for the patient

DIAGNOSIS

1. Symptoms
2. Physical examination
3. *Digital rectal examination*; note that 50% of all colorectal cancers are detected in this manner (See Figure 3-3)
    - Should be done on an annual basis for anyone over the age of 50
4. *Proctosigmoidoscopy*
    - Should be done every 3 to 5 years for anyone over the age of 50 or as directed by physician

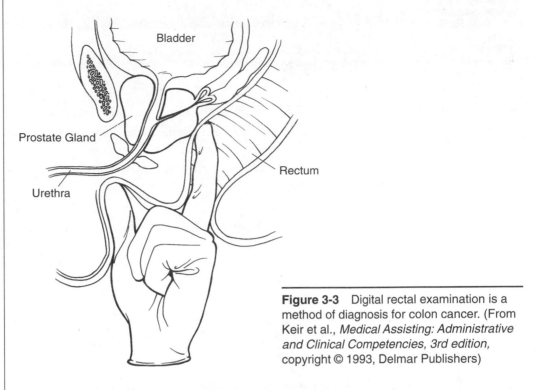

Figure 3-3 Digital rectal examination is a method of diagnosis for colon cancer. (From Keir et al., *Medical Assisting: Administrative and Clinical Competencies, 3rd edition,* copyright © 1993, Delmar Publishers)

5. *Fiberoptic colonoscopy*
   * Many physicians will substitute this test for a proctosigmoidoscopy and should be done every 3 to 5 years for anyone over the age of 50 or as directed by physician

6. *Stools checked for occult blood (Hemoccult®)* (See Figure 3-4)
   * Should be done on an annual basis for anyone over the age of 50

7. *Barium enema*
   * Indicates obstruction and possible tumor

8. *Hemoglobin*
   * Used to determine anemia

9. *Intravenous pyelography*
   * Used to determine metastasis

10. *CEA (carcinoembryonic antigen)*
    * Used to determine metastasis or recurrence

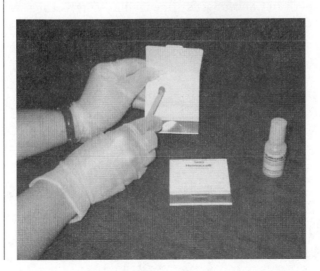

Figure 3-4 Hemoccult® test to check stools for the presence of blood

Colectomy – surgical removal of a portion of the colon or all of the colon

Resection – partial surgical removal of an organ or other part of the body

Colostomy – surgical creation of an opening between the colon and the abdomen as a method of excreting feces

Radiation – therapy for the treatment of malignancies and certain other disorders through the use of specified amounts of radiation directed at the specific location of the body to be treated

Feces – solid waste passed from the intestinal tract; stool or bowel movement

Enterostomal therapist – person with specific training to aid clients with the care of stomas

11. *Biopsy*
    - Used to confirm the diagnosis

TREATMENT

1. Surgery
   - Used to remove the tumor and adjacent tissues as needed
   - The type of surgery depends on the location, size of the tumor, and the extent, if any, of metastasis
   - **Colectomy**, **resection**, or **colostomy**; with or without removal of adjacent tissues
2. *Radiation*
   - Used in conjunction with surgery, for the treatment of metastasis or recurrent cancer
   - May be used as a curative method or palliative method
3. *Chemotherapy*
   - Used in conjunction with surgery, for the treatment of metastasis or recurrent cancer
   - Medications include 5FU, vincristine, methotrexate, mitomycin, and lomustine

CARE OF COLOSTOMY

A colostomy is an opening between the colon and the abdominal wall for the purpose of expelling **feces**. The colostomy may be temporary or permanent. (See Figure 3-5.)

1. **Enterostomal therapist** should be contacted prior to surgery to assist with possible placement of the stoma and to assist with education for the patient and family
2. Educate patient and family regarding different types of appliances that are available for covering the stoma
3. Educate patient and family regarding foods that cause an increase in odor and intestinal gas, such as onions, spicy foods, carbonated beverages (including beer), foods from the cabbage family, and beans
4. Educate regarding the ability to continue a normal life style, including sexual relationships, sporting activities, hygiene practices, and employment
5. Educate regarding care of the colostomy, including irrigation and skin care
6. American Cancer Society often will have advocates available to visit with the patient who have ostomies themselves

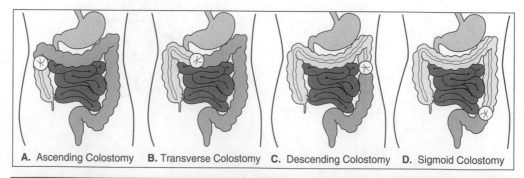

A. Ascending Colostomy   **B.** Transverse Colostomy   **C.** Descending Colostomy   **D.** Sigmoid Colostomy

Figure 3-5   Various colostomy positions related to the cancer sites and the amount of large intestine removed (shaded) (From Hegner, *Nursing Assistant: A Nursing Process Approach, 7th edition,* copyright © 1995, Delmar Publishers)

Nasogastric tubes (NG)
– tubes that are passed through the nose and into the stomach; option of using the tubes to drain stomach contents or instillation of fluids into the stomach

CONSIDERATIONS FOR CARE

1. Education regarding treatment options
2. Education regarding what to expect post-operatively when surgery is necessary, e.g. intravenous (IV) lines, **nasogastric tubes (NG)** (see Figure 3-6), deep-breathing exercises
3. Support group for patient and family
4. Educate regarding nutrition
5. Promote positive self-image by encouraging patient to assist with ADLs, offering choices and adjustment to life style
6. Colostomy care and education as required
7. Assess for pain post-operatively and treat accordingly
8. Encourage communication for the patient to discuss fears

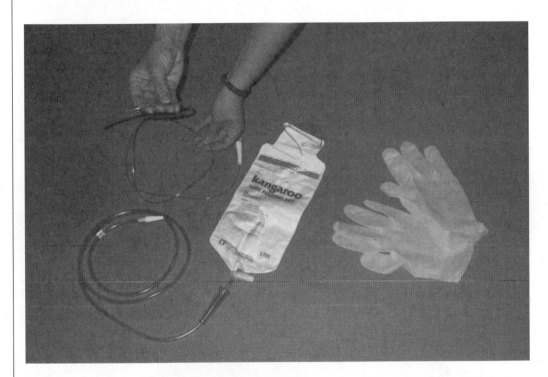

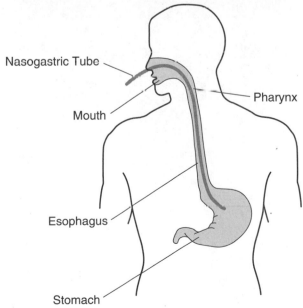

Figure 3-6   Nasogastric tube equipment and placement

9. Educate regarding symptoms to be aware of for recurrence or metastasis
10. Educate regarding need for follow-up care with physician
11. Educate regarding diet modifications

FOR MORE INFORMATION

American Cancer Society
1599 Clifton Road, NE
Atlanta, GA 30329

ASSIGNMENT SHEET: COLORECTAL CANCER

Short Answer

1. Describe the normal physiology and function of the colon and rectum.

2. Write a brief definition for colorectal cancer.

3. Describe the incidence of colorectal cancer.

4. List six (6) risk factors for colorectal cancer and describe what can be done to reduce or eliminate each of these factors.

5. List twenty-one (21) possible signs and symptoms for colorectal cancer. Describe the rationale for each and associated care for each.

6. Describe why people with hemorrhoids often ignore rectal bleeding. Why would it be important for anyone with rectal bleeding to be examined by a physician?

7. List and describe eleven (11) specific methods to aid in the diagnosis of colorectal cancer.

8. List the normal laboratory values for each of the following tests.
   a. Hemoglobin (Hg)
   b. Carcinoembryonic antigen (CEA)
   c. Hematocrit
   d. Sodium
   e. Potassium
   f. Chloride
   g. SGOT
   h. SGPT
   i. Bilirubin
   j. Albumin
   k. Alkaline phosphatase
   l. Prothrombin time

9. Describe three (3) specific methods used to treat colorectal cancer.

10. Write a definition for colostomy. Describe six (6) associated care measures to keep in mind when taking care of a patient with a colostomy.

11. Describe eleven (11) considerations for caring for a patient with colorectal cancer.

KNOWLEDGE INTO ACTION

1. Gary Harris, your 49-year-old uncle, confides in you that he hasn't had a bowel movement for 8 days and that he has been bloated and vomiting. He has abdominal pain and a fever of 100.2 degrees. He says, "I should probably just buy one of those enemas at the drugstore." What could be causing his symptoms? What will your response be? What would your recommendations for your uncle be?

2. Helena Andropolis, a 78-year-old patient who recently had surgery for colon cancer, is complaining of slight difficulty in breathing. The position of her bed is flat. What things could you do to assist in making her breathing less difficult? What symptoms would indicate that the breathing difficulty had become worse and that Mrs. Pearson had hypoxia?

3. Susan Graham, a 63-year-old patient admitted to the hospital to rule out cancer of the colon, is scheduled for a proctosigmoidoscopy. She says to you, "Can you tell me more about that test I'm having tomorrow? The doctor said something about a tube. What do they hope to prove by this thing?" What will your response be regarding the procedure itself and the purpose of the procedure?

4. Your 35-year-old neighbor, Marcie Klein, has just returned from a physical examination that she had scheduled as a result of her father being diagnosed with colon cancer. She says to you, "They sent these popsicle sticks home with me and some cardboard things. I think they want me to put some . . . you know . . . next time I go to the bathroom, they want me to smear some stool on one of the cardboards. How embarrassing! Is it really important that I do that?" What will your response be?

Lung Cancer

OBJECTIVES

Upon completion of this chapter, the student should be able to:

- Define the key terms listed throughout the chapter
- Describe the physiology of the respiratory system
- State a specific definition for lung cancer
- Describe the incidence of lung cancer
- List the risk factors associated with lung cancer
- Describe the signs and symptoms associated with lung cancer, the rationale for these symptoms, and associated care
- Identify specific methods for diagnosis of lung cancer
- Describe the categories and types of lung cancer
- Identify specific methods for treatment of lung cancer
- Describe considerations for caring for a patient with lung cancer

KEY TERMS

Pharynx – throat

Larynx – voice box, located at the base of the throat region

Trachea – airway that connects the larynx to the bronchial tubes

Bronchi – the two branches off the trachea; left and right bronchus

Bronchioles – the small branches off the bronchi within the lungs

Alveoli – small air sacks of the lungs in which carbon dioxide and oxygen exchange takes place during the process of respiration

Inspiration – process of drawing oxygen-rich air into the lungs

Carbon dioxide (CO_2) – waste product of cellular metabolism; excreted from the body during the process of respiration

INTRODUCTION

Lung cancer is defined as abnormal growth of cells that destroys lung tissue and impedes the function of the respiratory system.

PHYSIOLOGY OF THE RESPIRATORY SYSTEM

The respiratory system is made up of the nose and nasal cavity, sinuses, **pharynx**, **larynx**, **trachea**, **bronchi**, **bronchioles**, and **alveoli**. (See Figure 4-1.) The purpose of the respiratory system is to draw oxygen-rich air into the lungs (**inspiration**) to be transported to the body system through the blood vessels. The waste product, **carbon dioxide (CO_2)**, is then released through the lungs (**expiration**). The respiratory system is lined with mucous membrane, which moistens the respiratory tract and assists in trapping and removing foreign particles from entering the lungs. Also located along the respiratory system are **cilia**, tiny hairlike structures that also function to trap and remove foreign particles from the airway. Up to one quart of mucous is normally secreted daily by the mucous membranes of the respiratory tract.

STATISTICS

More than 170,000 cases of lung cancer are diagnosed each year in the United States with 149,000 people dying of lung cancer annually. Lung cancer accounts for approximately 15% of all cancers diagnosed in the United States annually and 25% of all cancer deaths annually. Lung cancer accounts for more cancer deaths than any other form of cancer. Over 90% of all lung cancers are preventable by abstaining from cigarette smoking or cessation of smoking. Secondhand smoke leads to 4,700 lung cancer deaths annually. Lung cancer occurs most often in people over the age of 50, with equal occurrence

Expiration – the process of breathing out during respiration (breathing)

Cilia – hairlike extensions found in the mucous membrane of the respiratory tract that aid in removing foreign bodies, e.g. dust or mucous, from the respiratory tract

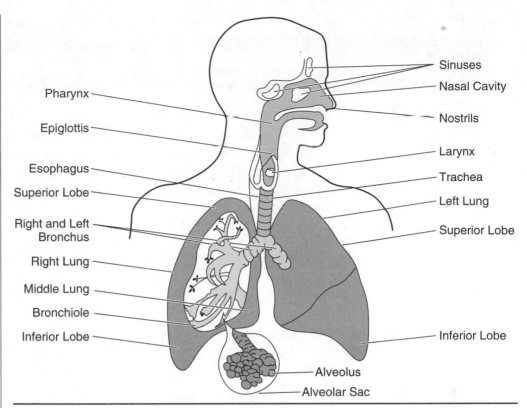

Figure 4-1   The respiratory system

between men and women. Lung cancer previously affected mostly men, but the incidence is more equal due to the increased number of women who smoke.

Lung cancer metastasizes by attacking adjacent tissue or spreads to distant parts of the body via the bloodstream or lymph system. The most common site for metastasis is the lymph nodes adjacent to the lungs. It can also metastasize to the kidneys, liver, bones, opposite lung, and brain. The five-year survival rate for lung cancer is approximately 13%.

RISK FACTORS

1. Smoking is the number one cause of cancer of the lung. Approximately 90% of people with lung cancer have a history of smoking, with only 10% of all cases occurring in people who do not smoke. When a person quits smoking, her risk decreases almost to that of a nonsmoker within 10 years. The risk of lung cancer is fifteen to twenty-five times higher for smokers than nonsmokers. People who are married to heavy smokers have a 70% chance of getting lung cancer.

2. Environmental factors are another major cause of lung cancer. Examples of this include asbestos, arsenic, radon, coal tar products, radioactive substances, general air pollution, and uranium.

    People who are exposed to asbestos routinely have a thirty times higher risk of getting lung cancer, with more than 5,500 cancer deaths annually associated with asbestos exposure.

    People who are exposed to radon routinely have a higher risk of getting lung cancer, with 5,000 to 20,000 cancer deaths annually associated with radon exposure.

Expectorants – medications or substances that promote the removal of fluids or phlegm from the respiratory tract

Postural drainage – procedure in which the patient is positioned in alternating positions to facilitate drainage and expectoration of secretions in the lung through the use of gravity

Hemoptysis – coughing up of blood from the respiratory tract

3. People who have close relatives with lung cancer have a slightly higher risk of having lung cancer.

SIGNS, SYMPTOMS, AND ASSOCIATED CARE

1. Chronic cough due to irritation of the lining of the bronchi
   - Encourage fluids to thin mucous secretions to cough up more easily
   - Administer **expectorants** as needed to aid in coughing up secretions
   - Splint chest to assist patient in coughing more effectively
   - Provide container for patient to cough secretions into
   - Dispose of tissues and sputum properly
   - Provide frequent mouth care
   - Employ meticulous hand washing by patient, visitors, and staff members
   - Administer *postural drainage* technique to facilitate drainage of mucous from lungs
   - Encourage patient to cover mouth when coughing
   - Observe sputum for signs of **hemoptysis** or infection
   - Educate regarding effective coughing techniques to facilitate productivity of cough
   - Provide humidified air
   - Employ universal precautions when handling any blood or body fluids (See Appendix C)

2. Hemoptysis due to irritation and bleeding of the cancerous area
   - Provide container for patient to cough secretions into
   - Observe phlegm for amount of blood present
   - Dispose of tissues and lung secretions properly
   - Provide frequent mouth care
   - Employ meticulous hand washing by patient and staff
   - Utilize universal precautions when handling any blood or body fluids

3. Dyspnea due to obstruction or partial obstruction of the bronchial tube which decreases air exchange
   - Assist with position for patient comfort
   - Administer oxygen as needed and as directed by physician (See Figure 4-2)
   - Avoid constrictive garments and undergarments
   - Provide fan in room to circulate air and assist in making breathing easier
   - Encourage frequent rest periods to conserve energy and arrange schedule of activities around patient rest periods
   - Assist with activities of daily living (ADLs) as necessary
   - Assess breath sounds on routine basis
   - Observe for signs of hypoxia such as cyanosis, diaphoresis, decreased level of consciousness, and confusion
   - Monitor ease of respirations and respiratory rate
   - Encourage to do as many activities as possible in a sitting position, e.g. dressing, bathing, cooking, and cleaning
   - Humidify air as needed
   - Provide reassurance to patient
   - Treat cause of dyspnea

Wheezing – whistling sound heard during the process of respirations due to constriction of the respiratory tract

Pleurisy – inflammation of the pleura of the lung

Insomnia – inability to fall asleep or stay asleep once sleep is achieved

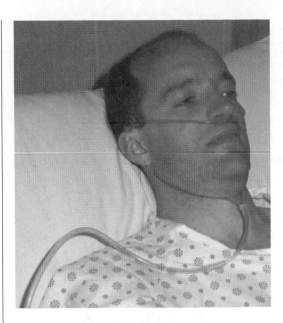

Figure 4-2   Correct placement of a nasal cannula for oxygen administration

4. **Wheezing** due to partial obstruction of the bronchial tube
   - Assist with position for patient comfort
   - Assess breath sounds routinely
   - Observe for signs of hypoxia, e.g. cyanosis, diaphoresis, confusion, and decreased level of consciousness
   - Administer oxygen as needed and as directed by physician
   - Provide reassurance to patient
   - Humidify air as needed
   - Monitor for breathing difficulty
   - Avoid constrictive clothing, undergarments, or linens

5. **Pleurisy** due to metastasis of the lung cancer into the ribs and muscle of the chest wall
   - Administer medications as directed for pain relief
   - Provide heating pad or other form of heat treatment as directed for pain relief
   - Observe for complications relating to the pain, such as **insomnia**, decreased appetite, or mood changes
   - Provide alternative methods of pain relief, such as relaxation techniques, imaging, and massage
   - Encourage rest periods as necessary
   - Monitor for adequate oxygenation
   - Monitor for increased respiratory distress

6. Recurrent respiratory infections due to: (1) partial obstruction that blocks mucous expectoration, (2) increased mucous production due to the irritation within the bronchial tube and lung, and (3) poor air exchange due to partial or complete obstruction of the airway due to the tumor
   - Educate patient and family regarding symptoms of respiratory infection, such as cough, phlegm production, chest pain, fever, chills, dyspnea, and diaphoresis
   - Educate patient and family to report symptoms of respiratory infection to physician

Influenza – acute viral respiratory infection characterized by fever, cough, chills, headache, and sore throat

Vaccinations – small amounts of an infectious agent given to a person to build up that person's immunity to the infectious agent

Hormone – substance secreted by certain organs or tissues in the body that stimulate the activity of other tissues or glands in the body

Sodium – mineral found in salt, cured meats, salted foods, and processed foods that is necessary for the maintenance of fluid balance within the body

- Educate patient regarding importance of completing medication prescribed for respiratory infection
- Encourage fluids to help in thinning secretions and making them easier to expel
- Prevent transmission of infection by hand washing and correctly disposing of tissues and phlegm
- Provide tissues and container to spit into and dispose of properly
- Avoid contact with people with respiratory infections
- Maintain optimal health to fight off infections
- Administer **influenza** and pneumonia **vaccinations** as directed by physician
- Avoid crowded areas, which increase the likelihood of contracting a respiratory infection

7. Hoarseness due to irritation of the larynx
   - Encourage patient to rest voice when possible
   - Provide alternate forms of communication, such as message board or writing messages
   - Offer liquids frequently to aid in reduction of hoarseness

8. Confusion due to an increase in **hormone** production that regulates sodium level in the body with subsequent decrease in serum *sodium* levels
   - Monitor serum sodium levels
   - Monitor for level of orientation
   - Provide protection from injury if the patient is confused
   - Offer emotional support to patient and family in the event of confusion
   - Provide calm, quiet environment for patient
   - Avoid startling patient
   - Allow family members or friends to stay with patient as much as needed if this is reassuring to patient
   - Monitor for changes in mental status
   - Assist patient with ADLs in the presence of decreased mental status

9. Fatigue due to the cancer growth in the body
   - Assist patient with ADLs as necessary
   - Schedule care, activities, and treatment around patient's rest schedule
   - Monitor phone calls and visitors around patient's energy level and rest schedule
   - Provide assistance as needed to prevent injury due to weakness
   - Provide method for patient to call for assistance
   - Encourage patient to set realistic goals of activities
   - Allow adequate time to do activities and procedures to avoid frustration or possible injury
   - Encourage exercise to maintain muscle strength
   - Provide cane or walker as necessary for ambulation and transfer
   - Provide private room as able for patient to promote rest periods

10. Loss of appetite and subsequent weight loss due to the cancer growth in the body
    - Obtain baseline weight and monitor weight on routine basis
    - Encourage patient to participate in dietary choices

Superior vena cava – one of the two main vessels that return blood from the body to the right atrium of the heart

Sputum – material that is coughed up from within the respiratory tract

Bronchoscopy – visualization of the bronchus using a flexible instrument; this procedure is used to aid in diagnosis of disease and also permits biopsy

- Offer nutritional supplements and vitamins as necessary
- Encourage family and friends to bring in food that is appealing to patient as their dietary restrictions allow
- Administer parenteral fluids as necessary
- Monitor intake and output (I and O)
- Encourage rest periods before and after meals
- Avoid unpleasant sights and odors in room to make meals more appealing
- Provide meticulous mouth care
- Monitor for skin breakdown due to loss of body tissue
- Encourage clothing styles that do not draw attention to weight loss
- Monitor for symptoms of dehydration, e.g. decreased urine output, constipation, dry skin, tenting of skin, dry mouth, dry eyes, concentrated urine, hypotension, and confusion

11. Edema of the face and neck due to lymph node involvement and **superior vena cava** involvement
    - Monitor for neurological symptoms of the face and neck
    - Restrict salt in diet as prescribed by physician
    - Monitor edema on routine basis
    - Monitor for skin breakdown in edematous areas
    - Monitor for symptoms of decreased circulation in edematous areas, e.g. cool to touch, cyanotic, and decreased sensation
    - Obtain baseline weight and monitor on routine basis
    - Monitor intake and output (I and O)

DIAGNOSIS

1. Symptoms
2. Physical examination
3. Medical history
4. *Chest x-ray* is used to locate abnormalities in the lung (See Figure 4-3)
5. **Sputum** specimen to determine the presence of malignant cells
6. *Bronchoscopy* to inspect the bronchial tubes and lungs; perform a biopsy as necessary

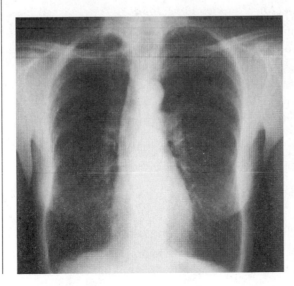

Figure 4-3 Radiography of the chest (chest x-ray) (From Carlton, *Principles of Radiographic Imaging: An Art and a Science*, copyright © 1992, Delmar Publishers)

Mediastinum – the area between the lungs in the chest

Pleural – refers to the pleura of the lung

Epidermoid – the epidermis (skin)

Manifests – makes itself known; usually refers to the appearance of symptoms

Carcinoma – cancerous tumor of the epithelium (lining of internal and external organs)

Lobectomy – surgical removal of the lobe of an organ; frequently refers to the lung or brain

Pneumonectomy – surgical removal of the lung

7. *Biopsy* of tissue removed to inspect for cancer cells; biopsy can be done using a needle or surgery

8. *Computerized tomography (CT scan)* to detect metastasis

9. *Mediastinoscopy* to detect metastasis to lymph nodes in **mediastinum**

10. Scans using radioisotope injection to detect metastasis

11. *Thoracentesis* to check **pleural** fluid for the presence of malignant cells

TYPES OF LUNG CANCER

Lung cancer can be divided into two specific groups: small cell lung cancer and nonsmall cell lung cancer.

1. Small cell lung cancer, also referred to as oat cell cancer, accounts for 20 to 25% of all reported cases of lung cancer. This cancer grows rapidly, is prone to metastasis, and is frequently found in heavy smokers.

2. Nonsmall cell lung cancer can be further divided into three groups depending on the type of the cancer cells:

   • **Epidermoid** cancer, also referred to as squamous cell carcinoma, accounts for 33% of all reported cases of lung cancer. This cancer usually begins in the bronchi and rarely metastasizes.

   • Adenocarcinoma accounts for 25% of all reported cases of lung cancer. It **manifests** itself along the edges of the lung and the lining of the bronchi.

   • Large cell **carcinomas** account for 16% of all reported cases of lung cancer and are generally located in the bronchioles.

TREATMENT

There are three specific forms of treatment for lung cancer: surgery, chemotherapy, and radiation therapy. The type of treatment depends on the type of cancer cell present as well as the presence of metastasis.

1. Small cell lung cancer generally metastasizes to distant parts of the body. Treatment for this form of cancer is generally a combination of *radiation* to the chest as well as *chemotherapy*.

2. Nonsmall cell lung cancer treatment is divided into three specific groups for treatment:

   • Lung cancer confined to the lung can be treated with surgery, e.g. *lobectomy* or *pneumonectomy*

   • Lung cancer that has spread to adjacent tissue or lymph nodes can be treated with radiation therapy to the chest

   • Lung cancer that has metastasized to distant parts of the body will be treated by a combination of radiation therapy and chemotherapy to relieve symptoms by reducing tumor size, e.g. chemotherapy: Cyclophosphamide (Cytoxan), Methotrexate, Vincristine (Oncovin), Doxorubicin (Adriamycin)

CONSIDERATIONS FOR CARE

1. Educate patient and family regarding the disease.

2. Educate patient and family regarding treatment options as well as possible side effects of specific treatments.

3. Educate patient and family regarding need to quit smoking and offer opportunities to obtain assistance with smoking cessation.

4. Provide opportunities for patient and family to communicate feelings and concerns regarding the cancer and course of treatment.

5. Acknowledge patient's and family's feelings in a nonjudgmental manner.

6. Provide patient opportunities to make decisions regarding treatment and care schedule.

7. Educate patient and family regarding importance of follow-up care by physician.

8. Provide information to patient and family regarding community resources that are available while hospitalized and upon discharge.

9. Provide information to patient and family regarding support groups in the area.

10. Provide information regarding resources to obtain financial assistance in the event of difficulty paying medical bills or in the event the patient is unable to return to work.

11. Assist the patient and family to set realistic goals regarding adjustment to possible life style changes.

12. Professional counseling may be necessary for the patient and family to deal with emotions brought on by the diagnosis or treatment.

13. Assist patient and family to arrange for home oxygen therapy if necessary.

14. Instruct patient and family regarding post-operative care if necessary.

15. Educate patient and family regarding nutritional guidelines for weight maintenance; diet should be high in calories and protein.

16. Educate patient regarding technique to cough effectively and productively.

FOR MORE INFORMATION

American Cancer Society
1599 Clifton Road, NE
Atlanta, GA 30329
(404) 320-3333

American Lung Association
1740 Broadway
New York, NY 10019
(212) 315-8700

ASSIGNMENT SHEET: LUNG CANCER

Short Answer

1. Describe the physiology of the respiratory system.

2. Write a brief definition for lung cancer.

3. Describe the incidence of lung cancer.

4. List and describe three (3) risk factors for lung cancer.

5. List eleven (11) signs and symptoms for lung cancer and describe the rationale and associated care for each.

6. List eleven (11) specific methods used to diagnose lung cancer.

7. Write the normal range for sodium.

8. List nine (9) specific symptoms of dehydration.

9. List seven (7) specific symptoms of a respiratory infection.

10. Describe the four (4) specific categories of lung cancer and the specific treatment as related to each type of lung cancer.

11. List sixteen (16) considerations for caring for a patient with lung cancer.

KNOWLEDGE INTO ACTION

1. James L. Porter, a 63-year-old diagnosed with lung cancer, is admitted to the hospital with extreme fatigue. Describe some methods you could take to ensure that Mr. Porter is able to obtain adequate rest in the hospital.

2. Maria Amone is scheduled for a bronchoscopy. She asks you what *bronchoscopy* means and what the procedure involves. What will your response be?

3. Art Pearson, a 58-year-old construction worker, is being discharged from the hospital following a pneumonectomy. He has edema of the face and neck as well as a weight loss of approximately 45 pounds from his normal weight. What would you suggest to him regarding his diet once he gets home?

4. Jenni Lamberts is being discharged from the hospital. Prior to her discharge, she says to you, "The doctor says I need to be careful about getting an infection in my lungs. How will I know if I have a respiratory infection?" What will your response be?

Uterine Cancer

OBJECTIVES

Upon completion of this chapter, the student should be able to:

- Define the key terms listed throughout the chapter
- Describe the physiology of the uterus
- State a specific definition for uterine cancer
- Describe the incidence of uterine cancer
- List risk factors for uterine cancer
- List specific methods to decrease the risk of uterine cancer
- Describe specific signs and symptoms of uterine cancer, the rationale for the symptoms, and associated care
- Identify specific methods for diagnosis of uterine cancer
- Identify specific methods for treatment of uterine cancer
- Describe specific considerations for caring for a patient with uterine cancer

KEY TERMS

Cervix – opening to the vagina located at the base of the uterus

Corpus uteri – the main body of the uterus

Uterus – female organ that holds the developing fetus during pregnancy

Fetus – refers to an unborn child during the last two trimesters (6 months) in the uterus

Postmenopausal – after cessation of the menstrual cycle (menopause)

Fatal – resulting in death

Heredity – genetic characteristics or traits that are passed from parents to their offspring

INTRODUCTION

Uterine cancer is a general category that covers cancer of the **cervix** as well as cancer of the body of the uterus, the **corpus uteri**.

PHYSIOLOGY OF THE UTERUS

The **uterus** is located in the pelvic region of the female. It is normally pear-shaped and the size of a small fist. The uterus is lined with a special tissue called endometrium. The function of the uterus and endometrium is to nourish the fertilized egg until the **fetus** reaches maturity and is ready to be delivered. (See Figure 5-1.)

STATISTICS

Cancer of the uterus is the fourth most common cancer among females. It is most common in **postmenopausal** women, generally occurring after the age of 55. Approximately 33,000 cases of uterine cancer are diagnosed annually in the United States, of which 5,000 will be **fatal**. The five-year survival rate is approximately 55% with an overall cure rate of 29%.

RISK FACTORS

1. Obesity
2. Hypertension
3. Estrogen therapy
4. **Heredity**
5. Late menopause

Polyps – growths originating in a mucous membrane

Genital – the reproductive organs of the male or female

Anovulation – temporary or permanent cessation of female ovulation

Vaginal – relating to the external opening to the cervix and uterus; birth canal

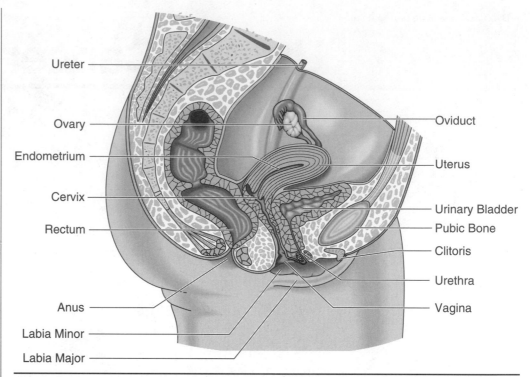

Figure 5-1   Side view of the female pelvic region (From Layman, *The Medical Language*, copyright © 1995, Delmar Publishers)

6. More than three sexual partners
7. History of uterine **polyps**
8. No children
9. Sexual relationships prior to age 20
10. Poor **genital** hygiene
11. Hormonal imbalance
12. **Anovulation**

METHODS TO DECREASE RISK FACTORS

1. Maintain normal weight
2. Annual physical examination to include *Pap smear* and pelvic examination
3. Alternative form of birth control rather than birth control pills for women at increased risk for uterine cancer, as directed by physician
4. Report unusual bleeding or discharge promptly to physician
5. Maintain meticulous genital hygiene
6. Control blood pressure
7. Monitor hormone therapy with physician as directed
8. Limit number of sexual partners

SIGNS, SYMPTOMS, AND ASSOCIATED CARE

1. Abnormal bleeding—either postmenopausal, between regular menstrual cycles, or longer or heavier bleeding during menstrual cycles due to hormonal abnormalities and tumor growth or irritation involving the endometrium
   - Monitor amount, color, consistency, and odor of **vaginal** discharge
   - Provide meticulous skin care to perineal area

Dysfunction – abnormal
function

- Monitor discharge for signs of bleeding or infection
- Utilize universal precautions at all times when coming in contact with blood or body fluids (See Appendix C)
- Provide sanitary napkins as necessary for patient use
- Dispose of sanitary napkins in appropriate manner
- Change clothing and bedding as necessary due to vaginal discharge

2. Uterine enlargement due to neoplastic growth and hormonal changes
   - Monitor for size of uterus through the use of *ultrasound*
   - Provide comfort measures as necessary due to pain associated with uterine enlargement
   - Provide pain control methods, such as relaxation techniques, massage, imaging, and pain medications as prescribed by physician

3. Abdominal or pelvic pain due to uterine enlargement or metastasis
   - Adjust position for patient comfort
   - Avoid constrictive garments and undergarments
   - Provide methods to promote comfort, such as relaxation techniques, imaging, massage, and warm baths
   - Monitor for level of pain and offer comfort measures as necessary
   - Administer medications as necessary and as prescribed by physician for the control of pain
   - Encourage patient to request pain relief methods before pain becomes too severe

4. Anemia due to bleeding
   - Administer blood transfusions and iron supplements as necessary to treat anemia
   - Monitor *hemoglobin* and *hematocrit*
   - Monitor for weakness associated with anemia, assist with activities of daily living (ADLs) as necessary, and protect from possible injury due to weakness
   - Monitor physical symptoms of anemia, such as pallor, weakness, and vertigo

5. Bowel or bladder **dysfunction** due to metastasis
   - Assess for bladder control and observe for incontinence
   - Provide meticulous skin care, especially in the presence of incontinence
   - Observe for and educate family to observe for and report symptoms of urinary tract infection, such as burning with urination, frequency, urgency, pain, fever, cloudy urine, malodorous urine, hematuria, and dysuria
   - Encourage fluid intake
   - Encourage urination schedule
   - Be aware of nonverbal clues a patient may give as to a need to use the bathroom
   - Prevent odors in the room by changing linens as needed and washing off chairs and other items that become wet or soiled
   - Use mild soap to cleanse the patient's skin and pat dry
   - Provide privacy for the patient when she is using the bathroom
   - Offer reassurance to the patient
   - Monitor for anemia in the presence of bloody stools
   - Check for the presence of blood (*Hemoccult*® *stools*)

Ovarian – relating to the female reproductive glands that store the ovum and produce estrogen and progesterone

---

Table 5-1 Intake and Output Measurement

INTAKE—includes all fluid taken into the body.

　a. **Oral intake** includes anything that is liquid at room temperature and includes the following examples: gelatin, water, juice, pudding, soup, cooked cereal, and coffee.

　b. **Parenteral intake** includes liquids taken into the body other than by mouth and includes the following examples: nasogastric tube feeding, intravenous (IV) fluids, blood, and blood products.

OUTPUT—includes all fluid that leaves the body and includes the following examples: urine, vomit, wound drainage, nasogastric suction or drainage, diarrhea stools, and perspiration.

- Monitor amount, frequency, and consistency of stools
- Provide meticulous skin care to the anal area
- Avoid foods that increase intestinal gas formation
- Control odors in patient room with ventilation and room deodorizers
- Provide private room as necessary
- Prevent embarrassment for the patient

6. Fever due to metastasis

- Monitor temperature at routine intervals
- Provide comfort measures for patient with elevated temperature, such as cool cloth to forehead, partial or complete bath as needed, clothing and bedding changed frequently due to diaphoresis, and encourage fluids to prevent dehydration. Symptoms of dehydration include decreased urine output, dry skin, dry mouth, dry eyes, constipation, tenting of skin, concentrated urine, confusion, and hypotension.
- Avoid exposing patient to a draft
- Cover with blankets as necessary
- Monitor intake and output (I and O) (See Table 5-1)
- Maintain comfortable room temperature for patient
- Avoid plastic mattresses and plastic bed protectors as they increase perspiration
- Use antiperspirant/deodorant to minimize sweating and odor

DIAGNOSIS

1. Symptoms
2. Physical examination
3. Pelvic examination would indicate uterine or **ovarian** enlargement
4. *Colposcopy* used for visual examination of the vagina and cervix
5. *Biopsy* of tissue from endometrium or cervix
6. *Conization* to remove large piece of tissue from cervical canal for biopsy
7. *Dilation and curettage (D and C)* to remove tissue from the body of the uterus
8. *Pap smear*
9. *Hysteroscopy* to view the endometrium
10. *Aspiration curettage* to suction tissue samples from the endometrium
11. Tests to determine metastasis, e.g. *CT scan*, *bone scan*, and *cystoscopy*
12. *Schiller's test*—healthy tissues turn brown when iodine is applied to the cervix while cancerous tissues do not accept the stain and remain pink

Hysterectomy – surgical removal of the uterus

Oophorectomy – surgical removal of the ovary

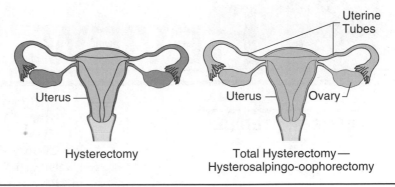

Figure 5-2   Examples of hysterectomies (From Smith et al., *Medical Terminology: A Programmed Text, 7th edition*, copyright © 1995, Delmar Publishers)

TREATMENT

1. *Hysterectomy* (See Figure 5-2)
2. *Chemotherapy*, e.g. Cisplatin, Doxorubicin, Methotrexate, Bleomycin
3. *Radiation therapy*
4. Hormonal therapy, e.g. Tamoxifen
5. Surgical removal of involved ovaries (**oophorectomy**), lymph nodes, or other tissues

CONSIDERATIONS FOR CARE

1. Educate patient and family regarding the disease process
2. Educate patient and family regarding forms of treatment as well as side effects of treatment
3. Provide emotional support to patient and family
4. Nonjudgmental acceptance of emotions and behavior of patient and family
5. Assess level of comfort and offer methods of pain control, such as relaxation, imaging, massage, heat treatment, and medications
6. Psychological counseling may be necessary post-hysterectomy for women of child-bearing age
7. Hormonal replacement may be necessary for women post-oophorectomy
8. Education for patient in the event of surgery regarding post-operative care, e.g. coughing and deep-breathing exercises, nasogastric tube (NG), intravenous (IV) line, urinary catheter, and vital signs (See Appendix D)

FOR MORE INFORMATION

American Cancer Society
1599 Clifton Road, NE
Atlanta, GA 30329
1-800-ACS-2345

ASSIGNMENT SHEET: UTERINE CANCER

Short Answer

1. Write a brief definition for the terms listed throughout the chapter.

2. Describe the normal physiology and function of the uterus.

3. Write a brief definition for uterine cancer.

4. Describe the incidence of uterine cancer.

5. List twelve (12) risk factors for uterine cancer.

6. Describe eight (8) methods to decrease or eliminate risk factors associated with uterine cancer.

7. List six (6) signs and symptoms of uterine cancer and the rationale and associated care for each of the symptoms.

8. List twelve (12) specific methods used to aid in the diagnosis of uterine cancer.

9. Describe five (5) specific methods used to treat uterine cancer.

10. Describe eight (8) considerations for caring for a patient with uterine cancer.

11. Describe the following procedures used to diagnose or treat uterine cancer.

    a. Pap smear
    b. Colposcopy
    c. Biopsy
    d. Conization
    e. Dilation and curettage (D and C)
    f. Hysteroscopy
    g. Aspiration curettage
    h. CT scan
    i. Bone scan
    j. Hysterectomy
    k. Cystoscopy
    l. Ultrasound
    m. Pelvic examination
    n. Blood transfusion
    o. Schiller's test
    p. Chemotherapy
    q. Radiation therapy
    r. Hemoccult® stools

12. Write the normal range for each of the following laboratory tests.

    a. Hemoglobin (Hg)
    b. Hematocrit (Hct)

KNOWLEDGE INTO ACTION

1. Yeu-Sheng Chang, a 72-year-old with uterine cancer that has metastasized, has incontinence of the bowel and bladder. Describe what you could do to assist this patient in the following areas:

   a. Skin integrity
   b. Maintenance of bedding and the environment
   c. Promotion of self-esteem
   d. Promoting continence

2. Yeu-Sheng Chang also has a fever of 102 degrees. Describe what you could do to make her more comfortable due to the fever and the diaphoresis that accompanies her fever.

3. Hannah Jensen, a 28-year-old who just had a hysterectomy, is in her room crying. She says to you, "My husband and I wanted to have children so badly. I just don't know what to do." What will your response be?

6 Prostate Cancer

KEY TERMS

Testosterone – male hormone that is responsible for secondary sex characteristics production in men; produced in the testes

Testicles – male reproductive glands located in the scrotum directly adjacent to the penis

Semen – thick, white fluid that is discharged from the urethra of the penis of the male during sexual arousal and climax

Ejaculation – forcible expulsion of semen from the penis

Sperm – male reproductive cells that are released in the semen during sexual arousal and climax

Penis – male sex organ used for the purpose of urination and sexual intercourse

INTRODUCTION

Prostate cancer is a malignant tumor of the prostate gland, most often (85%) located in the posterior portion of the prostate. Most prostatic tumors can be detected by doing a rectal examination. Prostate cancer can spread to adjacent tissues or metastasize by way of the bloodstream or lymph system. The growth of prostate cancer is stimulated by **testosterone**, a male hormone produced by the **testicles**.

PHYSIOLOGY OF THE PROSTATE GLAND

The prostate is a walnut-sized male gland located directly below the bladder. It surrounds the urethra. The urethra is the tube leading from the bladder that carries urine to be excreted as well as the expulsion of **semen** during **ejaculation**. The function of the prostate is to secrete a milky-white substance, which is carried to the urethra through ducts and helps to transport **sperm** during ejaculation through the **penis**. It also nourishes the sperm once it reaches the vaginal canal. (See Figure 6-1.)

STATISTICS

Prostate cancer accounts for 160,000 new cases of cancer each year in men and 25,000 deaths annually. Prostate cancer accounts for 18% of all male cancer deaths. It is the second leading cause of cancer death in males and is the most common cancer in males over the age of 65. Over 80% of prostate cancer occurs in males over the age of 65. Only 2% of all prostate cancers occur in men under the age of 50. The five-year survival rate is 78% if the tumor is localized and decreases to 35% if the tumor has metastasized. The most frequent site of metastasis is to the bones, lymph nodes, and lungs. Prostate cancer occurs most often among African-Americans and males with Type A blood. It possibly occurs in African-Americans more frequently due to decreased health care availability and, therefore, decreased detection. Prostate cancer is responsible for 22% of all cancers in the United States and will occur in 10% of all men in the United States.

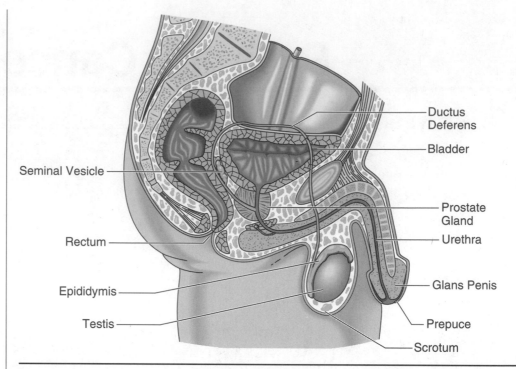

Figure 6-1 Side view of male pelvic region (From Layman, *The Medical Language*, copyright © 1995, Delmar Publishers)

RISK FACTORS

The following are risk factors and methods to reduce those risk factors associated with prostate cancer.

1. High intake of dietary fat

    • Decrease dietary fat intake. Fat should account for 30% or less of total caloric intake.

2. Obesity

    • Maintain normal body weight. Prostate cancer is 2.5 times more common in overweight males.

3. Smoking

    • Cease smoking or abstain from smoking; avoid secondhand smoke.

4. Exposure to cadmium

    • Avoid exposure to cadmium, which is used in industry for the purpose of electroplating as well as for atomic reactors.

SIGNS, SYMPTOMS, AND ASSOCIATED CARE

Signs and symptoms occur generally only in the later stages of the disease after the tumor has metastasized.

1. Frequent urination due to enlargement of the prostate gland. The bladder muscle needs to work harder to force urine through the urethra causing the bladder muscle to thicken, which causes increased frequency of urination.

    • Provide the patient opportunity to use the restroom, urinal, or commode on a frequent basis

    • Provide a night light for the patient who needs to urinate during the night

    • Watch for signals that a confused patient needs to urinate

Retention – holding something in the body that usually is excreted from the body; often refers to fluid within the cells of the body

- Change bedding or briefs frequently and provide meticulous skin care for the patient who may be incontinent
- Assist patient to bathroom as needed
- Be aware of urination frequency when planning treatments or when travelling
- Provide method for patient to contact staff if assistance is needed
- Respond promptly to patient request for assistance

2. Nocturia due to enlargement of the prostate gland
   - Assist patient to bathroom as needed
   - Monitor patient during night while going to the bathroom
   - Provide night light if patient is in new surroundings or is confused
   - Provide a urinal or commode for patient use
   - Provide a method for the patient to call for help if needed during the night

3. Urgency of urination due to enlargement of the prostate gland
   - Be aware of a place where the patient can urinate when out of his own environment
   - Respond to the patient's request promptly when he signals the need to go to the bathroom
   - Have equipment on hand and ready for the patient when he signals the need to go to the bathroom
   - Provide a method for the patient to contact staff if assistance is needed
   - Encourage a frequent urination schedule to avoid urgency and possible incontinence

4. Dribbling of urine due to enlargement of the prostate gland
   - Assess for bladder control and observe for incontinence
   - Provide meticulous skin care especially in the presence of incontinence
   - Observe for and educate family to observe for and report symptoms of urinary tract infection, e.g. burning with urination, frequency, urgency, pain, fever, cloudy urine, malodorous urine, bloody urine, and dysuria
   - Encourage fluid intake
   - Encourage a urination schedule (See Table 6-1)
   - Be aware of nonverbal clues a patient may give as to his need to use the bathroom
   - Prevent odors in the room by changing linens as needed and washing off chairs and other items that become wet or soiled
   - Prevent embarrassment to the patient
   - Avoid teasing or belittling the patient
   - Use mild soap to cleanse the patient's skin and pat dry
   - Provide privacy for the patient when he is using the bathroom
   - Provide protection as needed for bedding and clothing with waterproof pad or undergarment (See Figure 6-2)

5. Difficulty initiating a stream of urine due to enlargement of the prostate gland
   - Provide privacy
   - Utilize techniques, such as the sound of water running or warm water poured over the perineal area, which often aid in starting the urinary stream

6. Urinary **retention** due to enlargement of the prostate gland
   - Catheterization may be necessary to drain the urine from the bladder

Table 6-1   Urination Schedule

Patient: Date: Room: Time:	Voided (Y or N)	Leaking Amount (LA=Large, SA=Small)	Dry (Y or N)	Amount Voided (cc)	Fluid Intake (cc and type)
12–1 A.M.					
1–2 A.M.					
2–3 A.M.					
3–4 A.M.					
4–5 A.M.					
5–6 A.M.					
6–7 A.M.					
7–8 A.M.					
8-hour Total (I/O)					
8–9 A.M.					
9–10 A.M.					
10–11 A.M.					
11 A.M.–12 P.M.					
12–1 P.M.					
1–2 P.M.					
2–3 P.M.					
3–4 P.M.					
8-hour Total (I/O)					
4–5 P.M.					
5–6 P.M.					
6–7 P.M.					
7–8 P.M.					
8–9 P.M.					
9–10 P.M.					
10–11 P.M.					
11 P.M.–12 A.M.					
8-hour Total (I/O)					
24-hour Total (I/O)					

Signature: _____ Date:_____ Shift:_____

Signature: _____ Date:_____ Shift:_____

Signature: _____ Date:_____ Shift:_____

Suprapubic – located
above the pubic region

Cystitis – inflammation of
the urinary bladder

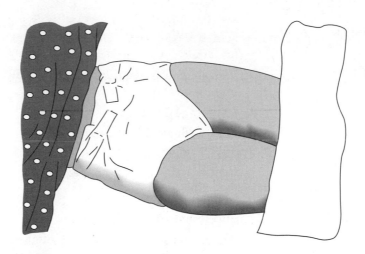

Figure 6-2   Adult incontinence brief

- If catheterization and other medical methods fail, surgery may be
  necessary, e.g. *TURP* or ***suprapubic*** *catheter placement*
7. Complete blockage of the urine due to enlargement of the prostate gland
   - Catheterization may be necessary to drain the urine from the bladder
     (See Figure 6-3)
   - TURP may be necessary
   - Suprapubic catheter may be necessary
8. Frequent **cystitis** due to enlargement of the prostate gland and retention of
   urine in the bladder after urination

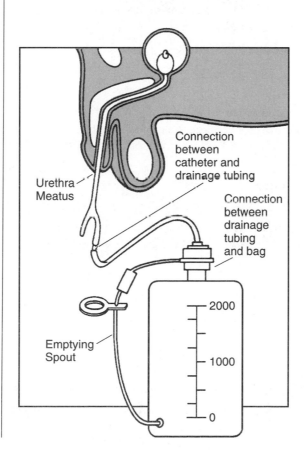

Urethra
Meatus

Connection
between
catheter and
drainage tubing

Connection
between
drainage
tubing
and bag

Emptying
Spout

— 2000

— 1000

— 0

Figure 6-3   Urinary catheter
placement (From Hegner, *Nursing
Assistant: A Nursing Process
Approach, 7th edition,* copyright
© 1995, Delmar Publishers)

Platelet – disklike structure in the blood that is important for the clotting of blood; also known as thrombocyte

- Monitor for symptoms of cystitis. Symptoms of cystitis include dysuria, hematuria, lower abdominal pain, urgency, frequency, burning with urination, cloudy urine, malodorous urine, pelvic pressure, and fever.
- Educate patient regarding need to complete antibiotic regimen as prescribed by physician for cystitis
- Encourage fluids
- Provide meticulous hygiene

9. Low back, hip, and leg pain due to metastasis
   - Encourage patient to report pain before it gets too severe
   - Monitor appetite due to pain
   - Encourage activity as able
   - Assist with activities of daily living (ADLs) as needed due to pain
   - *Radiation therapy* may be used to shrink tumor thereby relieving symptoms
   - Adjust patient position to relieve or reduce pain as possible
   - Avoid constrictive garments
   - Offer comfort measures, such as heat, massage, relaxation techniques, and medications to relieve pain

10. Hematuria due to irritation from the tumor, or metastasis to bladder or urethra
    - Monitor for anemia
    - Avoid blood-thinning medications
    - Provide reassurance for patient
    - Monitor for hematuria
    - Save ongoing urine specimens to monitor for improving or worsening hematuria
    - Avoid use of aspirin and aspirin-containing products as they interfere with normal ***platelet*** function

11. Anemia due to hematuria
    - Administer blood transfusions and iron supplements as necessary to treat anemia
    - Monitor *hemoglobin* and *hematocrit*
    - Monitor for weakness associated with anemia, assist with ADLs as necessary, and protect from possible injury due to weakness
    - Monitor physical symptoms of anemia, such as pallor, weakness, and vertigo

12. Leg edema due to decreased venous return from lymph node involvement
    - Avoid constrictive clothing or undergarments
    - Restrict salt in diet as prescribed by physician
    - Utilize elastic stockings or Jobst stockings to reduce swelling
    - Monitor edema on routine basis
    - Encourage patient to elevate edematous extremity above the level of the heart to reduce swelling
    - Monitor for skin breakdown in edematous areas
    - Monitor for symptoms of decreased circulation in edematous areas, e.g. skin cool to touch, cyanosis, and decreased sensation
    - Obtain baseline weight and monitor on a routine basis
    - Monitor intake and output (I and O)

Bladder – muscular organ that stores urine until it is ready to be excreted from the body

13. Dysuria due to irritation of the urethral lining
    - Offer comfort to patient experiencing pain
    - Encourage fluid intake to 3000 milliliters (ml) per day

DIAGNOSIS

1. Symptoms
2. Physical examination
3. *Digital rectal examination* is used to detect the presence of prostatic enlargement. Examination should be performed annually in males over the age of 40. (See Figure 6-4.)
4. *Biopsy* is used to confirm the diagnosis
5. Elevated serum *acid phosphatase* can be used after treatment to detect recurrence of the cancer or metastasis
6. *Bone scan* is used to detect metastasis to the bones
7. *Chest x-ray* is used to detect metastasis to the lungs
8. Serum *prostate-specific antigen (PSA)* is elevated in the presence of prostatic tumor; can also be used after treatment to detect recurrence of the cancer or metastasis; performed annually in men over the age of 50
9. *Transrectal prostatic ultrasonography* is a procedure in which an instrument is placed in the rectum to obtain ultrasound of prostate and surrounding tissues and organs
10. *CT scan* and *MRI* used to determine the presence of tumor and the extent of metastasis (See Figure 6-5)
11. *IVP (intravenous pyelogram)* is an x-ray of kidneys, ureters, and **bladder** to determine involvement or metastasis
12. *Lymphadenectomy* is the surgical removal of lymph nodes adjacent to prostate gland to determine cancerous involvement of lymph nodes

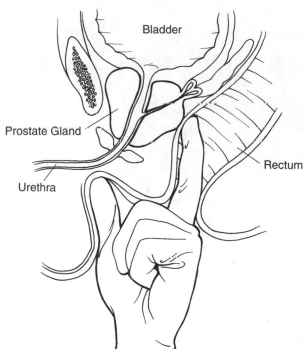

Figure 6-4   Side view of a digital rectal examination of a male (From Keir et al., *Medical Assisting: Administrative and Clinical Competencies, 3rd edition,* copyright © 1993, Delmar Publishers)

Prostatectomy – surgical removal of the prostate gland

Orchiectomy – surgical removal of the testicle

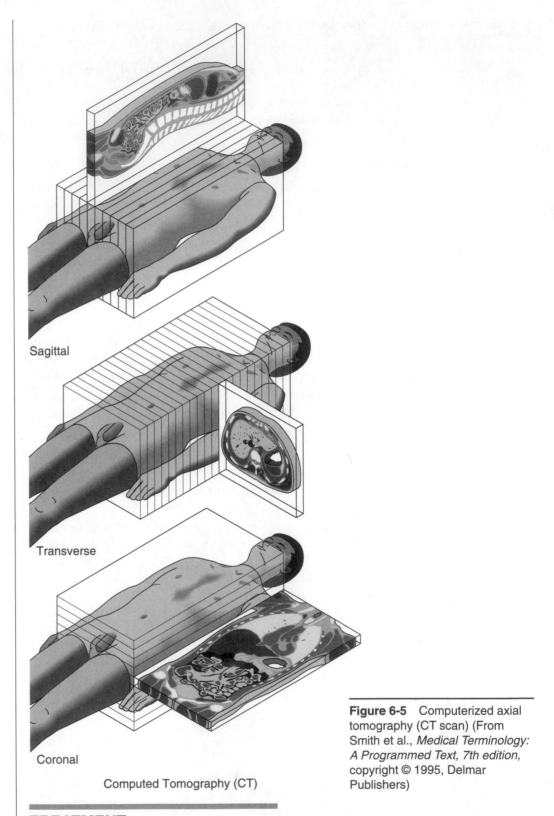

Sagittal

Transverse

Coronal

Computed Tomography (CT)

Figure 6-5   Computerized axial tomography (CT scan) (From Smith et al., *Medical Terminology: A Programmed Text, 7th edition*, copyright © 1995, Delmar Publishers)

TREATMENT

Since prostatic cancer generally affects older men, who often have co-existing diseases or disorders, some patients may choose to forego curative treatment and choose palliative care only.

1. *Prostatectomy*—removal of prostate and any other involved tissues

2. *Orchiectomy*—reduces the production of androgens (primarily testosterone), thereby slowing the growth rate of the tumor

Interstitially – relating to the spaces between the cells and tissues of the body

Luteinizing hormone – hormone secreted by the anterior pituitary gland that regulates ovulation and the endometrium in response to pregnancy

Impotence – incapability of the male to achieve an erection during sexual arousal

Antispasmodics – substances that prevent or treat spasms

3. *Radiation therapy*—externally or **interstitially**

4. Hormonal therapy (Diethylstilbestrol or DES)—suppresses the release of **luteinizing hormone**, which decreases androgen (testosterone) levels

5. *Chemotherapy*, e.g. Vinblastine, Bleomycin, Cisplatin, Cyclophosphamide, Doxorubicin, 5FU, Vindesine

6. *Transurethral resection of the prostate (TURP)*—may be used in the early stages of the disease; this procedure involves removing obstructing tissue or tumor through a tube inserted into the urethra. Procedure is not a cure for prostate cancer but is used for reduction of symptoms associated with an enlarged prostate.

CONSIDERATIONS FOR CARE

1. Educate patient and family regarding the disease process.

2. Educate patient and family regarding forms of treatment as well as side effects of treatment.

3. Provide emotional support to patient and family.

4. Nonjudgmental acceptance of emotions and behavior of patient and family.

5. Monitor for hematuria.

6. Educate regarding the importance of follow-up care with physician.

7. Educate regarding post-operative expectations if patient undergoes surgery, e.g. coughing and deep-breathing exercises, pain, incision, drainage, and intravenous (IV) fluids.

8. Educate patient regarding possibility of **impotence** following treatment. Radical surgery will produce impotence in the majority of males. Approximately 40 to 50% of males will be impotent after radiation therapy.

9. Educate regarding exercises that may diminish incontinence. As many as 7% of patients may experience incontinence following surgery.

10. Educate patient and family to be aware of symptoms of cystitis, e.g. dysuria, hematuria, lower abdominal pain, urgency, frequency, burning with urination, cloudy urine, malodorous urine, pelvic pressure, and fever.

11. Encourage fluid intake and monitor intake and output.

12. Meticulous skin care, especially if incontinent.

13. Monitor drainage in the presence of a catheter.

14. **Antispasmodics** may be necessary preoperatively and post-operatively for bladder spasms.

15. Assist in lining up home care as necessary, e.g. Hospice care, public health care, home health care agency, and Meals on Wheels.

FOR MORE INFORMATION

American Cancer Society
1599 Clifton Road
Atlanta, GA 30329
1-800-ACS-2345

ASSIGNMENT SHEET: PROSTATE CANCER

Short Answer

1. Write a brief definition for the terms listed throughout the chapter.

2. Describe the physiology and function of the prostate gland.

3. Write a brief definition for prostate cancer.

4. Describe the incidence of prostate cancer.

5. List thirteen (13) symptoms for prostate cancer. Describe the rationale for the symptoms and associated care.

6. List twelve (12) specific methods used to aid in the diagnosis of prostate cancer.

7. List six (6) specific methods used in the treatment of prostate cancer.

8. Describe fifteen (15) considerations for caring for a patient with prostate cancer.

9. Describe the following procedures used to diagnose or treat prostate cancer.

    a. Transurethral resection of the prostate (TURP)
    b. Suprapubic catheter
    c. Bone scan
    d. Chest x-ray
    e. Prostatectomy
    f. Orchiectomy
    g. CT scan
    h. MRI
    i. Intravenous pyelogram (IVP)
    j. Lymphadenectomy
    k. Radiation therapy
    l. Digital rectal examination
    m. Biopsy
    n. Transrectal prostatic ultrasonography
    o. Chemotherapy

10. List ten (10) symptoms of cystitis.

11. Name the normal range for each of the following laboratory tests.

    a. Hemoglobin (Hg)
    b. Hematocrit (Hct)
    c. Acid phosphatase
    d. Prostate-specific antigen (PSA)
    e. Platelet count

KNOWLEDGE INTO ACTION

1. Lee Wang, a 72-year-old male, is being discharged from the hospital with a diagnosis of prostate cancer. He has chosen not to go through treatment for the cancer since he has a history of heart disease and diabetes. The physician has told Mr. Carlson that he is at increased risk for cystitis. Mr. Carlson says to you, "The doctor told me that I might get cystitis. What does that mean? How would I know if I had cystitis?" How will you explain what cystitis means? What will you describe as symptoms of cystitis?

2. Jacob Smith, a 59-year-old male, is admitted to your facility with a diagnosis of hematuria, which has been going on for the past 2 weeks. Describe how you would monitor whether the hematuria was getting worse, staying the same, or improving. List two tests that could be done to determine if Mr. Smith was becoming anemic due to the hematuria.

3. Mike Christianson is being discharged from the hospital after a prostatectomy. Both legs are edematous. He asks you prior to his discharge, "What can I do about this edema? It's terribly uncomfortable." What will your response be?

Hodgkin's Disease

OBJECTIVES

Upon completion of this chapter, the student should be able to:

- Define the key terms listed throughout the chapter
- Describe the physiology of the immune system
- State a specific definition for Hodgkin's disease
- Describe the incidence of Hodgkin's disease
- List the risk factors for Hodgkin's disease
- Describe the signs and symptoms associated with Hodgkin's disease and the rationale and associated care for these symptoms
- Identify specific methods for diagnosis of Hodgkin's disease
- Identify specific methods for treatment of Hodgkin's disease
- Describe the method used for staging the progression of Hodgkin's disease
- List possible side effects of radiation therapy and associated care for these side effects
- List possible side effects of chemotherapy and associated care for these side effects
- Describe specific considerations for caring for a patient with Hodgkin's disease

KEY TERMS

Lymphomas – tumors of the lymph tissues

Neoplasm – new growth or formation of abnormal tissue often crowding out healthy tissue

Proliferation – ability for rapid multiplication or reproduction

Eosinophils – granular white blood cells; play an important part in the immune response of the body as well as during allergic reactions

Plasma – liquid portion of the blood

Histiocyte – cell that carries on the process of phagocytosis

Reed-Sternberg cells – cells present in the connective tissue with Hodgkin's disease

INTRODUCTION

Cancers of the immune system are called **lymphomas**. The most common of the lymphomas is Hodgkin's disease. Other lymphomas are non-Hodgkin's lymphomas. The **neoplasm** generally follows along the lymph node system, spreading to different regions of lymph nodes and can eventually involve the liver, spleen, bone marrow, and lungs. Hodgkin's disease involves the **proliferation** of **eosinophils**, **plasma** cells, **histiocytes**, lymphocytes, and **Reed-Sternberg cells**. Reed-Sternberg cells differentiate Hodgkin's disease from the non-Hodgkin's lymphomas. Hodgkin's disease involves a painless enlargement of the lymph nodes due to this proliferation of cells.

PHYSIOLOGY OF THE IMMUNE SYSTEM

The immune system, also referred to as the lymph system, provides the body's defense against infections. (See Figure 7-1.) The lymph system develops **white blood cells (WBCs)** which are transported to the entire body by way of the lymph system. Organs of the lymph system include tonsils, spleen, bone marrow, **thymus gland**, lymph nodes, appendix, and **Peyer's patches** in the small intestine.

Immature **lymphocytes**, or stem cells, are produced in the bone marrow of the long bones of the body. Some of these **stem cells** travel to the thymus gland to mature as **T-cells**, and others mature in the bone marrow or other lymph glands as **B-cells**. B-cells are necessary for the production of **antibodies** in response to a specific **antigen**. T-cells

White blood cells (WBCs) – responsible for fighting infection within the body; divided into granular white blood cells (basophils, eosinophils, and neutrophils) and nongranular white blood cells (lymphocytes and monocytes); also known as leukocytes

Thymus gland – gland located in the mediastinum; part of the lymph system; responsible for the maturation of T-cells (lymphocytes) that have been produced in the bone marrow

Peyer's patches – lymph nodes located in the ileum of the small intestine

Lymphocyte – one of the two nongranular leukocytes; responsible for providing immunity for the body against diseases

Stem cells – cells capable of reproducing cells for specific tissues in the body

T-cells – lymphocytes that are manufactured in the bone marrow and travel to the thymus gland of the body to mature; part of the immune system of the body; able to recognize antigens in the body and either destroy the antigens themselves or signal phagocytes to destroy the foreign substance

B-cells – lymphocytes produced in the bone marrow and maturing in the spleen and lymph nodes; sensitive to only a specific antigen

Antibodies – proteins formed within the body in response to an invading antigen

Antigen – foreign substance in the body that stimulates the body to produce antibodies

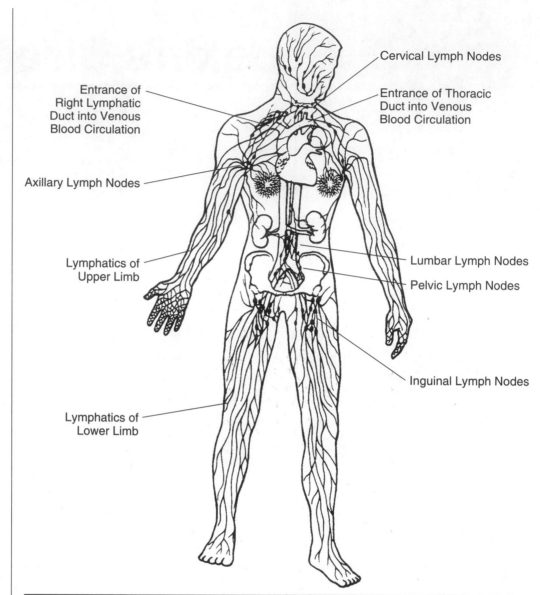

Figure 7-1   Lymphatic circulation (From Burke, *Human Anatomy and Physiology in Health and Disease, 3rd edition*, copyright © 1992, Delmar Publishers)

are categorized into "helper cells," which stimulate the B-cells, and "suppressor cells," which deactivate the B-cells.

The lymph system transports a clear fluid, which contains WBCs, to every part of the body. The lymph nodes are located along the path of the lymph vessels. The lymph nodes are responsible for filtering out foreign substances from the lymph vessels. (See Figure 7-2.)

STATISTICS

Approximately 30,000 new cases of lymphoma are diagnosed annually in the United States with one-third of these being Hodgkin's disease. Hodgkin's disease is most common in young adults, with a peak incidence rate in the 15 to 35 age group and another peak occurring in the over 50 age group. The disease is most common in the Caucasian race with a 2:1 higher incidence in males than females. Untreated Hodgkin's disease is invariably fatal whereas treatment leads to a 90% survival rate at 5 years.

Retrovirus – special group of viruses

Epstein-Barr virus – virus that causes mononucleosis

Mononucleosis – disease affecting the lymph system; often referred to as "kissing disease"

Groin – the area located at the junction of the abdomen and thighs

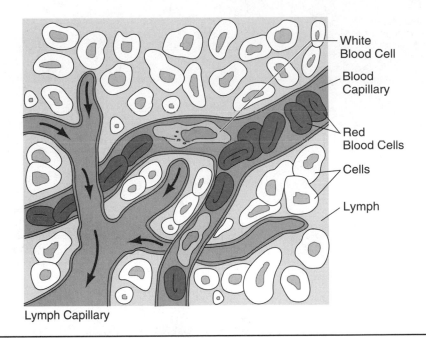

White Blood Cell

Blood Capillary

Red Blood Cells

Cells

Lymph

Lymph Capillary

Figure 7-2   Lymphatic circulation within the body

RISK FACTORS

Although the exact cause of Hodgkin's disease is unknown, the following have been shown to be risk factors for the disease:

1. History of tonsillectomy
2. Damaged immune system due to immune disorders or immunosuppressive drugs
3. Survivors of atomic bomb explosion
4. **Retrovirus** (RNA virus or type-C virus)
5. **Epstein-Barr virus**, the virus that causes infectious **mononucleosis**
6. HTLV-1 virus (human T-cell leukemia-lymphoma virus)
7. Occupations in the woodworking and chemistry field
8. Heredity

SIGNS, SYMPTOMS, AND ASSOCIATED CARE

1. Painless swelling of lymph glands, often in the neck, axillary region, or **groin**, due to neoplastic infiltration of the lymph nodes (See Figure 7-3)
   - Monitor for lymphadenopathy
   - Adjust position for patient comfort
   - Provide comfort measures as necessary due to lymphadenopathy
2. Persistent or recurrent fever due to lymph node involvement and infections
   - Monitor temperature at routine intervals
   - Provide comfort measures for patient with elevated temperature, such as cool cloth to forehead, partial or complete bath as needed, clothing and bedding changed frequently due to diaphoresis, and encourage fluids to prevent dehydration. Symptoms of dehydration include decreased urine output, constipation, dry skin, tenting of skin, dry mouth, dry eyes, concentrated urine, hypotension, and confusion.

Malaise – feeling of fatigue and vague discomfort

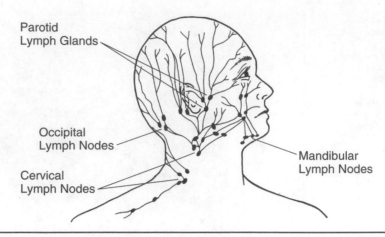

Parotid Lymph Glands

Occipital Lymph Nodes

Cervical Lymph Nodes

Mandibular Lymph Nodes

Figure 7-3   Lymphatic circulation of the head and neck (From Fong et al., *Body Structures and Functions, 8th edition,* copyright © 1993, Delmar Publishers)

- Avoid exposing patient to a draft
- Cover with blankets as necessary
- Monitor intake and output (I and O)
- Maintain comfortable room temperature for patient
- Avoid plastic mattresses and plastic bed protectors as they increase perspiration
- Use antiperspirant or deodorant to minimize sweating and odor

3. Nerve pain due to enlarged lymph nodes pressing on nerves
   - Encourage rest to decrease strain
   - Encourage patient to decrease weight-bearing to painful extremities
   - Provide heat or other methods of pain control, such as massage, relaxation techniques, distraction, and medications
   - Administration of *radiation* to involved lymph nodes may be necessary to relieve pressure

4. Jaundice due to liver damage as a result of obstructed bile ducts
   - Monitor skin color for presence of jaundice
   - Monitor serum liver function tests, e.g. *SGOT, SGPT, bilirubin, albumin, alkaline phosphatase,* and *prothrombin time*
   - Offer low-fat diet

5. Fatigue and **malaise** due to anemia
   - Assist patient with activities of daily living (ADLs) as necessary
   - Schedule care, activities, and treatment around patient's rest schedule
   - Monitor phone calls and visitors around patient's energy level and rest schedule
   - Encourage frequent rest periods
   - Provide assistance as needed to prevent injury due to weakness
   - Provide method for patient to call for assistance
   - Encourage patient to set realistic goals of activities
   - Allow adequate time to do activities and procedures to avoid frustration or possible injury
   - Encourage exercise to maintain muscle strength
   - Offer cane or walker to provide additional assistance for ambulation and transfer
   - Provide private room for patient to promote rest periods

Metabolic – refers to metabolism

Pruritus – itchiness of the skin

Antihistamines – substances that counteract the effect of histamines, which are amino acids normally present in the body and released into the bloodstream in response to injury to the tissues; histamines are also released during allergic reactions when the body is in contact with a substance to which it is sensitive

Splenomegaly – enlargement of the spleen

6. Weight loss due to fatigue and increased **metabolic** needs of the proliferating WBCs causing deprivation of normal body cells
   - Obtain baseline weight and monitor weight on routine basis
   - Encourage patient to participate in dietary choices
   - Offer nutritional supplements and vitamins
   - Encourage family and friends to bring in food that is appealing to patient as dietary restrictions allow
   - Administration of parenteral fluids may be necessary
   - Monitor intake and output (I and O)
   - Encourage rest periods before and after meals
   - Avoid unpleasant sights and odors in room to make meals more appealing
   - Provide meticulous mouth care
   - Monitor for skin breakdown due to loss of body tissue
   - Encourage clothing styles that do not draw attention to weight loss
   - Monitor for symptoms of dehydration. Symptoms of dehydration include decreased urine output, constipation, dry skin, tenting of skin, dry mouth, dry eyes, concentrated urine, hypotension, and confusion.

7. **Pruritus** (cause is unknown)
   - Provide meticulous skin care with mild, unscented soap
   - Avoid use of tapes and other adhesives on skin
   - Administration of medications or creams to prevent itching
   - Provide protective mittens, to prevent scratching and damage to skin for confused patients
   - Encourage fluid intake
   - Pat skin gently dry
   - Avoid harsh soaps or bleach in clothing and linens
   - Avoid clothing and bedding that is irritating
   - Assess skin redness and irritation on routine basis
   - Observe for open areas and signs of infection
   - Avoid use of scented lotions and cosmetics
   - Administer **antihistamines** as necessary to relieve itching

8. Bone pain due to neoplastic infiltration of the bone marrow
   - Decrease weight-bearing on bones as able
   - Provide heat or other methods of pain control, such as massage, relaxation techniques, and distraction
   - Administer medications as prescribed by physician for pain control
   - Assess for level of comfort and offer pain control methods
   - Encourage patient to ask for pain control methods before pain becomes too severe

9. Hepatomegaly and **splenomegaly** due to neoplastic involvement
   - Monitor for splenomegaly and hepatomegaly
   - Avoid abdominal injury in the presence of splenomegaly
   - Monitor for signs of internal bleeding in the presence of splenomegaly and hepatomegaly such as abdominal pain, tachycardia, hypotension, and abdominal distention
   - Monitor *hemoglobin* and *hematocrit*

Antiseptic – substance used to disinfect a specific area; may refer to the skin, mucous membranes, or an inanimate object

Erythrocytes – red blood cells; biconcave disc-shaped cells; function in the body to transport oxygen and carbon dioxide within the bloodstream; average of 5 million per cubic millimeter of blood

- Avoid abdominal injury in the presence of hepatomegaly and splenomegaly
- Monitor liver function with serum laboratory tests
- Monitor for bleeding tendencies in the presence of hepatomegaly
- Educate to avoid the use of alcohol and medications metabolized in the liver
- Monitor for jaundice

10. Increased susceptibility to infections due to impairment of immune system
    - Monitor for signs of infection and educate patient and family to observe for signs of infection and report promptly to medical staff, e.g. fever, chills, redness, swelling, pain, phlegm, skin rash, cough, dyspnea, flushed skin, diaphoresis, dysuria, and sore throat
    - Avoid people who have infections
    - Utilize meticulous hand and skin care on the part of the patient, staff, and visitors
    - Educate patient regarding the need to complete entire regimen of antibiotics
    - Restrict staff members who have taken care of patients with infectious disease from caring for the patient who has increased risk of infections
    - Avoid possible routes of infection when possible, such as urinary catheters and intravenous (IV) lines
    - Monitor temperature on a routine basis
    - Utilize protective isolation or private room as necessary during hospitalization (See Table 7-1)
    - Avoid crowded areas, which increase chances of being exposed to an infection
    - Provide meticulous mouth care, frequent dental checks, and **antiseptic** mouthwash
    - Avoid injury to skin and mucous membranes

11. Anemia due to shortened life span of **erythrocytes**
    - Administer blood transfusions and iron supplements as necessary to treat anemia
    - Monitor hemoglobin and hematocrit
    - Monitor for weakness associated with anemia; assist with ADLs as necessary due to weakness; protect from possible injury due to weakness
    - Monitor physical symptoms of anemia, such as pallor, weakness, and vertigo

12. Upper respiratory tract infections due to lymph node involvement in mediastinum as well as lung involvement
    - Educate patient and family regarding symptoms of respiratory infection, such as cough, phlegm production, chest pain, fever, chills, dyspnea, and diaphoresis
    - Educate patient and family to report symptoms of respiratory infection to physician

Table 7-1   Protective Isolation
1. *Hands* before and after
2. *Gowns* to enter
3. *Gloves* if contact
4. *Masks* to enter

- Educate patient regarding importance of completing medication prescribed for respiratory infection
- Encourage fluids to thin secretions and make them easier to expel
- Prevent transmission of infection by hand washing and correctly disposing tissues and phlegm
- Avoid people with respiratory infections
- Maintain optimal health to fight off infections
- Administer influenza and pneumonia vaccinations as directed by physician
- Avoid crowded areas, which increase the likelihood of contracting a respiratory infection

13. Edema due to pressure on blood vessels from enlarged lymph nodes causing decreased venous return

- Avoid constrictive clothing or undergarments
- Restrict salt in diet as prescribed by physician
- Utilize elastic stockings or Jobst stockings as necessary to reduce swelling
- Monitor edema on routine basis
- Encourage patient to elevate edematous extremity above the level of the heart to reduce swelling
- Monitor for skin breakdown in edematous areas
- Monitor for symptoms of decreased circulation in edematous areas, e.g. skin cool to touch, cyanosis, and decreased sensation
- Obtain baseline weight and monitor on routine basis
- Monitor intake and output (I and O)

DIAGNOSIS

1. Symptoms
2. Physical examination
3. *Lymph node biopsy* to determine presence of Reed-Sternberg cells
4. *Bone marrow aspiration*
5. *Chest x-ray* to determine involvement of lymph nodes in mediastinum
6. *Liver biopsy* to determine liver involvement
7. *Spleen biopsy* to determine spleen involvement
8. *CT scan* of abdomen to determine extent of lymph node biopsy
9. *Bone scan*
10. Serum *alkaline phosphatase* elevation would indicate liver or bone involvement
11. *CBC* to determine anemia
12. *Lymphangiogram* to determine size of lymph nodes as well as extent of lymph node involvement

STAGES OF HODGKIN'S DISEASE

Hodgkin's disease is categorized into stages. These stages are used to determine the form of treatment that will be used.

Stage 1: Single lymph node involvement

Stage 2: Multiple lymph node region involvement on the same side of the diaphragm

Oophoropexy – repair of an ovary that is not in the correct position

Esophagitis – inflammation of the esophagus

Stage 3:   Lymph nodes on both sides of the diaphragm; spleen may also be involved

Stage 4:   Includes widespread lymph node involvement as well as involvement of bone marrow, liver, and other organs of the lymph system

TREATMENT

The form of treatment used depends on the stage of Hodgkin's disease to which the patient has progressed.

Stage 1:   Radiation

Stage 2:   Radiation

Stage 3:   Radiation and chemotherapy

Stage 4:   Chemotherapy

Radiation therapy involves delivery of high-intensity localized radiation to the involved lymph node regions.

Chemotherapy involves combination anti-neoplastics. These combinations may in-clude one of the following combination groups:

1. MOPP—Mechlorethamine (nitrogen mustard), Oncovin (vincristine), Procarbazine, and Prednisone (Deltasone)
2. ABVD—Adriamycin, Bleomycin, Vinblastine, and DTIC (Dacarbazine)

SIDE EFFECTS OF RADIATION THERAPY

1. Sterility
   - Provide counseling for couples of child-bearing age
   - Educate men regarding option of placing sperm in a sperm bank
   - Educate women regarding option of an **oophoropexy**
2. **Esophagitis**
   - Provide meticulous mouth care at frequent intervals through the day (See Figure 7-4)
   - Offer food and beverages that are nonabrasive, e.g. spicy foods, acidic fruits and juices, carbonated beverages, highly salted foods, and foods that are extremely hot or cold
   - Offer ice chips and fluids frequently according to patient preference

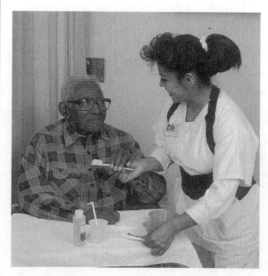

Figure 7-4   Equipment for the administration of mouth care (From Hegner, *Nursing Assistant: A Nursing Process Approach, 7th edition,* copyright © 1995, Delmar Publishers)

Antacids – substances used to neutralize stomach acid

- Monitor intake and output (I and O)
- Elevate head while sleeping
- Administer **antacids** as necessary
- Administer nasogastric (NG) or parenteral fluids as necessary
- Administer medications as prescribed by physician to treat any accompanying infection
- Observe for sores in the mouth
- Offer foods that are easy to chew and swallow
- Utilize antiseptic mouthwash and a soft-bristled toothbrush
- Provide moisture to lips with lip balm, mineral oil, or petroleum jelly
- Humidify air as necessary
- Avoid use of harsh toothpaste

3. Diarrhea
   - Monitor number, amount, and consistency of stools
   - Monitor intake and output to avoid dehydration
   - Monitor serum electrolytes (*sodium*, *potassium*, and *chloride*)
   - Provide meticulous skin care, especially if incontinent
   - Monitor for presence of hemorrhoids
   - Monitor for rectal discomfort and offer sitz baths, warm soaks, and topical ointments or suppositories
   - Administer antidiarrheal medications as prescribed by physician
   - Provide frequent skin care, especially to anal area, to prevent skin breakdown
   - Monitor for presence of blood (*Hemoccult*®)
   - Offer reassurance to patient
   - Avoid foods that are too hot or too cold as they increase peristalsis

4. Numbness and tingling to extremities
   - Assist with ADLs as needed due to numbness and tingling
   - Provide safety measures, e.g. handrails, walker, or cane

5. Nausea and vomiting
   - Administer antiemetics before meals as prescribed by physician
   - Offer food as tolerated by patient and according to patient preference
   - Control odors and unpleasant sights in room
   - Offer fluids frequently to prevent dehydration
   - Monitor intake and output to avoid dehydration
   - Monitor serum electrolytes
   - Offer frequent, small meals as tolerated
   - Plan rest periods after meals
   - Avoid foods that are spicy, rich, or previously disagreeable to patient
   - Provide receptacle for patient to vomit into as needed and clean whenever used
   - Provide meticulous mouth care
   - Prevent aspiration of emesis
   - Utilize universal precautions at all times when coming in contact with blood or body fluids (See Appendix C)
   - Avoid greasy foods as they tend to stay in the stomach a long period of time
   - Avoid cooking food if possible due to increased nausea with odors of foods

Dysphagia – difficulty with swallowing

Heimlich maneuver – technique used to remove an obstruction caused by a foreign body in the respiratory tract; technique consists of inward and upward abdominal thrusts, which cause pressure on the diaphragm

Anorexia – loss of appetite

- Avoid hot foods as necessary due to the increased odors of hot foods
- Encourage to eat in well-ventilated area to decrease the accumulation of odors of foods while eating

6. Dry mouth
   - Provide meticulous mouth care
   - Frequently offer ice chips and fluids according to patient preference
   - Utilize humidifier at bedside to moisturize air
   - Offer hard candies as patient desires

7. **Dysphagia**
   - Offer foods that are easy to chew according to patient preference
   - Avoid fresh fruits and vegetables as these are often more difficult to chew
   - Alternate liquids and solids during meals
   - Monitor for choking
   - Instruct family members on the **Heimlich maneuver** should choking occur while they are with the patient and for when the patient returns home
   - Utilize suction equipment in the event of choking
   - Encourage to concentrate on chewing food thoroughly
   - Educate that food may need to be cut into smaller pieces, ground, or pureed
   - Provide method, such as a warming plate, to keep food warm during entire length of time needed for patient to eat
   - Obtain baseline weight and monitor on routine basis
   - Encourage patient to take as much time as necessary during meals
   - Avoid outside distractions during mealtime to avoid choking
   - Encourage patient to sit upright to eat
   - Be alert for symptoms of dehydration
   - Use a syringe to feed liquids in small amounts

8. Fatigue
   - Assist patient with ADLs as necessary
   - Schedule care, activities, and treatments around patient's rest schedule
   - Monitor phone calls and visitors around patient's energy level and rest schedule
   - Encourage frequent rest periods
   - Provide assistance as needed to prevent injury due to weakness
   - Provide method for patient to call for assistance
   - Encourage patient to set realistic goals of activities
   - Allow adequate time to do activities and procedures to avoid frustration or possible injury
   - Encourage exercise to maintain and promote muscle strength
   - Utilize cane or walker to provide additional assistance for ambulation and transfer

9. Decreased taste
   - Provide meticulous mouth care
   - Offer foods and fluids according to patient preference

10. **Anorexia**
    - Obtain baseline weight and monitor on routine basis
    - Offer small, frequent meals as tolerated
    - Encourage patient to participate in dietary choices

Enema – introduction of fluid into the rectum to stimulate a bowel movement; fluid may also be introduced for the purpose of treatments or testing (x-ray)

Leukopenia – decreased number of white blood cells

- Administer nutritional supplements and vitamins
- Monitor for signs of dehydration, such as decreased urine output, concentrated urine, dry skin, tenting of skin, dry mucous membranes, dry mouth, dry eyes, confusion, and constipation
- Encourage family and friends to bring in food that is appealing to the patient as dietary restrictions allow
- Administer parenteral fluids as necessary
- Monitor intake and output (I and O)
- Encourage fluids to prevent dehydration
- Avoid unpleasant sights and odors in room to make meals more appealing
- Provide meticulous mouth care
- Maintain social atmosphere for mealtimes to encourage the patient to eat
- Encourage clothing that enhances patient appearance
- Utilize exercise program as tolerated to increase appetite

11. Skin reaction, e.g. redness and peeling
    - Provide meticulous skin care with mild, unscented soap
    - Avoid use of tapes and other adhesives on skin as able
    - Use medications or creams to prevent itching
    - Utilize protective mittens for confused patients to prevent scratching and damage to skin
    - Encourage fluid intake
    - Pat skin gently dry
    - Avoid harsh soaps or bleach in clothing and linens
    - Avoid clothing and bedding that is irritating
    - Assess skin redness and irritation on routine basis
    - Observe for open areas and signs of infection
    - Avoid use of scented lotions and cosmetics
    - Administer antihistamines as necessary to relieve itching

SIDE EFFECTS OF CHEMOTHERAPY

1. Constipation
   - Encourage fluids
   - Encourage high-fiber diet
   - Increase exercise as tolerated
   - Administer **enemas**, suppositories, stool softeners, and laxatives as prescribed by physician
   - Monitor frequency, number, and consistency of stools
   - Monitor for possible bowel obstruction
   - Encourage fresh fruits and vegetables
   - Establish regular bowel routine
   - Provide privacy for bowel routine as able

2. **Leukopenia**
   - Monitor for signs of infection and educate patient and family to observe for signs of infection and report promptly to medical staff, e.g. fever, chills, redness, swelling, pain, phlegm, skin rash, cough, dyspnea, flushed skin, diaphoresis, dysuria, and sore throat

Thrombocytopenia – decrease in the number of platelets in the blood, which could predispose the patient to abnormal bleeding

Central nervous system (CNS) – the voluntary and involuntary nerves of the brain and spinal column

Stomatitis – inflammation of the mouth

- Avoid people who have infections
- Provide meticulous hand and skin care on the part of the patient, staff, and visitors
- Educate patient regarding need to complete entire regimen of antibiotics
- Provide a private room if possible
- Restrict staff members who have taken care of patients with infectious disease from caring for the patient who has increased risk of infections
- Avoid possible routes of infection when possible, such as urinary catheters and IVs
- Monitor temperature on a routine basis
- Utilize protective isolation as necessary during hospitalization
- Avoid crowded areas, which increase chances of being exposed to an infection
- Provide meticulous mouth care, dental checks, and antiseptic mouthwash
- Avoid injury to skin and mucous membranes

3. **Thrombocytopenia**
   - Observe for signs of abnormal bleeding and educate patient and family to observe and report any signs promptly to physician, e.g. hemoptysis, bloody emesis, bloody or tarry stools, nose bleeds, vaginal bleeding between menstrual cycles or post-menopausal, bleeding gums, or hematuria
   - Observe for signs of **central nervous system (CNS)** bleeding and educate patient and family to observe and report symptoms promptly to physician, e.g. altered level of consciousness, headache, vision changes, and vertigo
   - Prevent injury to patient who has thrombocytopenia, e.g. soft toothbrush, electric razor rather than straight-edge razor, wear seat belts in the car, elevate siderails, avoid straining with bowel movements, avoid vigorous nose-blowing, avoid intramuscular injections, avoid rectal temperatures, avoid use of tampons, and seek physician advice prior to vaginal or anal intercourse
   - Avoid products that contain aspirin, which alters normal platelet function
   - Monitor *platelet* count
   - Monitor *hemoglobin* and *hematocrit*
   - Apply pressure at sites of injection or blood drawing sites for minimum of 5 minutes or until bleeding stops

4. Anemia
   - Administer blood transfusions and iron supplements as necessary to treat anemia
   - Monitor *hemoglobin* and *hematocrit*
   - Monitor for weakness associated with anemia, assist with ADLs as necessary due to weakness, and protect from possible injury due to weakness
   - Monitor physical symptoms of anemia, such as pallor, weakness, and vertigo

5. **Stomatitis**
   - Provide meticulous mouth care at frequent intervals through the day
   - Offer food and beverages that are nonabrasive, e.g. avoid spicy foods, acidic fruits and juices, carbonated beverages, highly salted foods, and foods that are extremely hot or cold

- Frequently offer ice chips and fluids according to patient preference
- Humidify air as necessary
- Monitor intake and output (I and O)
- Elevate head while sleeping
- Administer antacids as necessary
- Administer NG or parenteral fluids as necessary
- Administer medications as prescribed by physician to treat any accompanying infection
- Observe for sores in the mouth
- Offer foods that are easy to chew and swallow
- Utilize soft bristled toothbrush and antiseptic mouthwash
- Maintain proper fit of dentures
- Provide moisture to lips with lip balm, mineral oil, or petroleum jelly
- Avoid use of harsh toothpaste

6. Nausea and vomiting
   - Administer antiemetics before meals as prescribed by physician
   - Offer choices according to patient preference
   - Control odors and unpleasant sights in room
   - Frequently offer fluids to prevent dehydration
   - Monitor intake and output to avoid dehydration
   - Monitor serum electrolytes
   - Offer frequent, small meals as tolerated
   - Encourage rest periods after meals
   - Avoid foods that are spicy, rich, or previously disagreeable to patient
   - Provide receptacle for patient to vomit into as needed; this should be cleaned whenever used and changed on a frequent basis
   - Provide meticulous mouth care
   - Prevent aspiration of vomit
   - Utilize universal precautions at all times when coming in contact with blood or body fluids (See Appendix C)
   - Avoid greasy foods as they tend to stay in the stomach for long periods
   - Avoid cooking food if possible due to increased nausea with food odors
   - Avoid hot foods as necessary due to the increased hot food odors
   - Encourage to eat in well-ventilated area to decrease the accumulation of food odors while eating

7. Diarrhea
   - Monitor number, amount, and consistency of stools
   - Monitor intake and output to avoid dehydration
   - Monitor serum electrolytes
   - Provide meticulous skin care, especially if incontinent
   - Monitor for presence of hemorrhoids
   - Monitor for rectal discomfort and offer sitz baths, warm soaks, and topical ointments or suppositories
   - Administer antidiarrheal medications as prescribed by physician
   - Provide frequent skin care, especially to anal area to prevent skin breakdown
   - Monitor for presence of blood (*Hemoccult*®)

Alopecia – hair loss

- Offer reassurance to patient
- Avoid foods that are too hot or too cold as they increase peristalsis

8. Anorexia
   - Obtain baseline weight and monitor on routine basis
   - Encourage patient to participate in dietary choices
   - Offer nutritional supplements and vitamins
   - Monitor for signs of dehydration, such as decreased urine output, concentrated urine, dry skin, tenting of skin, dry mucous membranes, dry mouth, dry eyes, confusion, and constipation
   - Encourage family and friends to bring in food that is appealing to patient as dietary restrictions allow
   - Encourage frequent, small meals as tolerated
   - Administer parenteral fluids as necessary
   - Encourage fluids to prevent dehydration
   - Avoid unpleasant sights and odors in room to make meals more appealing
   - Provide meticulous mouth care
   - Maintain social atmosphere for mealtimes to encourage the patient to eat
   - Encourage clothing that enhances patient appearance
   - Utilize exercise program as tolerated to increase appetite

9. **Alopecia**
   - Provide emotional support for patient
   - Assist to obtain wigs, scarves, or head-covering as patient desires
   - Avoid use of white linens as this may make hair loss more noticeable and distressing to the patient
   - Avoid use of harsh shampoos, chemicals, colors, or permanents in hair
   - Avoid using blowdriers or curling irons in hair
   - Encourage to cut hair in a style that is easy to maintain

CONSIDERATIONS FOR CARE

1. Educate patient and family regarding the disease process.
2. Educate patient and family regarding forms of treatment as well as side effects of treatment.
3. Provide emotional support to patient and family.
4. Provide nonjudgmental acceptance of emotions and behavior of patient and family.
5. Assist patient to reduce or eliminate side effects of the treatments.
6. Assess patient level of comfort and offer measures to increase comfort such as relaxation techniques, heat treatments, massage, imaging, and medications.
7. Observe for signs of infection and educate patient and family to observe for signs of infection and report promptly to physician, e.g. fever, chills, redness, swelling, pain, phlegm, dysuria, skin rash, cough, dyspnea, flushed skin, and diaphoresis.
8. Educate patient and family to observe for signs of advancing Hodgkin's disease.
9. Educate patient and family regarding importance of follow-up care with physician.

10. Observe for signs of abnormal bleeding and educate patient and family to observe and report symptoms promptly to physician, e.g. hemoptysis, bloody emesis, bloody or black tarry stools, nose bleeds, vaginal bleeding between menstrual cycles or post-menopausal bleeding, bleeding gums, hematuria, and bruising.

11. Observe for signs of CNS bleeding and educate patient and family to observe and report symptoms promptly to physician, e.g. altered level of consciousness, headache, vision changes, and vertigo.

12. Prevent injury to patient who has thrombocytopenia, e.g. soft toothbrush, electric razor rather than straight-edge razor, wear seat belts in the car, elevate siderails, avoid straining with bowel movements, avoid vigorous nose-blowing, avoid intramuscular injections, and avoid rectal temperatures.

FOR MORE INFORMATION

American Cancer Society
1599 Clifton Road
Atlanta, GA 30329

ASSIGNMENT SHEET: HODGKIN'S DISEASE

Short Answer

1. Write a brief definition for the terms listed throughout the chapter.

2. Describe the physiology of the immune (lymph) system.

3. List the seven (7) organs that make up the immune system.

4. Write a brief definition for Hodgkin's disease.

5. Describe the incidence of Hodgkin's disease.

6. List eight (8) risk factors for Hodgkin's disease.

7. List thirteen (13) symptoms for Hodgkin's disease. Describe the rationale and associated care for each symptom.

8. Describe twelve (12) specific methods used to aid in the diagnosis of Hodgkin's disease.

9. Describe the four (4) stages of Hodgkin's disease according to the spread of the disease.

10. Describe the specific treatment for Hodgkin's disease according to the four stages of the disease.

11. List eleven (11) side effects of radiation and associated care for each of the side effects.

12. Describe nine (9) side effects of chemotherapy and associated care for each of the side effects.

13. List twelve (12) specific considerations for caring for a patient with Hodgkin's disease.

14. Describe the following procedures used in the diagnosis or treatment of Hodgkin's disease.
    a. Biopsy
    b. Bone marrow aspiration
    c. Chest x-ray
    d. Liver biopsy
    e. Spleen biopsy
    f. CT scan
    g. Bone scan
    h. Lymphangiogram
    i. Chemotherapy
    j. Radiation therapy
    k. Hemoccult® stools

15. Write the normal range for each of the following laboratory tests.
    a. Alkaline phosphatase
    b. Sodium
    c. Potassium
    d. Chloride
    e. White blood cell count (WBC)
    f. Platelet count
    g. SGOT
    h. SGPT
    i. Bilirubin
    j. Albumin
    k. Hematocrit
    l. Prothrombin time
    m. Hemoglobin

KNOWLEDGE INTO ACTION

1. Andrea Schmidt is taking her husband home from the hospital today. Mr. Schmidt has been diagnosed with Hodgkin's disease and has extreme pruritus, which is a symptom of Hodgkin's disease. What can you tell Mrs. Schmidt that she can do to help her husband to ease the pruritus?

2. Shamika Hill has been diagnosed with Hodgkin's disease. Her physician has told her that she may be more prone to infections due to Hodgkin's disease. She says to you, "Why would I have more of a chance of infection? What do I need to watch for? What can I do to prevent an infection?" What will your response be regarding the reason for her increased risk of infection? What will your response be regarding possible symptoms of infection? What will your response be regarding methods for her to reduce her risk of getting an infection?

3. Eric Heller has been diagnosed with Hodgkin's disease and is undergoing radiation treatment for the disease. He says to you, "I have a friend who had Hodgkin's disease and they did radiation and chemotherapy on him. What's the difference? Maybe my doctor isn't doing everything he can for me." What can you tell him regarding the

difference between his treatment and his friend's?

4. You are helping to train a new staff member at your facility. One of the patients you are caring for that day is Shawnda Preston, a 37-year-old female who is receiving chemotherapy for Hodgkin's disease. Describe five (5) possible side effects of the chemotherapy you may tell the new staff member to be alert for and two methods of assisting Ms. Preston should the side effects occur.

5. Shari Hammond is taking her husband, who has recently been diagnosed with Hodgkin's disease, home from the hospital. She says to you, "The doctor said my husband has thrombo-something (thrombocytopenia). What did he mean by that? Is it serious?" How can you describe thrombocytopenia? What are specific considerations for care due to the thrombocytopenia?

Acute Myelogenous Leukemia

OBJECTIVES

Upon completion of this chapter, the student should be able to:

■ Define the key terms listed throughout the chapter

■ Describe the basic blood facts

■ State a specific definition for acute myelogenous leukemia

■ Describe the incidence of acute myelogenous leukemia

■ List the risk factors for acute myelogenous leukemia

■ Describe the signs and symptoms of acute myelogenous leukemia and associated care to assist a patient who has these symptoms

■ Describe the cause of the symptoms associated with acute myelogenous leukemia

■ Identify specific methods for diagnosis of acute myelogenous leukemia

■ Identify specific methods for treatment of acute myelogenous leukemia

■ Describe specific considerations for caring for a patient with acute myelogenous leukemia

KEY TERMS

Acute – sudden onset of symptoms with a short duration

Granulocytes – the granular leukocytes (basophils, eosinophils, and neutrophils)

Monocytes – nongranular white blood cells (lymphocytes are the other nongranular white blood cells)

Thrombocytes – disklike structures in the blood that are important for the clotting of blood

Leukocytes – white blood cells; divided into two groups: granular (basophils, eosinophils, neutrophils) and nongranular (lympho-cytes, monocytes)

Basophils – one of the three granular white blood cells (granular white blood cells are basophils, eosinophils, and neutro-phils); make up 1 to 3% of the total number of white blood cells

INTRODUCTION

Acute myelogenous leukemia (AML) is characterized by the proliferation of immature white blood cells, with lymphocytes, **granulocytes**, and **monocytes** involved in the disease. This proliferation of WBCs accumulates in the organs, bone marrow, and bloodstream.

PHYSIOLOGY

There are four basic components of blood. (See Figure 8-1.)

1. Plasma—liquid portion of the blood
2. Platelets (**thrombocytes**)—portion of the blood necessary for clot formation
3. White blood cells (WBCs or **leukocytes**)—portion of the blood necessary for fighting infection within the body; includes granular WBCs and nongranular WBCs
   • Granular WBCs: **basophils**, eosinophils, and **neutrophils**
   • Nongranular WBCs: lymphocytes and monocytes
4. Red blood cells (also known as RBCs or erythrocytes)—portion of the blood necessary for transporting oxygen (O_2) and carbon dioxide (CO_2)

STATISTICS

AML usually develops in people between the ages of 30 and 60 with men having a slightly higher risk than women. The leukemias are the twentieth most common cause of cancer-related deaths for people of all ages in the United States. More than 11,000 people develop a type of leukemia annually.

Neutrophils – one of the three granular white blood cells or leukocytes (granular leukocytes include basophils, eosinophils, and neutrophils)

Genetic – heredity or reproduction

RED BLOOD CELLS

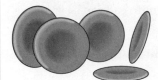

PLATELETS

WHITE BLOOD CELLS
(leukocytes)

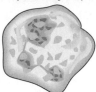

Neutrophil

Basophil

Eosinophil

Granular Leukocytes

Lymphocyte

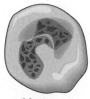

Monocyte

Nongranular Leukocytes

Figure 8-1 Blood cells of the human body (Adapted from Layman, *The Medical Language*, copyright © 1995, Delmar Publishers)

RISK FACTORS

The exact cause for leukemia is unknown, though the following factors have been shown to increase the incidence:

1. Environmental carcinogens including exposure to radiation and certain chemicals
2. Retrovirus
3. **Genetic** factors, such as familial predisposition and certain chromosomal abnormalities; e.g. Down syndrome
4. Long-term exposure to Benzene. Benzene is a hydrocarbon chemical used as a solvent for thinning and cleaning.

SIGNS, SYMPTOMS, AND ASSOCIATED CARE

1. Fatigue/malaise due to anemia
   - Assist patient with activities of daily living (ADLs) as necessary
   - Schedule care, activities, and treatment around patient's rest schedule
   - Screen phone calls and visitors based on patient's energy level and rest schedule
   - Encourage activity as able

Arthralgia – joint pain

- Provide assistance as needed to prevent injury due to weakness
- Provide method for patient to call for assistance
- Encourage patient to set realistic goals of activities
- Allow adequate time to do activities and procedures to avoid frustration or possible injury
- Encourage exercise to maintain muscle strength
- Provide a cane or walker for ambulation and transfer
- Utilize a private room for patient to promote rest periods

2. Pallor due to anemia
   - Administer blood transfusion as necessary if pallor due to anemia
   - Encourage clothing and makeup to enhance skin coloring as patient desires

3. **Arthralgia** due to accumulation of leukemic cells in the bones
   - Provide heat or other methods of pain control, such as massage, relaxation, and imaging
   - Administer medications as prescribed by physician for pain control
   - Monitor level of comfort
   - Protect joints, immobilize joints, and decrease weight-bearing
   - Assist with ADLs as necessary due to pain
   - Adjust position for patient comfort
   - Encourage patient to keep as active as possible
   - Allow frequent rest periods to provide joint rest and pain relief
   - Allow adequate time to do as much as possible for themselves, even though it may take longer
   - Use pillows to support extremities

4. Bone pain due to accumulation of leukemic cells in the bones
   - Promote decreased weight-bearing on bones as able
   - Provide heat or other methods of pain control such as massage, relaxation techniques, and distraction
   - Administer medications as prescribed by physician for pain control
   - Assess for level of comfort and offer pain control methods
   - Encourage patient to ask for pain control methods before pain becomes too severe

5. Bleeding tendencies due to thrombocytopenia
   - Observe for signs of abnormal bleeding and educate patient and family to observe and report any signs promptly to physician, e.g. hemoptysis, bloody emesis, bloody or tarry stools, nose bleeds, vaginal bleeding between menstrual cycles or postmenopausal, bleeding gums or hematuria
   - Observe for signs of central nervous system (CNS) bleeding and educate patient and family to observe and report symptoms promptly to physician. For example, altered level of consciousness, headache, vision changes, and vertigo.
   - Prevent injury to patient who has thrombocytopenia, e.g. soft toothbrush, electric razor rather than straight-edge razor, wear seat belts in the car, elevate siderails, avoid straining with bowel movements, avoid vigorous nose-blowing, avoid intramuscular injections, avoid rectal temperatures, avoid use of tampons, and seek physician advice prior to vaginal or anal intercourse
   - Avoid products that contain aspirin, which alters normal platelet function

- Monitor *platelet* count

- Monitor *hemoglobin* and *hematocrit*

- Apply pressure at sites of injection or blood drawing sites for minimum of 5 minutes or until bleeding stops

6. Fever due to leukopenia

- Monitor temperature at routine intervals

- Administer comfort measures for patient with elevated temperature, such as a cool cloth to the forehead, partial or complete bath as needed, clothing and bedding changed frequently due to diaphoresis, and encourage fluids to prevent dehydration. Symptoms of dehydration include decreased urine output, dry skin, dry mouth, dry eyes, constipation, tenting of skin, concentrated urine, confusion, and hypotension.

- Avoid exposing patient to a draft

- Cover with blankets as necessary

- Monitor intake and output (I and O)

- Maintain comfortable room temperature for patient

- Avoid plastic mattresses and plastic bed protectors as they have a tendency to increase perspiration

- Use antiperspirant and deodorant to minimize sweating and odor

7. Increased tendency towards infection due to leukopenia

- Monitor for signs of infection and educate patient and family to observe for signs of infection and report promptly to medical staff, e.g. fever, chills, redness, swelling, pain, phlegm, skin rash, cough, dyspnea, flushed skin, diaphoresis, dysuria, and sore throat

- Avoid people with infections

- Employ meticulous hand and skin care on the part of the patient, staff, and visitors

- Educate patient regarding need to complete entire regimen of antibiotics indicated for infection

- Utilize a private room if necessary

- Avoid exposure to staff members who have taken care of patients with infectious disease

- Avoid possible routes of infection when possible, such as urinary catheters and intravenous (IV) lines

- Monitor temperature on a routine basis

- Initiate protective isolation if necessary during hospitalization (See Figure 8-2)

- Avoid crowded areas, which increase chances of being exposed to an infection

- Provide frequent dental checks, meticulous mouth care, and antiseptic mouthwash

- Avoid injury to skin and mucous membranes

8. Lymphadenopathy due to infiltration from leukemic cells

- Monitor for lymphadenopathy

- Adjust position for patient comfort

- Provide comfort measures as necessary due to lymphadenopathy

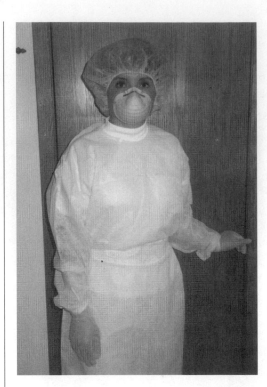

Figure 8-2 Garments used in the isolation room

9. Splenomegaly and hepatomegaly due to infiltration from leukemic cells
    - Monitor for hepatomegaly and splenomegaly
    - Avoid abdominal injury in the presence of hepatomegaly and splenomegaly
    - Monitor for signs of internal bleeding in the presence of hepatomegaly, such as abdominal pain, tachycardia, hypotension, and abdominal distention
    - Monitor liver function with serum laboratory tests, e.g. *SGOT*, *SGPT*, *bilirubin*, *albumin*, *alkaline phosphatase*, and *prothrombin time*
    - Monitor for bleeding tendencies in the presence of hepatomegaly
    - Educate to avoid the use of alcohol and medications metabolized in the liver
    - Monitor for jaundice
    - Monitor for signs of internal bleeding in the presence of splenomegaly such as abdominal pain, tachycardia, hypotension, and abdominal distention
    - Monitor hemoglobin and hematocrit

10. Abdominal pain due to organ involvement
    - Adjust position for patient comfort
    - Avoid constrictive garments and undergarments
    - Employ methods to promote comfort such as relaxation techniques, imaging, massage, and warm baths
    - Monitor for level of pain and offer comfort measures as necessary
    - Administer medications as necessary and as prescribed by physician for the control of pain
    - Encourage patient to request pain relief methods before pain becomes too severe

11. CNS symptoms due to leukemic cell invasion of CNS
    - Monitor for symptoms of CNS involvement, e.g. altered level of consciousness, headache, vision changes, and vertigo

Remission – period of diminished or absent symptoms of a disease or illness

- Protect patient from injury in the event of CNS symptoms and changes
- Assist patient with ADLs as necessary in the event of CNS symptoms and changes

CAUSE OF SYMPTOMS

1. Proliferation of immature WBCs which depletes normal WBCs needed to fight infection
2. Due to the increased number of WBCs, the erythrocytes and thrombocytes are decreased in number for lack of space
3. Abnormal WBCs accumulate in the organs, CNS, lymph nodes, bone marrow, and, occasionally, the skin
4. Nutrients are used to provide energy for the metabolic needs of the proliferating WBCs causing deprivation of normal body cells

DIAGNOSIS

1. Symptoms
2. Physical examination
3. *Serum WBC* elevation, which shows proliferation of immature WBCs
4. *Bone marrow* examination, which shows a proliferation of immature WBCs
5. *Chest x-ray* used to determine involvement of lymph nodes or lungs
6. *Lymph node biopsy*
7. *Platelet count*—shows thrombocytopenia
8. *Serum RBC count*
9. *CT scan* could detect organ involvement

TREATMENT

1. *Chemotherapy*—goal is to obtain **remission** and continue with chemotherapy to prevent relapse, e.g. Daunorubicin, Cytarabine, Cyclophosphamide, Vincristine, Methotrexate
2. *Radiation* therapy to prevent CNS invasion
3. *Bone marrow transplant*
4. *Platelet transfusion* to prevent/treat bleeding tendencies due to thrombocytopenia
5. RBC transfusion for treatment of anemia
6. Treat infections promptly according to causative agent, e.g. bacterial, viral, or fungal

If left untreated, acute leukemia is fatal due to complications involving the bone marrow and body organs. Even with treatment, survival time is 1 to 2 years, although half of affected children may have a remission of up to one year.

CONSIDERATIONS FOR CARE

1. Educate patient and family regarding the disease process.
2. Educate patient and family regarding forms of treatment as well as side effects of treatment.
3. Provide emotional support to patient and family.

Uricemia – accumulation of uric acid in the blood

4. Provide nonjudgmental acceptance of emotions and behavior of patient and family.

5. Encourage proper nutrition.

6. Observe for signs of infection and educate patient and family to observe for signs of infection and report promptly to physician, e.g. fever, chills, redness, swelling, pain, phlegm, skin rash, cough, dyspnea, flushed skin, diaphoresis, dysuria, and sore throat.

7. Observe for signs of abnormal bleeding and educate patient/family to observe and report any signs promptly to physician, e.g. hemoptysis, bloody emesis, bloody or black tarry stools, nose bleeds, vaginal bleeding between menstrual cycles or post-menopausal, bleeding gums, hematuria, and bruising.

8. Observe for signs of CNS bleeding or leukemic cell infiltration and educate patient and family to observe and report symptoms promptly to physician, e.g. altered level of consciousness, headache, vision changes, and vertigo.

9. Prevent injury to patient who has thrombocytopenia, e.g. soft toothbrush, electric razor rather than straight-edge razor, wear seat belts in the car, elevate siderails, avoid straining with bowel movements, avoid vigorous nose-blowing, avoid intramuscular injections, and avoid rectal temperatures.

10. Avoid products that contain aspirin, which alters normal platelet function.

11. Educate patient to avoid people who have infections.

12. Meticulous handwashing on the part of the staff.

13. Protective isolation may be necessary while in the hospital.

14. Assess level of comfort and offer methods of pain control, such as relaxation, imaging, massage, heat treatment, and medications.

15. Prevent skin breakdown due to increased risk of infection and bleeding, e.g. reposition frequently; meticulous skin care; linen and clothing should be clean, dry, and wrinkle-free; and encourage fluid intake.

16. Monitor fluid intake especially with chemotherapy; due to destruction of leukemic cells, **uricemia** may result.

17. Monitor laboratory results, especially WBC count.

18. Educate patient and family regarding methods to control bleeding, such as direct pressure, elevation, and ice packs to the area.

FOR MORE INFORMATION

American Cancer Society
1599 Clifton Road, NE
Atlanta, GA 30329
1-800-ACS-2345

Leukemia Society of America
733 Third Avenue
New York, NY 10017
(212) 573-8484

ASSIGNMENT SHEET: ACUTE MYELOGENOUS LEUKEMIA

Short Answer

1. Write a brief definition for the terms located throughout the chapter.

2. List the four (4) basic components of blood and describe the function of each.

3. List the granular and nongranular white blood cells.

4. Write a brief definition for acute myelogenous leukemia.

5. Describe the incidence of acute myelogenous leukemia.

6. List four (4) risk factors for acute myelogenous leukemia.

7. List eleven (11) signs and symptoms of acute myelogenous leukemia. Describe the rationale and associated care for each of the symptoms.

8. Describe the cause of the symptoms associated with acute myelogenous leukemia.

9. List nine (9) specific methods used to diagnose acute myelogenous leukemia.

10. Write the normal laboratory value for each of the following lab tests.
    a. WBC
    b. Platelet count
    c. RBC
    d. Hemoglobin (Hg)
    e. Hematocrit (Hct)
    f. SGOT
    g. SGPT
    h. Bilirubin
    i. Albumin
    j. Alkaline phosphatase
    k. Prothrombin time

11. Describe six (6) specific methods of treatment used for acute myelogenous leukemia.

12. List eighteen (18) specific considerations for caring for a patient with acute myelogenous leukemia.

13. List nine (9) specific symptoms of dehydration.

KNOWLEDGE INTO ACTION

1. Dennis Doyle has been admitted to your facility with acute myelogenous leukemia. He complains of extreme fatigue. Describe the rationale behind the fatigue and five (5) methods of associated care for Mr. Doyle.

2. Craig Dennison, an 82-year-old diagnosed with AML, was found on the floor by his bed. You notice a bruise on his left hip and abdomen and notice his face is scraped. He doesn't remember what happened. X-rays reveal no broken bones. You recall reading in Mr. Dennison's chart that he was admitted with hepatomegaly, splenomegaly, and thrombocytopenia. List seven (7) symptoms of complications you would monitor for due to Mr. Dennison's admitting diagnosis and the fall that he just experienced.

3. Amy Wong, a 53-year-old female diagnosed with AML, is scheduled for a CT scan in the morning. She says to you, "My doctor has ordered this test tomorrow because he wants to check my liver and spleen and other organs. Why would he do that? I thought leukemia was cancer of the lymph nodes. Does he think something else is wrong with me? Did he make a mistake about my diagnosis?" How would you explain the diagnostic testing?

Acute Lymphocytic Leukemia

OBJECTIVES

Upon completion of this chapter, the student should be able to:

■ Define the key terms listed throughout the chapter

■ State a specific definition for acute lymphocytic leukemia

■ Describe the incidence of acute lymphocytic leukemia

■ List the risk factors associated with acute lymphocytic leukemia

■ Describe the signs and symptoms associated with acute lymphocytic leukemia, the rationale for these symptoms, and associated care

■ Identify specific methods for diagnosis of acute lymphocytic leukemia

■ Identify specific methods for treatment of acute lymphocytic leukemia

■ Describe specific considerations for caring for a patient with acute lymphocytic leukemia

KEY TERMS

Blast – an immaturely developed cell

Neutropenia – decrease in the total number of neutrophils

Red blood cells (RBCs) – biconcave cells present in the blood; combine with hemoglobin to transport oxygen and carbon dioxide throughout the body; normal accumulation of 5,000,000 per cubic millimeter in the human body; also known as erythrocytes

Prognosis – projected outcome of a disease or illness

INTRODUCTION

Acute lymphocytic leukemia (ALL) is a disease in which immature WBCs (**blasts**) replace the normal elements of the bone marrow, which results in thrombocytopenia, anemia, and **neutropenia**. Nongranular leukocytes are involved in the disease.

PHYSIOLOGY

There are four basic components of blood. (See Figure 9-1.)

1. Plasma—liquid portion of the blood
2. Platelets (thrombocytes)—portion of the blood necessary for clot formation
3. White blood cells (WBCs or leukocytes)—portion of the blood necessary for fighting infection within the body; divided into granular WBCs and non-granular WBCs
   - Granular WBCs: basophils, eosinophils, and neutrophils
   - Nongranular WBCs: lymphocytes and monocytes
4. **Red blood cells (RBCs** or erythrocytes)—portion of the blood necessary for transporting oxygen (O_2) and carbon dioxide (CO_2)

STATISTICS

Acute lymphocytic leukemia is the most common childhood cancer with 4 of every 100,000 children under the age of 15 affected by the disease. Caucasian children are affected more frequently by the disease than other races and incidence is higher in males than in females. Between 90 and 95% of children with this disease can expect a remission (with treatment) with a five-year survival rate of 50%. Approximately 65% of adults can expect a remission after treatment with an average survival time of 1 to 2 years. With consecutive relapses, the **prognosis** worsens.

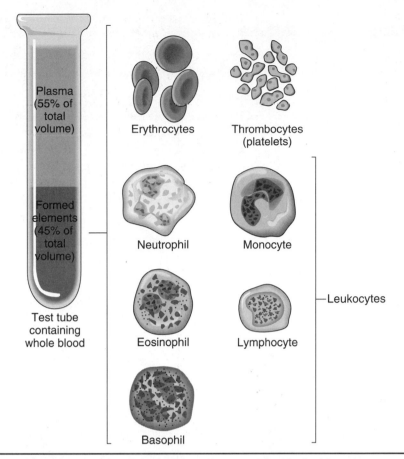

Figure 9-1   Components of whole blood (From Layman, *The Medical Language,* copyright © 1995, Delmar Publishers)

RISK FACTORS

While the exact cause of acute lymphocytic leukemia is unknown, following are several of the theories:

1. Environmental carcinogens
2. Infectious agents, especially viruses
3. Genetic factors
4. Chromosomal abnormalities

SIGNS, SYMPTOMS, AND ASSOCIATED CARE

1. Fatigue/malaise due to anemia from decreased RBCs
    - Assist patient with activities of daily living (ADLs) as necessary
    - Schedule care, activities, and treatment around patient's rest schedule
    - Monitor phone calls and visitors around patient's energy level and rest schedule
    - Encourage frequent rest periods
    - Provide assistance as needed to prevent injury due to weakness
    - Provide method for patient to call for assistance
    - Encourage patient to set realistic goals of activities
    - Allow adequate time to do activities and procedures to avoid frustration or possible injury
    - Encourage exercise to maintain muscle strength

- Provide cane or walker to provide additional assistance for ambulation and transfer
- Provide private room for patient to promote rest periods

2. Fever due to leukopenia

- Monitor temperature at routine intervals
- Provide comfort measures for patient with elevated temperature, such as cool cloth to forehead, partial or complete bath as needed, clothing and bedding changed frequently due to diaphoresis, and encourage fluids to prevent dehydration. Symptoms of dehydration include decreased urine output, dry skin, dry mouth, dry eyes, constipation, tenting of skin, confusion, concentrated urine, and hypotension.
- Avoid exposing patient to a draft
- Cover with blankets as necessary
- Monitor intake and output (I and O)
- Maintain comfortable room temperature for patient
- Avoid plastic mattresses and plastic bed protectors as they have a tendency to increase perspiration
- Use antiperspirant or deodorant to minimize sweating and odor

3. Bone pain and arthralgia due to accumulation of leukemic cells in the bone marrow

- Provide heat or other methods of pain control, such as massage, relaxation, and imaging
- Administer medications as prescribed by physician for pain control
- Monitor level of comfort
- Protect joints, immobilize joints, and decrease weight-bearing
- Assist with ADLs as necessary due to pain
- Assist with position for patient comfort
- Encourage patient to keep as active as possible
- Encourage frequent rest periods to provide joint rest and pain relief
- Allow adequate time to do as much as possible for themselves, even though it may take longer
- Use pillows to support extremities

4. Bleeding tendencies due to thrombocytopenia

- Observe for signs of abnormal bleeding and educate patient and family to observe and report any signs promptly to physician, e.g. hemoptysis, bloody emesis, bloody or tarry stools, nose bleeds, vaginal bleeding between menstrual cycles or postmenopausal, bleeding gums, or hematuria
- Observe for signs of central nervous system (CNS) bleeding and educate patient and family to observe and report symptoms promptly to physician, e.g. altered level of consciousness, headache, vision changes, and vertigo
- Prevent injury to patient who has thrombocytopenia, e.g. soft toothbrush, electric razor rather than straight-edge razor, wear seat belts in the car, elevate siderails, avoid straining with bowel movements, avoid vigorous nose-blowing, avoid intramuscular injections, avoid rectal temperatures, avoid use of tampons, and seek physician advice prior to vaginal or anal intercourse
- Avoid products that contain aspirin, which alters normal platelet function
- Monitor *platelet* count
- Monitor *hemoglobin* and *hematocrit*

- Apply pressure at sites of injection or blood drawing sites for minimum of 5 minutes or until bleeding stops

5. Lymphadenopathy due to infiltration of leukemic cells in the lymph nodes
   - Monitor for lymphadenopathy
   - Assist with position for patient comfort
   - Offer comfort measures as necessary due to lymphadenopathy

6. Abdominal pain due to infiltration of leukemic cells in the organs of the body
   - Assist with position for patient comfort
   - Avoid constrictive garments and undergarments
   - Provide methods to promote comfort, such as relaxation techniques, imaging, massage, and warm baths
   - Monitor for level of pain and offer comfort measures as necessary
   - Administer medications as necessary and as prescribed by physician for the control of pain
   - Encourage patient to request pain relief methods before pain becomes too severe

7. Recurrent infections due to decreased number of normal WBCs
   - Monitor for signs of infection and educate patient and family to observe for signs of infection and report promptly to medical staff, e.g. fever, chills, redness, swelling, pain, phlegm, skin rash, cough, dyspnea, flushed skin, diaphoresis, dysuria, and sore throat
   - Encourage to avoid people who have infections
   - Utilize meticulous hand and skin care for the patient, staff, and visitors (See Figure 9-2)
   - Educate patient regarding need to complete entire regimen of antibiotics
   - Provide private room as necessary
   - Restrict staff members who have taken care of patients with infectious disease

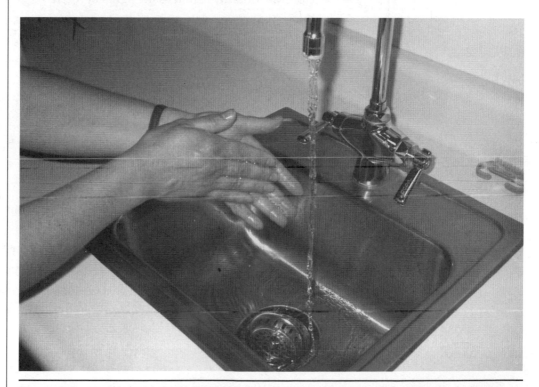

Figure 9-2   Handwashing is an important aspect in the prevention of the spread of infection in a health care facility.

Photophobia – increased
sensitivity to light

- Avoid possible routes of infection when possible, such as urinary catheters and intravenous (IV) lines
- Monitor temperature on a routine basis
- Utilize protective isolation as necessary during hospitalization
- Avoid crowded areas, which increase chances of being exposed to an infection
- Utilize meticulous mouth care
- Provide frequent dental checks and antiseptic mouthwash
- Avoid injury to skin and mucous membranes

8. Pallor due to anemia from decreased RBCs
    - Administer blood transfusion as necessary if pallor due to anemia
    - Encourage clothing and makeup to enhance skin coloring as patient desires

9. Headache due to infiltration of leukemic cells in the CNS
    - Provide dim lights if **photophobia** accompanies headache
    - Provide quiet, relaxed atmosphere
    - Assist with position for patient comfort
    - Administer pain control methods, such as relaxation techniques, massage, imaging, and pain medications as prescribed by physician
    - Encourage patient to avoid eye strain during periods of headache
    - Encourage frequent rest periods as necessary
    - Monitor phone calls and visitors to promote rest periods

10. Vomiting due to infiltration of leukemic cells in the CNS
    - Administer antiemetics before meals as prescribed by physician
    - Offer food choices according to patient preference and tolerance
    - Control odors and unpleasant sights in room
    - Offer fluids frequently to prevent dehydration
    - Monitor intake and output (I and O) to avoid dehydration
    - Monitor serum electrolytes (*sodium*, *potassium*, and *chloride*)
    - Encourage rest periods after meals
    - Avoid foods that are spicy, rich, or previously disagreeable to patient
    - Utilize receptacle for patient to vomit into as needed; this should be cleaned whenever used and changed on a frequent basis
    - Provide meticulous mouth care
    - Prevent aspiration of emesis
    - Utilize universal precautions at all times when coming in contact with blood or body fluids (See Appendix C)
    - Avoid greasy foods as they tend to stay in the stomach a long period of time
    - Avoid cooking food if possible due to increased nausea with odors of foods
    - Avoid hot foods as necessary due to the increased odors of hot foods
    - Eat in well-ventilated area to decrease the accumulation of odors of foods while eating

11. Hepatomegaly and splenomegaly due to infiltration of leukemic cells in the liver and spleen
    - Monitor for hepatomegaly and splenomegaly
    - Avoid abdominal injury in the presence of hepatomegaly and splenomegaly

- Monitor for signs of internal bleeding in the presence of hepatomegaly and splenomegaly, such as abdominal pain, tachycardia, hypotension, and abdominal distention
- Monitor liver function with serum laboratory tests, e.g. *SGOT, SGPT, bilirubin, albumin, alkaline phosphatase,* and *prothrombin time*
- Monitor for bleeding tendencies in the presence of hepatomegaly
- Educate to avoid the use of alcohol and medications metabolized in the liver
- Monitor for jaundice
- Monitor *hemoglobin* and *hematocrit*

12. Weight loss and anorexia due to the increased metabolic needs of the proliferating WBCs causing deprivation of normal body cells
- Obtain baseline weight and monitor on routine basis
- Encourage patient to participate in dietary choices
- Provide nutritional supplements and vitamins
- Monitor for signs of dehydration, such as decreased urine output, concentrated urine, dry skin, tenting of skin, dry mucous membranes, dry mouth, dry eyes, confusion, and constipation
- Encourage family and friends to bring in food that is appealing to patient as dietary restrictions allow
- Encourage frequent, small meals as tolerated
- Administer parenteral fluids as necessary
- Monitor intake and output (I and O)
- Encourage fluids to prevent dehydration
- Avoid unpleasant sights and odors in room to make meals more appealing
- Provide meticulous mouth care
- Maintain social atmosphere for mealtimes to encourage the patient to eat
- Encourage clothing that enhances patient appearance
- Encourage exercise program as tolerated to increase appetite

DIAGNOSIS

1. Symptoms
2. Physical examination
3. Laboratory studies may show decreased *hemoglobin*, decreased *RBCs*, decreased *platelet count*, and decreased *hematocrit*
4. *WBCs* may be normal, increased, or decreased
5. *Bone marrow aspiration* and examination will show proliferation of lymphoblasts and lymphocytes
6. Liver function tests to determine liver involvement, e.g. *SGOT, SGPT, bilirubin, albumin, alkaline phosphatase,* and *prothrombin time*
7. *Lumbar puncture* to determine CNS involvement

TREATMENT

1. *Chemotherapy*—goal is to obtain remission and continue with chemotherapy to prevent relapse, e.g. Vincristine (Oncovin), Cytarabine, Daunorubicin, Methotrexate, Cyclophosphamide (Cytoxan)
2. *Bone marrow transplant*

CONSIDERATIONS FOR CARE

1. Educate patient and family regarding the disease process.

2. Educate patient and family regarding forms of treatment as well as side effects of treatment.

3. Provide emotional support to patient and family.

4. Provide nonjudgmental acceptance of emotions and behavior of patient and family.

5. Encourage proper nutrition and rest.

6. Observe for signs of infection and educate patient and family to observe for signs of infection and report promptly to physician, such as fever, chills, redness, swelling, pain, phlegm, skin rash, cough, dyspnea, flushed skin, diaphoresis, dysuria, and sore throat.

7. Observe for signs of abnormal bleeding and educate patient and family to observe and report any signs promptly to physician, such as hemoptysis, bloody emesis, bloody or black tarry stools, nose bleeds, vaginal bleeding between menstrual cycles or postmenopausal, bleeding gums, hematuria, and bruising.

8. Observe for signs of CNS bleeding or leukemic cell infiltration and educate patient and family to observe and report symptoms promptly to physician, e.g. altered level of consciousness, headache, vision changes, and vertigo.

9. Prevent injury to patient who has thrombocytopenia, e.g. soft toothbrush, electric razor rather than straight-edge razor, wear seat belts in the car, elevate siderails, avoid straining with bowel movements, avoid vigorous noseblowing, avoid intramuscular injections, and avoid rectal temperatures.

10. Avoid products that contain aspirin, which alters normal platelet function.

11. Educate patient to avoid people who have infections.

12. Encourage meticulous handwashing on the part of the staff.

13. Protective isolation may be necessary while in the hospital.

14. Assess level of comfort and offer methods of pain control, such as relaxation, imaging, massage, heat treatments, and medications.

15. Prevent skin breakdown due to increased risk of infection and bleeding, e.g. reposition frequently; meticulous skin care; linen and clothing should be clean, dry, and wrinkle-free; and encourage fluid intake.

16. Monitor and encourage fluid intake; leukemic cell destruction from chemotherapy may cause uricemia.

17. Monitor laboratory results, especially WBC count.

18. Educate patient and family regarding methods to control bleeding, such as direct pressure, elevation, and ice packs to the area.

FOR MORE INFORMATION

American Cancer Society
1599 Clifton Road, NE
Atlanta, GA 30329
1-800-ACS-2345

Leukemia Society of America
733 Third Avenue
New York, NY 10017

ASSIGNMENT SHEET: ACUTE LYMPHOCYTIC LEUKEMIA

Short Answer

1. Write a brief definition for the terms listed throughout the chapter.

2. Write a brief definition for acute lymphocytic leukemia.

3. Describe the incidence of acute lymphocytic leukemia.

4. List the granular and nongranular WBCs.

5. List four (4) risk factors for acute lymphocytic leukemia.

6. List twelve (12) signs and symptoms for acute lymphocytic leukemia. Describe the rationale and associated care for each of the symptoms.

7. Write the normal ranges for each of the following laboratory tests.
    a. WBC
    b. RBC
    c. Platelet count
    d. Hemoglobin (Hg)
    e. Hematocrit (Hct)
    f. SGOT
    g. SGPT
    h. Bilirubin
    i. Albumin
    j. Alkaline phosphatase
    k. Prothrombin time

8. List eight (8) specific avenues of bleeding that would be symptoms of thrombocytopenia.

9. Describe eight (8) methods to prevent bleeding in a patient who is prone to bleeding due to thrombocytopenia.

10. List thirteen (13) possible signs and symptoms of an infection.

11. Describe the following procedures used in the diagnosis or treatment of acute lymphocytic leukemia.
    a. Bone marrow aspiration
    b. Lumbar puncture (spinal tap)
    c. Bone marrow transplant

12. List seven (7) specific methods used to aid in the diagnosis of acute lymphocytic leukemia.

13. Describe the two (2) specific methods of treatment used in acute lymphocytic leukemia.

14. List five (5) specific methods to prevent skin breakdown in a patient.

15. List eighteen (18) considerations for caring for a patient with acute lymphocytic leukemia.

KNOWLEDGE INTO ACTION

1. Stephanie Lorenz, an 11-year-old patient who has been diagnosed with ALL, has been vomiting frequently for the past few days. Her mother, Mrs. Lorenz, asks you for some suggestions to help reduce Stephanie's nausea and vomiting. What suggestions could you make to Mrs. Lorenz?

2. Stephanie is scheduled for a lumbar puncture to determine whether the central nervous system has been infiltrated with leukemic cells. Mrs. Lorenz was not in the room when the physician explained the procedure and is asking you what a lumbar puncture is. What will your response be?

3. Stephanie is scheduled to go home in the morning. During her admission, she has had a platelet count of 73,000 cubic millimeters. Mrs. Lorenz asks if Stephanie has any restrictions regarding going back to school and playing with her friends. She also mentions to you that Stephanie occasionally will get a leg ache and would it be okay to "give her a couple of aspirin?" What will your response be regarding activity restrictions for Stephanie? What will your response be regarding administering aspirin to Stephanie?

4. You are walking in the hall when you notice Laurie Kellogg, a 22-year-old patient with ALL, bleeding profusely from a cut on her arm. Describe the steps you would take to control Laurie's bleeding and any special considerations you would keep in mind while caring for Laurie's bleeding.

Chronic Myelogenous Leukemia

OBJECTIVES

Upon completion of this chapter, the student should be able to:

■ Define the key terms listed throughout the chapter

■ State a specific definition for chronic myelogenous leukemia

■ Describe the incidence of chronic myelogenous leukemia

■ Describe the signs and symptoms of chronic myelogenous leukemia, the rationale for these symptoms, and associated care

■ Identify specific methods for diagnosis of chronic myelogenous leukemia

■ Describe the importance of the presence of the Philadelphia chromosome in the diagnosis of chronic myelogenous leukemia and differentiating between other types of leukemias

■ Identify specific methods for treatment of chronic myelogenous leukemia

■ Describe specific considerations for caring for a patient with chronic myelogenous leukemia

KEY TERMS

Philadelphia chromosome – abnormality in chromosome 9 or 22; commonly found in patients with chronic myelocytic leukemia

Bone marrow – tissue located in the bones of the body and refers either to yellow bone marrow (located in the medullary cavity) or red bone marrow, which is located in the spongy bone

INTRODUCTION

Chronic myelogenous leukemia (CML) is characterized by proliferation of granulocytes, monocytes, platelets, and RBCs. The proliferation of these cells causes them to accumulate in the bone marrow, body organs, and bloodstream.

PHYSIOLOGY

There are four basic components of blood. (See Figure 9-1.)

1. Plasma—liquid portion of the blood
2. Platelets (thrombocytes)—portion of the blood necessary for clot formation
3. White blood cells (WBCs or leukocytes)—portion of the blood necessary for fighting infection within the body, divided into granular WBCs and nongranular WBCs

   • Granular WBCs: basophils, eosinophils, and neutrophils

   • Nongranular WBCs: lymphocytes and monocytes
4. Red blood cells (RBCs or erythrocytes)—portion of the blood necessary for transporting oxygen (O_2) and carbon dioxide (CO_2)

STATISTICS

Chronic myelogenous leukemia most often occurs in the 40 to 60 age group. Approximately 90% of all patients have the **Philadelphia chromosome** present in **bone marrow** cells. Chronic myelogenous leukemia constitutes approximately 20% of all leukemias. Approximately 2,000 to 4,000 people in the United States develop CML annually. The disease is always fatal with the average survival time estimated as 3 months to 4 years.

Distention – state of being swollen or distended

SIGNS, SYMPTOMS, AND ASSOCIATED CARE

1. Fatigue due to anemia
   - Assist patient with activities of daily living (ADLs) as necessary
   - Schedule care, activities, and treatment around patient's rest schedule
   - Monitor phone calls and visitors around patient's energy level and rest schedule
   - Encourage frequent rest periods
   - Provide assistance as needed to prevent injury due to weakness
   - Provide method for patient to call for assistance
   - Encourage patient to set realistic goals of activities
   - Allow adequate time to do activities and procedures to avoid frustration or possible injury
   - Encourage exercise to maintain muscle strength
   - Utilize cane or walker to provide additional assistance for ambulation and transfer
   - Provide private room for patient to promote rest periods

2. Weakness due to increased metabolic needs of the proliferating WBCs causing deprivation of normal body cells
   - Assist patient with ADLs as necessary
   - Schedule care, activities, and treatment around patient's rest schedule
   - Monitor phone calls and visitors around patient's energy level and rest schedule
   - Encourage frequent rest periods
   - Provide assistance as needed to prevent injury due to weakness
   - Provide method for patient to call for assistance
   - Encourage patient to set realistic goals of activities
   - Allow adequate time to do activities and procedures to avoid frustration or possible injury
   - Encourage exercise to maintain muscle strength
   - Utilize cane or walker to provide additional assistance for ambulation and transfer
   - Provide private room for patient to promote rest periods

3. Pain in long bones due to infiltration of leukemic cells in the bone marrow
   - Encourage rest to decrease stress on bones
   - Decrease weight-bearing on bones
   - Provide heat or other methods of pain control, such as massage, relaxation techniques, and distraction
   - Administer medications as prescribed by physician for pain control
   - Assess for level of comfort and offer pain control methods
   - Encourage patient to ask for pain control methods before pain becomes too severe

4. Splenomegaly due to infiltration of leukemic cells in the spleen
   - Monitor for splenomegaly
   - Avoid abdominal injury in the presence of splenomegaly
   - Monitor for signs of internal bleeding in the presence of splenomegaly, such as abdominal pain, tachycardia, hypotension, and abdominal **distention**
   - Monitor *hemoglobin* and *hematocrit*

Palpitations – unusually strong, bounding pulse of the heart that is often felt or noticed by the patient

5. Pallor due to anemia
   - Administer blood transfusion if pallor is due to anemia
   - Encourage clothing and makeup to enhance skin coloring as patient desires

6. Dyspnea due to anemia
   - Assist with position for patient comfort
   - Administer oxygen as needed and as directed by physician
   - Avoid constrictive garments and undergarments
   - Utilize fan in room to circulate air and assist in making breathing easier
   - Encourage frequent rest periods to conserve energy
   - Arrange schedule of activities around patient rest periods
   - Assist with ADLs as necessary
   - Assess breath sounds on routine basis
   - Observe for signs of hypoxia, such as cyanosis, diaphoresis, decreased level of consciousness, and confusion
   - Monitor ease of respirations and respiratory rate
   - Do as many activities as possible in a sitting position, e.g. dressing, bathing, cooking, and cleaning
   - Humidify air as needed
   - Provide reassurance to patient
   - Treat cause of dyspnea

7. **Palpitations** due to anemia
   - Monitor heart rhythm and pulse rate
   - Instruct patient to report periods of palpitations
   - Educate patient and family regarding method to take patient's pulse rate
   - Assess heart rate and rhythm changes with exertion and rest
   - Instruct regarding relaxation techniques for patient use
   - Provide calm, quiet, relaxed atmosphere for patient

8. Weight loss and anorexia due to the increased metabolic needs of the proliferating WBCs causing depravation of normal body cells as well as splenomegaly
   - Obtain baseline weight and monitor weight on a routine basis
   - Encourage patient to participate in dietary choices
   - Provide nutritional supplements and vitamins
   - Encourage family and friends to bring in food that is appealing to patient as dietary restrictions allow
   - Administer parenteral fluids as necessary
   - Monitor intake and output (I and O)
   - Encourage rest periods before and after meals
   - Avoid unpleasant sights and odors in room to make meals more appealing
   - Provide meticulous mouth care
   - Monitor for skin breakdown due to loss of body tissue
   - Encourage clothing styles that do not draw attention to weight loss
   - Monitor for symptoms of dehydration, such as decreased urine output, constipation, dry skin, tenting of skin, dry mouth, dry eyes, concentrated urine, hypotension, and confusion

Thrombocytosis –
increase in the number of
platelets in the blood

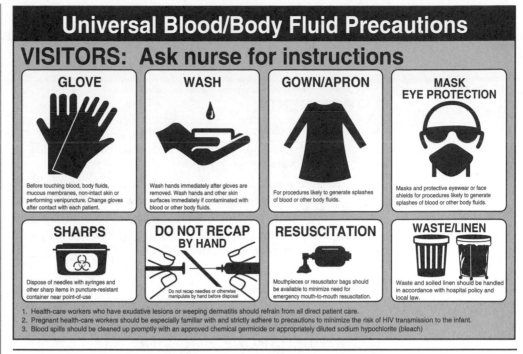

Figure 10-1   Universal precautions (From Shapiro, *Basic Maternal/Pediatric Nursing*, copyright © 1994, Delmar Publishers)

9. Bleeding tendencies due to **thrombocytosis**—an increase in immature platelets
    - Observe for signs of abnormal bleeding and educate patient and family to observe and report any signs promptly to physician, such as hemoptysis, bloody emesis, bloody or tarry stools, nose bleeds, vaginal bleeding between menstrual cycles or post-menopausal, bleeding gums, or hematuria
    - Observe for signs of central nervous system (CNS) bleeding and educate patient and family to observe and report symptoms promptly to physician, such as altered level of consciousness, headache, vision changes, and vertigo
    - Prevent injury to patient who has thrombocytopenia, e.g. soft toothbrush, electric razor rather than straight-edge razor, wear seat belts in the car, elevate siderails, avoid straining with bowel movements, avoid vigorous nose-blowing, avoid intramuscular injections, avoid rectal temperatures, avoid use of tampons, and seek physician advice prior to vaginal or anal intercourse
    - Avoid products that contain aspirin, which alters normal platelet function
    - Monitor *platelet* count
    - Monitor *hemoglobin* and *hematocrit*
    - Apply pressure at sites of injection or blood drawing sites for minimum of 5 minutes or until bleeding stops
    - Utilize universal precautions (See Figure 10-1)

DIAGNOSIS

1. Symptoms
2. Physical examination
3. Leukocytosis
4. Thrombocytosis—increase in immature platelets

Hemorrhage – extreme
bleeding or blood loss;
may be internal or
external

5. Increased granulocyte count
6. Presence of Philadelphia chromosome* in bone marrow cells
7. *CT scan* used to detect organ involvement.

TREATMENT

1. *Chemotherapy* used to treat splenomegaly and treat symptoms, and return WBC count to a normal range, e.g. Busulfan, Hydroxyurea (Hydrea), Chlorambucil (Leukeran)
2. Initial remission will generally lead to a "blast crisis" during which the patient has symptoms resembling acute leukemia; terminal for the majority of patients. Initial remission generally is induced by chemotherapy. Complete remission generally only lasts approximately 2 to 4 years. Death is generally due to infection or **hemorrhage**.
3. *Leukapheresis*
4. *Bone marrow transplant*

CONSIDERATIONS FOR CARE

1. Educate patient and family regarding the disease process.
2. Educate patient and family regarding forms of treatment as well as side effects of treatment.
3. Provide emotional support to patient and family.
4. Provide nonjudgmental acceptance of emotions and behavior of patient and family.
5. Encourage proper nutrition.
6. Observe for signs of infection and educate patient and family to observe for signs of infection and report promptly to physician, such as fever, chills, redness, swelling, pain, phlegm, skin rash, cough, dyspnea, flushed skin, and diaphoresis.
7. Observe for signs of abnormal bleeding and educate patient and family to observe and report any signs promptly to physician, e.g. hemoptysis, bloody emesis, bloody or black tarry stools, nose bleeds, vaginal bleeding between menstrual cycles or postmenopausal, bleeding gums, hematuria, and bruising.
8. Observe for signs of CNS bleeding and educate patient and family to observe and report symptoms promptly to physician, e.g. altered level of consciousness, headache, vision changes, and vertigo.
9. Prevent injury to patient who has thrombocytosis, e.g. soft toothbrush, electric razor rather than straight-edge razor, wear seat belts in the car, elevate siderails, avoid straining with bowel movements, avoid vigorous nose-blowing, avoid intramuscular injections, and avoid rectal temperatures.
10. Avoid products that contain aspirin, which alters normal platelet function.
11. Educate patient to avoid people who have infections.
12. Encourage meticulous handwashing for the staff, patient, and family.
13. Protective isolation may be necessary while in the hospital.
14. Assess level of comfort and offer methods of pain control, such as relaxation, imaging, massage, heat treatments, and medications.

---

* Philadelphia chromosome is an abnormality occurring in chromosome pairs 9 and 22. The problem is not an inherited genetic problem but occurs in patients with chronic myelogenous leukemia and occasionally in chronic lymphocytic leukemia as well as the acute leukemias.

15. Prevent skin breakdown due to increased risk of infection and bleeding; reposition frequently; meticulous skin care; linen and clothing should be clean, dry, and wrinkle-free; and encourage fluid intake.

16. Educate patient and family regarding symptoms of anemia. Symptoms of anemia include pallor, fatigue, diaphoresis, decreased tolerance to exercise or exertion, dizziness, and chest pain.

MORE INFORMATION

American Cancer Society
1599 Clifton Road, NE
Atlanta, GA 30329
1-800-ACS-2345

Leukemia Society of America
733 Third Avenue
New York, NY 10017

CHAPTER 10 REVIEW

ASSIGNMENT SHEET: CHRONIC MYELOGENOUS LEUKEMIA

Short Answer

1. Write a brief definition for the terms listed throughout the chapter.

2. Write a brief definition for chronic myelogenous leukemia.

3. Describe the incidence of chronic myelogenous leukemia.

4. List the granular and nongranular WBCs.

5. List nine (9) signs and symptoms for chronic myelogenous leukemia and the rationale and associated care for each symptom.

6. List seven (7) specific methods used to aid in the diagnosis of chronic myelogenous leukemia.

7. List four (4) specific methods of treatment used in chronic myelogenous leukemia.

8. Describe the importance of the presence of the Philadelphia chromosome in the diagnosis of chronic myelogenous leukemia as well as differentiating between other types of leukemias.

9. List sixteen (16) considerations for care when taking care of a patient with chronic myelogenous leukemia.

10. Write the normal range for each of the following laboratory tests.
    a. WBC
    b. Platelet
    c. Granular white blood cells
       • Basophil
       • Eosinophil
       • Neutrophil
    d. Hemoglobin (Hg)
    e. Hematocrit (Hct)

11. Describe each of the following procedures used for the diagnosis or treatment of chronic myelogenous leukemia.
    a. Leukapheresis
    b. Bone marrow transplant
    c. CT scan
    d. Chemotherapy

KNOWLEDGE INTO ACTION

1. Yolanda Lander, a 42-year-old grade school teacher, has been diagnosed with CML. She has come into the hospital with extreme exhaustion and much of the day has been in the radiology department for a CT scan. A teacher from her school calls and tells you, "We want to surprise Kathy and bring all her students up this afternoon. Will that be okay?" What will your response be?

2. Later that same evening, Mrs. Lander calls you into her room and says to you, "Why am I so tired all of the time? No matter how much sleep I get, I'm still tired. I'm so frustrated!" What will your response be regarding her constant fatigue? What methods could you employ to help Mrs. Lander rest?

3. Rita Prescott, a 61-year-old diagnosed with CML, is being discharged from the hospital. She has been having dyspnea during her hospitalization. While you are helping her get her belongings packed, she asks you for "helpful hints" to help her out at home due to the dyspnea. What would you suggest?

4. You have been asked to assist Mr. Murphy, a 57-year-old newly diagnosed with CML, with his bath and personal cares. While you are gathering the necessary supplies, you drop the washcloth on the floor. Mr. Murphy yells at you, saying, "I certainly hope you don't plan on using that washrag on me. You are the most incompetent person that works here! Tell them to send in someone that knows what's going on!" What will your response be? What is probably the reason behind Mr. Murphy's outburst?

Chronic Lymphocytic Leukemia

OBJECTIVES

Upon completion of this chapter, the student should be able to:

- Define the key terms listed throughout the chapter
- State a specific definition for chronic lymphocytic leukemia
- Describe the incidence of chronic lymphocytic leukemia
- Describe the signs and symptoms associated with chronic lymphocytic leukemia, the rationale, and associated care for these symptoms
- Identify specific methods for diagnosis of chronic lymphocytic leukemia
- Identify specific methods for treatment of chronic lymphocytic leukemia
- Describe considerations for caring for a patient with chronic lymphocytic leukemia

KEY TERMS

Predisposition – presence of conditions that could increase the tendency toward developing a disease or illness

INTRODUCTION

Chronic lymphocytic leukemia (CLL) is characterized by proliferation of lymphocytes in the blood circulation as well as accumulation in the lymph organs of the body. Lymph organs in the body include the thymus gland, spleen, tonsils, appendix, bone marrow, lymph nodes, and Peyer's patches in the small intestine. There is also characteristic accumulation in the organs of the body.

PHYSIOLOGY

There are four basic components of blood. (See Figure 8-1.)

1. Plasma—liquid portion of the blood
2. Platelets (thrombocytes)—portion of the blood necessary for clot formation
3. White blood cells (WBCs or leukocytes)—portion of the blood necessary for fighting infection within the body; divided into granular WBCs and non-granular WBCs
   - Granular WBCs: basophils, eosinophils, and neutrophils
   - Nongranular WBCs: lymphocytes and monocytes
4. Red blood cells (RBCs or erythrocytes)—portion of the blood necessary for transporting oxygen (O_2) and carbon dioxide (CO_2)

STATISTICS

Chronic lymphocytic leukemia is the most common form of leukemia in Western nations. The average age at diagnosis is 60 years of age. This form of leukemia is two to three times more common in males than in females and has the highest genetic **predisposition** of all forms of leukemia. CLL accounts for greater than 30% of all new leukemia cases diagnosed annually in the United States.

Chromosomal – pertaining to chromosomes, which contain the DNA in the cell nucleus that transmits genetic information; the normal cell contains 46 chromosomes (23 pair)

Immunologic – condition of being immune

RISK FACTORS

1. Heredity
2. **Chromosomal** abnormalities
3. **Immunologic** disorders

No correlation has been shown to radiation exposure and the development of chronic lymphocytic leukemia.

SIGNS, SYMPTOMS, AND ASSOCIATED CARE

1. Anorexia and weight loss due to the increased metabolic needs of the prolifer-ating lymphocytes
   - Obtain baseline weight and monitor weight on routine basis
   - Encourage patient to participate in dietary choices
   - Provide nutritional supplements and vitamins
   - Encourage family and friends to bring in food that is appealing to patient as dietary restrictions allow
   - Administer parenteral fluids as necessary
   - Monitor intake and output (I and O)
   - Encourage rest periods before and after meals
   - Avoid unpleasant sights and odors in room to make meals more appealing
   - Provide meticulous mouth care
   - Monitor for skin breakdown due to loss of body tissue
   - Encourage clothing styles that do not draw attention to weight loss
   - Monitor for symptoms of dehydration, such as decreased urine output, constipation, dry skin, tenting of skin, dry mouth, dry eyes, concentrated urine, hypotension, and confusion
2. Weakness and fatigue due to anemia
   - Assist patient with activities of daily living (ADLs) as necessary
   - Schedule care, activities, and treatment around patient's rest schedule
   - Monitor phone calls and visitors around patient's energy level and rest schedule
   - Encourage frequent rest periods
   - Provide assistance as needed to prevent injury due to weakness
   - Provide a method for the patient to call for assistance
   - Encourage the patient to set realistic goals of activities
   - Allow adequate time to do activities and procedures to avoid frustration or possible injury
   - Encourage exercise to maintain muscle strength
   - Utilize cane or walker as necessary for additional assistance
   - Provide private room for patient to promote rest periods
3. Lymphadenopathy due to infiltration of lymphocytic cells in the lymph nodes
   - Monitor for lymphadenopathy
   - Assist with position for patient comfort
   - Provide comfort measures as necessary due to lymphadenopathy
4. Splenomegaly and hepatomegaly due to infiltration of lymphocytic cells in the spleen or liver
   - Monitor for hepatomegaly and splenomegaly

Lymphocytosis – increased number of lymphocytes

- Avoid abdominal injury in the presence of hepatomegaly and splenomegaly
- Monitor for signs of internal bleeding in the presence of hepatomegaly and splenomegaly, such as abdominal pain, tachycardia, hypotension, and abdominal distention
- Monitor liver function with serum laboratory tests, e.g. *SGOT, SGPT, bilirubin, albumin; alkaline phosphatase,* and *prothrombin time*
- Monitor for bleeding tendencies in the presence of hepatomegaly
- Educate to avoid the use of alcohol and medications metabolized in the liver
- Monitor for jaundice
- Monitor *hemoglobin* and *hematocrit*

5. Fever due to **lymphocytosis**
   - Monitor temperature at routine intervals
   - Provide comfort measures for patient with elevated temperature, such as a cool cloth to the forehead, partial or complete bath as needed, clothing and bedding changed frequently due to diaphoresis, and encourage fluids to prevent dehydration
   - Avoid exposing patient to a draft
   - Cover with blankets as necessary
   - Monitor intake and output (I and O)
   - Maintain comfortable room temperature for patient
   - Avoid plastic mattresses and plastic bed protectors as they have a tendency to increase perspiration
   - Use antiperspirant or deodorant to minimize sweating and odor

6. Anemia due to decreased RBCs
   - Administer blood transfusions and iron supplements as necessary to treat anemia
   - Monitor *hemoglobin* and *hematocrit*
   - Monitor for weakness associated with anemia; assist with ADLs as necessary due to weakness and protect from possible injury due to weakness
   - Treat anemia according to cause
   - Monitor physical symptoms of anemia, such as pallor, weakness, and vertigo

7. Thrombocytopenia due to decreased number of mature platelets
   - Observe for signs of abnormal bleeding and educate patient and family to observe and report any signs promptly to physician, e.g. hemoptysis, bloody emesis, bloody or tarry stools, nose bleeds, vaginal bleeding between menstrual cycles or post-menopausal, bleeding gums, or hematuria
   - Observe for signs of central nervous system (CNS) bleeding and educate patient and family to observe and report symptoms promptly to the physician, such as altered level of consciousness, headache, vision changes, and vertigo
   - Prevent injury to patient who has thrombocytopenia by using soft toothbrush, electric razor rather than straight-edge razor, wear seat belts in the car, elevate siderails, avoid straining with bowel movements, avoid vigorous nose-blowing, avoid intramuscular injections, avoid rectal temperatures, avoid use of tampons, and seek physician advice prior to vaginal or anal intercourse

- Avoid products that contain aspirin, which alters normal platelet function
- Monitor *platelet* count
- Monitor *hemoglobin* and *hematocrit*
- Apply pressure at sites of injection or blood drawing sites for minimum of 5 minutes or until bleeding stops

8. Frequent infections due to lymphocytosis

- Monitor for signs of infection, such as fever, chills, redness, swelling, pain, phlegm, skin rash, cough, dyspnea, flushed skin, diaphoresis, dysuria, and sore throat. Educate patient and family to observe for signs of infection and report promptly to medical staff.
- Avoid contact with people who have infections
- Utilize meticulous hand and skin care on the part of the patient, staff, and visitors
- Educate patient regarding need to complete entire regimen of antibiotics indicated for infection
- Provide private room as necessary
- Restrict staff members who have taken care of patients with infectious disease from caring for the patient who has an increased risk of infections
- Avoid possible routes of infection when possible, such as urinary catheters and intravenous (IV) lines
- Monitor temperature on a routine basis
- Utilize protective isolation as necessary during hospitalization
- Avoid crowded areas, which increase chances of being exposed to an infection
- Provide meticulous mouth care, antiseptic mouthwash, and frequent dental checks
- Avoid injury to skin and mucous membranes

DIAGNOSIS

1. Laboratory tests that include *CBC* and *liver function tests*, e.g. *SGOT*, *SGPT*, *bilirubin*, *albumin*, *alkaline phosphatase*, and *prothrombin time*
2. *Bone marrow aspiration* which indicates lymphocyte infiltration
3. *Lymph node biopsy*
4. Thrombocytopenia
5. Leukocytosis
6. Neutropenia

Chronic lymphocytic leukemia is frequently diagnosed during a routine examination that includes laboratory studies.

TREATMENT

1. The patient who is nonsymptomatic may not require treatment other than promotion of wellness with proper nutrition, exercise, and rest

Corticosteroids – hormones secreted from the adrenal gland; also refers to a medication given to reduce inflammation

Splenectomy – surgical removal of the spleen

2. The patient who is symptomatic may be treated by the following methods:

- *Chemotherapy* to relieve symptoms and treat splenomegaly and lymphadenopathy, e.g. Chlorambucil (Leukeran), Cyclophosphamide (Cytoxan)

- **Corticosteroids** increase the effectiveness of chemotherapy, e.g. Prednisone

- *Radiation* therapy is palliative by treating splenomegaly and lymphadenopathy

- *Blood transfusions* may be necessary to treat anemia

- *Splenectomy* may be done to treat painful splenomegaly

CONSIDERATIONS FOR CARE

1. Educate patient and family regarding the disease process.

2. Educate patient and family regarding forms of treatment as well as side effects of treatment.

3. Provide emotional support to patient and family.

4. Provide nonjudgmental acceptance of emotions and behavior of patient and family.

5. Encourage proper rest and nutrition.

6. Observe for signs of infection and educate patient and family to observe for signs of infection. Report promptly to physician symptoms such as fever, chills, redness, swelling, pain, phlegm, skin rash, cough, dyspnea, flushed skin, and diaphoresis.

7. Observe for signs of abnormal bleeding and educate patient and family to observe and report signs promptly to physician, e.g. hemoptysis, bloody emesis, bloody or black tarry stools, nose bleeds, vaginal bleeding between menstrual cycles or post-menopausal bleeding, bleeding gums, hematuria, and bruising.

8. Observe for signs of CNS bleeding and educate patient and family to observe and report symptoms promptly to physician, such as altered level of consciousness, headache, vision changes, and vertigo.

9. Prevent injury to patient who has thrombocytopenia by using a soft toothbrush, an electric razor rather than straight-edge razor, wear seat belts in the car, elevate siderails, avoid straining with bowel movements, avoid vigorous nose-blowing, avoid intramuscular injections, and avoid rectal temperatures.

10. Avoid products that contain aspirin, which alters normal platelet function.

11. Educate patient to avoid people who have infections.

12. Encourage meticulous handwashing for the staff, patient, and family.

13. Protective isolation may be necessary while in the hospital.

14. Assess level of comfort and offer methods of pain control, such as relaxation, imaging, massage, heat treatment, and medications.

15. Prevent skin breakdown due to increased risk of infection and bleeding. Reposition frequently; encourage meticulous skin care; provide clean, dry, and wrinkle-free linen and clothing; and encourage fluid intake.

16. Monitor laboratory results, especially WBCs.

17. Educate patient and family regarding methods to control bleeding, such as direct pressure, elevation, and ice packs to the area.

FOR MORE INFORMATION

American Cancer Society
1599 Clifton Road, NE
Atlanta, GA 30329
1-800-ACS-2345

Leukemia Society of America
733 Third Avenue
New York, NY 10017

ASSIGNMENT SHEET: CHRONIC LYMPHOCYTIC LEUKEMIA

Short Answer

1. Write a brief definition for the terms listed throughout the chapter.

2. Write a brief definition for chronic lymphocytic leukemia.

3. List the seven (7) organs included in the lymph system.

4. Describe the incidence of chronic lymphocytic leukemia.

5. List eight (8) symptoms for chronic lymphocytic leukemia. Describe the rationale and associated care for each symptom.

6. List six (6) specific methods used to aid in the diagnosis of chronic lymphocytic leukemia.

7. Describe the difference in the methods of treatment depending on whether the patient with chronic lymphocytic leukemia is symptomatic versus nonsymptomatic.

8. List seventeen (17) considerations for caring for a patient with chronic lymphocytic leukemia.

9. Write the normal ranges for each of the following laboratory tests.
   a. Platelet count
   b. Lymphocytes
   c. Hemoglobin
   d. Hematocrit
   e. SGOT
   f. SGPT
   g. Bilirubin
   h. Albumin
   i. Alkaline phosphatase
   j. Prothrombin time

10. Describe each of the following procedures used to diagnose or treat chronic lymphocytic leukemia.
    a. Bone marrow aspiration
    b. Lymph node biopsy
    c. Chemotherapy
    d. Radiation therapy
    e. Blood transfusion

11. List thirteen (13) specific signs and symptoms frequently related to an infection.

12. List eight (8) specific areas in which abnormal bleeding could be noticed in a patient with thrombocytopenia.

13. List nine (9) specific signs and symptoms of dehydration.

14. List four (4) specific signs and symptoms of central nervous system (CNS) bleeding.

15. List ten (10) specific considerations for care when taking care of a patient with thrombocytopenia to decrease the risk of abnormal bleeding.

KNOWLEDGE INTO ACTION

1. Dennis Lenz, a 67-year-old patient with a history of CLL, also has a diagnosis of thrombocytopenia. He is currently in the hospital and you are helping him with his personal cares due to his weakness. He asks you to help him shave and tells you he prefers to use the straight-edge razor and shaving cream in his bedside table. What will your course of action be? What complications could result?

2. Later in the day, Dennis Lenz tells you his "arthritis is acting up" and asks you to get him "a couple of aspirin." Would this medication be appropriate for Mr. Lenz? Why or why not?

3. Alan O'Leary, a 71-year-old male, has come to your clinic for an insurance physical. The physician tells you that after seeing Mr. O'Leary's laboratory results, he is quite certain Mr. O'Leary has CLL. When you look at Mr. O'Leary's chart, what laboratory results would you expect to see that have helped Mr. Peterson's physician make this diagnosis?

Eating Disorders

Bulimia

OBJECTIVES

Upon completion of this chapter, the student should be able to:

■ Define the key terms listed throughout the chapter

■ State a specific definition for bulimia

■ Describe the incidence of bulimia

■ List the risk factors associated with bulimia

■ Describe the signs and symptoms of bulimia

■ Identify specific methods for diagnosis of bulimia and the rationale for symptoms of bulimia

■ Identify specific methods for treatment of bulimia

■ Describe complications that may result due to bulimia, symptoms of these complications, and associated care

■ Describe specific considerations for caring for a patient with bulimia

KEY TERMS

Binge – as in bulimia; constituted by the consumption of large amounts of food and calories

Purge – emptying of the gastrointestinal tract by manually forcing oneself to vomit or through the use of laxatives

Diuretic – medication or substance that increases urine output and decreases the fluid level of tissues in the body

Cardiac arrest – cessation of the beating of the heart

INTRODUCTION

Bulimia is an eating disorder characterized by recurrent episodes of eating **binges** followed by induced vomiting, or the "binge-**purge**" syndrome. The patient may also use laxatives, *enemas*, **diuretics**, or excessive exercising to counteract the large amounts of food and calories they have consumed. A binge may consist of up to 20,000 calories at one time; generally, a binge is between 5,000 and 10,000 calories.

STATISTICS

Bulimia affects mainly females, with 2 to 6% of the female population between the ages of 14 and 30 affected by the disease. Females account for approximately 90% of all people in the United States who are affected by bulimia. An estimated 2.5 million teens in the United States have an eating disorder. High-risk periods for developing an eating disorder for females are upon entering high school (14 to 15 years old) as well as upon graduation from high school (17 to 18 years old). An estimated 5% of all college-age females in the United States are bulimic. "The consequences of eating disorders can be severe, with 1 in 10 cases leading to death from starvation, **cardiac arrest**, or suicide" (*Eating Disorders*, by Lee Hoffman, National Institute of Mental Health: Decade of the Brain).

RISK FACTORS

The cause of bulimia is unknown although there are several suggested theories.

1. Biological factors. Genetic studies suggest an inherited predisposition. An identical twin of a person with an eating disorder has a 50% chance of also having an eating disorder. A sibling of a person with an eating disorder has a 10 to 20% chance of also having an eating disorder.

Satiated – being full or satisfied

Serotonin – chemical that acts as a vasoconstrictor

Norepinephrine – hormone produced by the adrenal gland that acts as a vasoconstrictor

Neurotransmitters – substances that enable an impulse to travel from the axon of a neuron, across the synapse, and to the dendrite of another neuron

Caries – process of deterioration of the bones or teeth

Amenorrhea – absence of menstruation (menses)

Potassium – mineral found in bananas, potatoes, yellow vegetables, citrus fruits, and milk; necessary for the regulation of fluid balance in the body as well as muscle and nerve function

2. Psychological factors. Bulimia is often seen in individuals who are from a dysfunctional family. The disease is often preceded by a family disturbance or conflict of some sort. Many individuals come from homes in which there is drug or alcohol abuse or have had problems themselves with alcohol or drug abuse. The individual displays maladjustive behavior in other aspects of their lives and seems to be struggling for control or self-identity. Control seems to be the driving force in many cases. The individual that has been diagnosed with bulimia often suffers from low self-esteem and has had many perceived failures in life. Sexual abuse may also be a precipitating factor. Parental obesity has also been shown to be a contributing factor for the development of bulimia in the children of these parents.

3. Sociocultural factors (due to an overemphasis on physical appearance). Our society influences this emphasis through clothing styles, diet fads and pills, exercise videos, and increasing numbers of magazines that offer articles on losing weight and "tightening" muscles, food industries' use of slogans such as "low fat," movie and music stars, and, of course, peer pressure.

4. Physical factors. Possible central nervous system disorders prevent the person from feeling **satiated** even after consumption of large amounts of food.

5. **Serotonin** and **norepinephrine** (**neurotransmitters**), which have been shown to be decreased in clients with depression, have also been shown to be decreased in clients with eating disorders.

SIGNS AND SYMPTOMS

Signs and symptoms of bulimia include the following:

1. Excessive concern about weight and body image
2. Feeling out of control about eating habits
3. Strict dieting followed by eating binges
4. Overeating associated with periods of stress or conflict
5. Expressing shame or guilt for eating
6. Distorted body image
7. Binge episode that continues until the person experiences abdominal pain, sleep, or the presence of another person
8. Binge foods that are often high in calories and carbohydrates, with the person often consuming as many as 20,000 calories at one time
9. Secretive behavior about binges and vomiting
10. Disappearance after meals, especially to the bathroom
11. Periods of depression (chronic)
12. Dental **caries**, erosion of tooth enamel and gum infections
13. Frequent weighing
14. Scarring to fingers due to self-induced vomiting
15. Weight usually within normal limits
16. Others perceive the individual as a perfectionist
17. Competitive
18. **Amenorrhea**
19. Hyperactivity
20. Peculiar eating habits or rituals
21. Physical symptoms associated with *sodium* and ***potassium*** balance, such as muscle spasm, kidney problems, and cardiac arrest

Syrup of Ipecac –
medication used to induce
vomiting in certain cases
of poisoning

Parotid glands – salivary
glands in the mouth

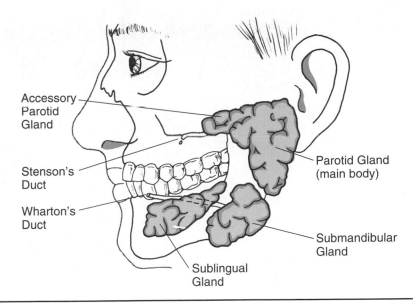

Accessory
Parotid
Gland

Stenson's
Duct

Wharton's
Duct

Parotid Gland
(main body)

Submandibular
Gland

Sublingual
Gland

Figure 12-1   Salivary glands (From Kinn, *Medical Terminology: Building Blocks for Health Careers*, copyright © 1990, Delmar Publishers)

22. Use of diuretics, laxatives, **Syrup of Ipecac**, or overuse of exercise
23. Increased isolation from family and friends
24. Compulsive exercising
25. Compulsive neatness
26. Low frustration level
27. Depression
28. Constipation
29. "Chipmunk cheeks" due to swollen **parotid glands** (See Figure 12-1)

ASSOCIATED CARE

Associated care for the signs and symptoms of this disease are aimed at treating the disease itself as well as the underlying cause(s) of the disease. Associated care for this disease is included in the Treatment and Considerations for Care sections of this chapter.

CAUSES FOR PHYSICAL SYMPTOMS

1. Inadequate fluid intake
2. Inadequate nutrition and fiber intake (See Table 12-1)
3. Fluid loss from vomiting and abuse of laxatives
4. Electrolyte imbalance from dehydration or inadequate nutrition
5. Inadequate intake of protein and carbohydrates
6. Absence of hormone production due to excessive exercising, loss of body fat, and stress or depression

DIAGNOSIS

1. Symptoms
2. Patient history
3. Physical examination

Hypokalemia – decreased amounts of potassium in the blood

Cardiac – refers to the heart

Table 12-1 Protein and Calcium Content in Foods

Food	Serving Size	Protein (grams)	Calcium (mg)
Whole milk	1 cup	9	288
Skim milk	1 cup	9	296
Cheddar cheese	1 oz	7	213
Cottage cheese	1 cup	34	180
Ice cream	1 cup	6	194
Eggs	1 large	80	27
Hamburger	3 oz (broiled)	21	9
Chicken	3 oz (breast)	20	8
White bread	1 slice	2	21
Tuna	3 oz (canned)	24	7
Whole wheat bread	1 slice	3	24
Peanuts	1 cup	37	107
Corn muffin	1 each	3	42
Asparagus	1 cup	3	30
Rhubarb	1 cup (cooked w/sugar)	1	212
Green beans	1 cup	2	63
Orange juice	1 cup	1	20
Broccoli	1 cup	5	136
Apple	1 medium	trace	8
Spinach	1 cup (cooked)	5	167

Recommended Daily Allowances: Protein = 45–55 grams; Calcium = 800–1200 mg

4. Laboratory analysis to include the following: *CBC, electrolytes,* liver function tests, *BUN, creatinine, amylase,* and *urinalysis*

5. Presence of dehydration. Symptoms of dehydration include decreased urine output, constipation, dry skin, tenting of skin, dry mouth, dry eyes, concentrated urine, hypotension, and confusion.

6. Dental work

7. History obtained from family members

COMPLICATIONS

Complications of bulimia include the following:

1. **Hypokalemia**

   Symptoms: weakness, and **cardiac** irregularities

   Associated care:

   - Monitor serum potassium levels as directed by a physician
   - Encourage foods high in potassium, such as bananas, yellow vegetables, dried fruits, citrus fruits, and potatoes
   - Administer potassium supplements as ordered by physician
   - Monitor intake and output (I and O)

2. Fat depletion

   Symptom: weight loss

Hypothermia – a body temperature that is abnormally low

Bradycardia – decreased heartbeat, generally less than 60 beats per minute

Apathy – absence of feelings or emotions

Renal failure – failure of the kidney to function

Turgor – the normal elasticity and characteristics of the skin

Associated care:

- Encourage clothing to enhance body size as desired by the patient
- Obtain baseline weight and monitor on routine basis

3. Loss of breast tissue

   Symptom: decreased breast size

   Associated care:

   - Encourage clothing to enhance breast size as desired by the patient
   - Assist in obtaining brassiere that fits

4. **Hypothermia**

   Symptoms: chills, **bradycardia**, hypotension, cyanosis, decreased sensation to extremities, and **apathy**

   Associated care:

   - Encourage to dress warmly in several layers of clothing
   - Avoid wearing wet clothing
   - Monitor vital signs (See Appendix D)
   - Monitor heart rate and rhythm
   - Monitor skin temperature and color
   - Avoid injury to extremities due to decreased sensation
   - Encourage activity and participation in activities of daily living (ADLs)

5. **Renal failure**

   Symptoms: nausea, vomiting, difficulty in voiding, fluid retention, weight gain, hypertension, fever, decreased tissue **turgor**, diarrhea, skin rash, and urinary tract infection

   Associated care:

   - Monitor adequate hydration
   - Monitor intake and output (I and O)
   - Avoid medications that are metabolized in the kidney
   - Avoid urinary tract infections and be aware of symptoms of urinary tract infection (UTI). Symptoms of UTI include pain with urination, fever, cloudy urine, malodorous urine, urgency or frequency of urination, pain in pelvis or low back, hematuria, and dysuria.
   - Monitor for nausea and vomiting and offer appropriate diet choices
   - Weigh patient on a daily basis
   - Monitor vital signs (See Appendix D)
   - Monitor skin color and integrity
   - Monitor for diarrhea
   - Monitor and care for skin rash
   - Monitor for electrolyte (*sodium*, *potassium*, and *chloride*) imbalance and *BUN* levels

6. Constipation

   Symptoms: inability or difficulty in having a bowel movement; stool that is extremely dry and formed

   Associated care:

   - Encourage fluids and high fiber
   - Increase exercise as tolerated
   - Administer enemas, suppositories, stool softeners, and laxatives as prescribed by a physician

Infertility – inability to become pregnant (female) or to cause a pregnancy (male)

Atrophy – reduction in size of tissue or organ within the body

Osteoporosis – refers to loss of bone tissue and skeletal mass

Kyphosis – curvature of the spine in the thoracic region; also known as hunchback

Pacemaker – instrument capable of delivering an electrical current to the heart to stimulate contraction of the heart muscle

- Monitor frequency, number, and consistency of stools
- Monitor for possible bowel obstruction. Symptoms of bowel obstruction include absence of bowel movements, diarrhea stools, abdominal pain, abdominal distention, and fever
- Encourage fresh fruits and vegetables
- Establish regular bowel routine
- Provide privacy for bowel routine as able

7. Muscle wasting

Symptoms: decrease in the amount of muscle mass and weakness

Associated care:

- Encourage activity as able
- Schedule activities, care, and treatments around rest periods
- Encourage a high-protein diet. Foods high in protein include meats, fish, milk, cheese, soybeans, and eggs.
- Encourage exercise program

8. Hormonal changes

Symptoms: amenorrhea, **infertility**, **atrophy** of vaginal lining, and mood changes

Associated care:

- Monitor for symptoms of hormonal changes
- Administer hormone supplements as prescribed by a physician

9. **Osteoporosis**

Symptoms: frequent fractures, x-rays that show osteoporosis, back and joint pain, and **kyphosis**

Associated care:

- Encourage increase of dietary calcium through foods or supplements. Foods high in calcium include dairy products and green leafy vegetables.
- Encourage adequate intake of Vitamin D through foods or supplements. Sources of Vitamin D include fortified dairy products and egg yolks.
- Prevent injury due to falls or trauma
- Increase exercise as tolerated

10. Bradycardia

Symptoms: low pulse rate and dizziness

Associated care:

- Monitor vital signs
- Monitor heart rate and rhythm
- Administer medications as needed and directed by physician to increase heart rate, e.g. Atropine
- **Pacemaker** may be needed if bradycardia severe

11. Anemia

Symptoms: pallor, fatigue, headache, dizziness, and dyspnea

Associated care:

- Monitor serum *CBC*
- Schedule activities, care, and treatment around rest periods
- Assist with position for comfort with dyspnea
- Monitor vital signs
- Monitor nutritional status
- Administer dietary and vitamin supplements as necessary

Esophagus – hollow muscular tube that connects the pharynx to the stomach; average of 10 to 12 inches in length; part of the gastrointestinal system

Hematemesis – presence of blood in emesis

Esophageal reflux – backing up of stomach acid into the esophagus

Tachypnea – rapid respiratory rate; generally refers to a respiratory rate greater than 40 breaths per minute

12. Heart failure

    Symptoms: dyspnea, weight gain, edema, hypertension, fatigue, and neck vein distention

    Associated care:

    - Adjust position for comfort with dyspnea
    - Weigh daily
    - Monitor intake and output (I and O)
    - Utilize a low-sodium diet. Foods that are high in sodium and should be avoided include processed foods, cured meats, salted chips and crackers, pickles, and table salt.
    - Elevate edematous extremities as necessary
    - Schedule activities, care, and treatment around rest periods
    - Monitor vital signs
    - Monitor edema

13. Hypotension

    Symptoms: low blood pressure readings and dizziness

    Associated care:

    - Monitor blood pressure
    - Treat underlying cause
    - Encourage changing positions slowly to avoid increased hypotension
    - Check blood pressure in lying, sitting, and standing positions to note changes due to patient position

14. **Esophagitis**

    Symptoms: heartburn, chest pain, dysphagia, **hematemesis**, and **esophageal reflux**

    Associated care:

    - Provide meticulous mouth care at frequent intervals through the day
    - Offer food and beverages that are nonabrasive; avoid spicy foods, acidic fruits and juices, carbonated beverages, highly salted foods, and foods that are extremely hot or cold
    - Offer ice chips and fluids frequently according to patient preference
    - Humidify air as necessary
    - Monitor intake and output (I and O)
    - Elevate patient's head while sleeping
    - Administer antacids as necessary
    - Administer nasogastric (NG) or parenteral fluids as necessary
    - Administer medications as prescribed by physician to treat any accompanying infection
    - Observe for sores in mouth
    - Offer foods that are easy to chew and swallow
    - Utilize antiseptic mouthwash and a soft-bristled toothbrush
    - Provide moisture to lips with lip balm, mineral oil, or petroleum jelly
    - Avoid use of harsh toothpaste

15. Aspiration pneumonia

    Symptoms: cough, dyspnea, fever, chills, chest pain, green or blood-tinged phlegm, and **tachypnea**

Antibiotics – substances used to destroy pathogens

Behavior modification – a method of controlling or encouraging change in a person's behavior with a reward system; positive behavior results in the granting of a reward or privilege, whereas negative behavior results in the loss of a reward or privilege

Antidepressants – medications used in the treatment of depression

Associated care:

- Administer **antibiotics** as directed by physician
- Encourage fluids
- Prevent transmission of infection by handwashing and correctly disposing of tissues and phlegm
- Utilize sponge baths as needed to reduce fever
- Maintain clean bedding and clothing
- Use antiperspirant or deodorant to minimize sweating and odor
- Provide medications, a heating pad, or other measures for chest pain
- Assist with position for patient comfort
- Monitor vital signs (See Appendix D)
- Educate patient and family regarding symptoms of respiratory infection, such as cough, phlegm production, chest pain, fever, chills, dyspnea, and diaphoresis
- Educate patient and family to report symptoms of respiratory infection to the physician
- Educate patient regarding importance of completing medication prescribed for respiratory infection
- Encourage fluids to thin secretions and make them easier to expel
- Avoid people with respiratory infections
- Maintain optimal health to fight off infections
- Administer influenza and pneumonia vaccinations as directed by the physician
- Avoid crowded areas, which increase the likelihood of contracting a respiratory infection

16. Syncope

    Symptoms: dizziness, lightheadedness, and temporary confusion

    Associated care:

    - Monitor for vertigo
    - Monitor vital signs
    - Assist with ambulation and transfer to prevent injury in the presence of vertigo
    - Educate patient to ask for assistance when out of bed in presence of syncope
    - Provide method for patient to call for assistance

TREATMENT

1. Treatment must address the underlying cause of personality dysfunction
   - **Behavior modification**
   - Private counseling
   - Group counseling
   - Family counseling
   - Long-term follow-up
   - **Antidepressants** if required
2. Patient needs to have control over his eating behavior
   - Behavior modification
   - Private, group, and family counseling

Calcium – mineral found in foods, such as dairy products and green leafy vegetables, which is necessary for the formation and strength of bones and teeth as well as the function of muscles and nerves; calcium is also stored in the bones of the body

- Education regarding nutrition
- Allow patient to make informed choices regarding diet and nutrition
- Long-term follow-up

3. Patient needs to be motivated to change for treatment to be effective
   - Behavior modification
   - Private, group, and family counseling
   - Educate patient regarding health risks placed on themselves by their disease and the associated eating behaviors
   - Long-term follow-up is necessary
   - Overeater's Anonymous

4. Dental care to treat dental problems due to vomiting, poor nutrition, and lack of **calcium**

5. Dietary counseling to educate regarding lifelong dietary habits

6. Antidepressants

CONSIDERATIONS FOR CARE

1. Educate patient and family regarding the disease process.
2. Educate patient and family regarding forms of treatment.
3. Provide emotional support to patient and family.
4. Provide nonjudgmental acceptance of emotions and behavior of patient and family.
5. Educate patient and family regarding importance of follow-up care.
6. Monitor patient's eating habits.
7. Monitor patient after eating to prevent purging.
8. Have patient keep daily diary of food consumed.
9. Obtain baseline weight and monitor on a routine basis.
10. Monitor patient for symptoms of complications.
11. Educate patient and family regarding nutrition.
12. Encourage support groups for patient and family.
13. Encourage ongoing counseling for patient and family.
14. Monitor for possible causes of the eating disorder, e.g. dysfunctional family.
15. Provide a calm, relaxed, and social atmosphere for meals.
16. Educate patient, family, and staff regarding behavior modification techniques that will be used to promote patient compliance while allowing control over choices.
17. Consider the use of a signed contract between the patient and staff regarding amounts to be eaten, weight gain goals, and behavior.
18. Allow the patient to ventilate feelings. Take threats of suicide seriously; threats of suicide should be dealt with promptly with referrals made to counselors, a physician, and therapists. Protect patient from harm. (See Table 12-2.)
19. Develop a trusting relationship with the patient and family by establishing open and honest communication, responding to requests as soon as possible, and following through with requests.
20. Provide alternate activities for the patient to take the place of binges.
21. Assist patient in making mealtime pleasant, the food attractive, and eating and tasting the food enjoyable.
22. Assist to identify strengths and build on these strengths.

Table 12-2 Suicide Precautions

The following list of precautions should be followed at all times when a hospitalized patient is at risk for attempting to commit suicide or if the patient has threatened to commit suicide.

1. Remove all cords and wires from the room, e.g. curtain cords, electrical cords, phone cords, hangers, and belts.

2. Remove all cleaning supplies and potentially toxic liquids from the room, e.g. cleaning solutions, mouthwash, and shaving lotion.

3. Utilize plastic, paper, or Styrofoam dishes and eating utensils for patient use rather than metal or glass dishes and utensils.

4. Provide patient with a first-floor room if possible. If the patient is on a floor other than the first floor, windows should be locked or barred.

5. The patient should be accompanied at all times if it is necessary to leave the room for any purpose, e.g. therapy, x-ray or other procedures, bathing, and toileting.

6. Remove patient's clothing and personal items from the room.

7. Remove all potentially harmful items from the room, e.g. mirrors, glass lamps, pens, pencils, nail files, matches, and lighters.

8. All electrical outlets should be covered.

23. Allow the patient to have control in as many aspects of her life as possible. Allow the patient to make decisions; offer choices whenever possible.

24. Help the patient develop methods to deal with conflict in positive ways.

FOR MORE INFORMATION

Center for the Study of Anorexia and Bulimia
1 West 91st Street
New York, NY 10024
(212) 595-3449

American Anorexia/Bulimia Association (AABA)
418 East 76th Street
New York, NY 10021
(212) 734-1114

Anorexia Nervosa and Related Eating Disorders
1255 Hiliard
P.O. Box 5102
Eugene, OR 97405
(503) 344-1144

National Association of Anorexia Nervosa and Associated Disorders (ANAD)
P.O. Box 7
Highland Park, IL 60035
(708) 831-3438

ASSIGNMENT SHEET: BULIMIA

Short Answer

1. Write a brief definition for the terms listed throughout the chapter.

2. Write a brief definition for bulimia.

3. Describe the incidence of bulimia.

4. List five (5) risk factors for bulimia.

5. List twenty-nine (29) possible signs and symptoms of bulimia.

6. Describe six (6) causes for the symptoms associated with bulimia.

7. Describe seven (7) specific methods used to aid in the diagnosis of bulimia.

8. List the normal range for each of the following serum laboratory tests used in the diagnosis of bulimia or associated risk factors.
   a. Hemoglobin
   b. Hematocrit
   c. WBC
   d. RBC
   e. Sodium (Na)
   f. Potassium (K)
   g. Chloride (Cl)
   h. BUN
   i. Creatinine
   j. Amylase

9. List nine (9) possible symptoms of dehydration.

10. List eight (8) possible symptoms of a urinary tract infection.

11. For each of the complications of bulimia, describe the symptoms as well as the associated care.
    a. Hypokalemia
    b. Fat depletion
    c. Loss of breast tissue
    d. Hypothermia
    e. Renal failure
    f. Constipation
    g. Muscle wasting
    h. Hormonal changes
    i. Osteoporosis
    j. Bradycardia
    k. Anemia
    l. Heart failure
    m. Hypotension
    n. Esophagitis
    o. Aspiration pneumonia
    p. Syncope

12. Describe six (6) specific treatments used for bulimia.

13. Describe twenty-four (24) considerations for caring for a patient with bulimia.

14. Describe the following vital signs and the normal range for each. (See Appendix D.)
    a. Temperature
    b. Pulse
    c. Respirations
    d. Blood pressure (BP)

KNOWLEDGE INTO ACTION

1. While in one of your classes, the student in front of you complains of feeling weak and dizzy. You check her pulse and find it is irregular. What could be the cause of these symptoms? What would an appropriate action be to help this student?

2. Helen Spencer, a 15-year-old diagnosed with bulimia, is in your facility. You notice her weight is up 5 pounds from the previous day and she has urinated only 275 ml compared to the 2150 ml of fluid she has taken in. You check her blood pressure and obtain a reading of 176/108. Her skin feels hot to touch and you notice her legs are edematous. What could be causing these symptoms? What care could you give this patient to assist in relieving her symptoms? What laboratory tests might her physician order to check her status?

3. Thomas Heller, a 17-year-old diagnosed with bulimia, is in your facility. One afternoon he complains of chest pain. He states he has been having difficulty swallowing the past several days and has been "burping up some acidy stuff" in the back of his throat. Shortly after he calls you into his room, he vomits and you notice there seems to be blood in the vomitus. Based on the signs and

symptoms you have just observed with Mr. Heller, what initial diagnosis could be made? What associated care items could be included to make your patient more comfortable?

4. The next day, as you are in Thomas Heller's room, he says to you, "I don't know why I've done this to myself and my family. What a loser! Last night was the worst! My parents came up and had this big fit about my bulimia. They just don't seem to understand. Maybe if I were gone, they would realize how sick I am." What will your initial response be regarding what Mr. Heller said to you? What precautions would be necessary to take regarding Mr. Heller's threats to harm himself?

Anorexia Nervosa

OBJECTIVES

Upon completion of this chapter, the student should be able to:

- Define the key terms listed throughout the chapter
- State a specific definition for anorexia nervosa
- Describe the incidence of anorexia nervosa
- Describe the risk factors for anorexia nervosa
- Describe the signs and symptoms of anorexia nervosa and the rationale for these signs and symptoms
- Describe the complications associated with anorexia nervosa, and the rationale and associated care for these complications
- Identify specific methods for diagnosis of anorexia nervosa
- Identify specific methods for treatment of anorexia nervosa
- Describe specific requirements for successful treatment of anorexia nervosa
- Describe specific considerations for caring for a patient with anorexia nervosa

KEY TERMS

Puberty – time when a person becomes able to reproduce; generally occurs during adolescence

INTRODUCTION

Anorexia nervosa is characterized by self-starvation with weight loss of up to 25% or more of total body weight. Even though the person generally experiences hunger, they deny these feelings due to an overwhelming fear of being fat.

STATISTICS

There are an estimated 2.5 million teenagers in the United States with an eating disorder. Approximately 90 to 95% of those affected are female. Approximately one out of every 250 adolescents in the United States has anorexia nervosa. The disease affects 5 to 10% of the total population of the United States. Approximately 10 to 20% of patients with anorexia nervosa will die from complications of the disease. Close to one-third of these deaths will result from suicide.

RISK FACTORS

1. History of emotional problems
2. Onset frequently at time of **puberty** due to changing body shape and normal weight gain
3. Perfectionist attitude
4. Poor expression of feelings
5. Low self-esteem
6. History of drug or alcohol abuse (as many as 25 to 50%)
7. Family member with chemical dependency
8. Adult daughters of alcoholics

Lanugo – fine hair that covers the body; generally seen in newborn infants and especially premature infants

9. Societal attitudes equating slimness with beauty and popularity, e.g. commercials on television and in magazines; clothing styles geared toward slim clients; increasing diet centers, diet foods, exercise and weight-loss videos; and peer pressure

10. Achievement-oriented families

11. Sexual abuse

12. Parental obesity

13. Serotonin and norepinephrine (neurotransmitters) which have been shown to be decreased in patients with depression, have also been shown to be decreased in patients with eating disorders

SIGNS AND SYMPTOMS

1. Weight loss of up to 25% or more of total body weight

2. Amenorrhea

3. Mood swings

4. Preoccupation with food, eating, and calories

5. Ritualistic eating habits

6. Compulsive behavior

7. Perfectionism

8. Excessive exercising

9. Complaints of feeling full after small amounts of food or complaints of bloating or nausea after eating

10. Distorted body image

11. Weighing frequently

12. Possible use of laxatives, diuretics, or vomiting to control weight

13. Isolation from family and friends

14. Plays with food at mealtimes, often eating very slowly

15. Frequent excuses to miss meals, e.g. over-involvement in work, school, or activities so will not have to eat

16. Excessive concern about appearance

17. Intolerant and oversensitive

18. Low self-esteem

19. Fantasizes about high-calorie foods

20. May feel in control over the eating aspect of life and feel out of control over other aspects of life

21. Constipation

22. Dry skin and dry hair

23. **Lanugo** over portions of the body

24. Irregular heartbeat

25. Cavities due to calcium depletion

26. Unhealthy look due to undernourishment

27. Muscle atrophy

28. Hypotension

29. Increased susceptibility to infection due to malnourishment

30. Pallor due to anemia

31. Alopecia

Libido – sexual desires

Pancreatitis – inflammation of the pancreas

Cardiac arrhythmia – abnormal rhythm of the beat of the heart

32. Diminished **libido**
33. Frequent complaints of feeling chilled
34. Anemia

ASSOCIATED CARE

Associated care for the signs and symptoms of this disease are aimed at treating the disease itself as well as the underlying cause(s) of the disease. Associated care for this disease is included in the Treatment and Considerations for Care sections of this chapter.

CAUSES FOR PHYSICAL SYMPTOMS

1. Inadequate fluid intake
2. Inadequate nutrition and fiber intake
3. Fluid loss from vomiting and abuse of laxatives
4. Electrolyte imbalance from dehydration or inadequate nutrition
5. Inadequate intake of protein and carbohydrates
6. Absence of hormone production due to excessive exercising, loss of body fat, and stress or depression

COMPLICATIONS

Complications of anorexia nervosa may need to be dealt with in an inpatient setting and, in approximately 20% of untreated cases, have led to the death of the patient.

1. Syncope due to electrolyte imbalance
   - Monitor electrolyte levels (*sodium*, *potassium*, and *chloride*)
   - Monitor for signs of syncope
   - Monitor vital signs (See Appendix D)
   - Assist with ambulation and transfer to prevent injury in the presence of syncope
   - Educate patient to ask for assistance when out of bed in presence of syncope
   - Provide method for patient to call for assistance
2. Renal insufficiency due to dehydration
   - Monitor kidney function tests
   - Monitor intake and output (I and O)
   - Monitor weight on routine basis
   - Monitor for signs of renal insufficiency, e.g. decreased urine output, weight gain, edema, hypertension, dyspnea, and crackles in lungs
3. **Pancreatitis** due to the body's use of stored fat for energy, which would cause hyperlipidemia (increase of circulating fat in the blood)
   - Monitor for signs and symptoms of pancreatitis, e.g. abdominal pain, nausea, vomiting, fever, decreased bowel sounds, and elevated serum amylase level
   - Monitor *amylase* levels
4. **Cardiac arrhythmias** due to electrolyte imbalance
   - Monitor heart rate and rhythm
   - Obtain baseline *EKG* and monitor on a routine basis
   - Monitor vital signs

Hypoalbuminemia – decreased amounts of albumin in the blood

Albumin – protein found in the blood that is important for maintaining fluid balance in the body (blood volume)

Endocrine – gland that secretes hormones directly into the bloodstream, such as adrenal, islets of Langerhans, ovaries, parathyroid, pineal, pituitary, testes, thymus, and thyroid

5. Osteoporosis due to hypocalcemia
   - Monitor *serum calcium* levels
   - Provide dietary calcium supplements
   - Encourage foods high in calcium, e.g. cheese, milk, and yogurt
   - Encourage fluid intake to reduce the risk of kidney stone formation
6. Increased susceptibility to infection
   - Monitor for signs of infection, such as fever, chills, redness, swelling, pain, phlegm, skin rash, cough, dyspnea, flushed skin, diaphoresis, dysuria, and sore throat. Educate patient and family to observe for signs of infection and report promptly to medical staff.
   - Avoid people who have infections
   - Employ meticulous hand and skin care for the patient, staff, and visitors
   - Educate patient regarding need to complete entire regimen of antibiotics indicated for infection
   - Provide private room if necessary
   - Restrict staff members who have taken care of patients with infectious disease from caring for the patient who has increased risk of infections
   - Avoid possible routes of infection when possible, such as urinary catheters and intravenous (IVs) lines
   - Monitor temperature on a routine basis
   - Utilize protective isolation as necessary during hospitalization
   - Avoid crowded areas, which increase chances of being exposed to an infection
   - Provide meticulous mouth care, frequent dental checks, and antiseptic mouthwash
   - Avoid injury to skin and mucous membranes
7. **Hypoalbuminemia** due to inadequate protein intake
   - Monitor intake and output (I and O)
   - Monitor for edema
   - Obtain baseline weight and monitor on routine basis
   - Administer **albumin** as needed, transfused intravenously
   - Monitor *serum albumin* levels
8. Death often due to cardiac arrest from electrolyte imbalance
   - Monitor electrolyte levels
   - Monitor vital signs (See Appendix D)
   - Monitor heart rate and rhythm
   - Perform CPR in the event of cardiac arrest

DIAGNOSIS

1. Symptoms
2. Physical examination
3. *EKG*
4. History of weight loss of 25% or more of body weight
5. Tests to rule out other causes of weight loss, such as **endocrine** malignancy, malabsorption, or metabolic disorders
6. Laboratory tests to include *electrolytes*, *blood glucose*, *calcium* levels and *urinalysis*, *creatinine* (elevated), *BUN* (decreased), *albumin* (decreased), *SGPT* (increased), *SGOT* (increased), and *amylase* (decreased)

Table 13-1   Behavior Modification

Behavior modification is the use of "rewards" or positive reinforcement to increase the frequency of a chosen behavior or "punishments" or negative reinforcement to decrease the frequency of a chosen behavior. Consistency among all staff members is important in behavior modification as is choosing rewards and/or punishments that are important to the person to whom the therapy is directed. Some examples of behavior modification, as related to specific behaviors involved with anorexia nervosa, include the following:

Behavior	Positive or Negative Reinforcement of Behavior
1. Weight loss	Remove privileges, e.g. withdraw privileges to attend field trips, withdraw pass to go home for a visit, or withdraw privileges for phone calls and letters.
2. Weight gain	Restore or add privileges, e.g. allow field trips, allow pass to go home for a visit, or allow phone calls and letters.
3. Not eating	Nasogastric tubes as directed by physician.
4. Tantrums or crying	Ignore the tantrums and crying. Isolate the patient during outbursts. Give attention to the patient during periods of "appropriate behavior."

TREATMENT

1. Promote weight gain
2. Individual, group, and family counseling
3. Behavior modification (See Table 13-1)
4. Activity restriction to conserve energy
5. Nutritional supplements and nutritional education (See Figure 13-1)

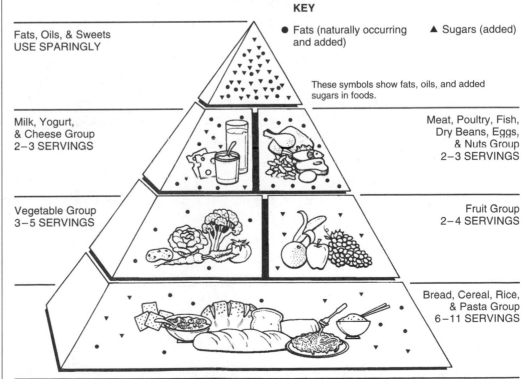

Figure 13-1   Food pyramid

6. Parenteral fluids may be necessary
7. Tube feeding may be necessary (Nasogastric—NG)
8. Dental treatment due to dental problems caused by inadequate calcium intake
9. Hospitalization becomes necessary in the presence of complications, risk of suicide, or for extreme weight loss
10. Antidepressants to treat accompanying or underlying depression

REQUIREMENTS FOR SUCCESSFUL TREATMENT

1. Diagnosis early in the course of the disease
2. Patient who seeks help has a higher chance of success
3. Patient demonstrates desire to overcome the eating disorder
4. Change in social situation may have triggered the eating disorder
5. Long-term counseling
6. Development of long-term, positive eating habits

CONSIDERATIONS FOR CARE

1. Encourage self-esteem for patient and family.
2. Realize that anorexia nervosa is a disease.
3. Obtain baseline weight and monitor on a routine basis.
4. Observation of patient while eating may be necessary due to hiding of food, manipulation, and possible purging.
5. Involve family in patient care and counseling.
6. Monitor intake and output (I and O).
7. Offer foods and fluids frequently according to patient preference.
8. Support group for patient and family.
9. Allow the patient to have control in as many aspects of life as possible. Allow the patient to make decisions and offer choices whenever possible.
10. Educate patient and family regarding the disease process.
11. Educate patient and family regarding treatment options.
12. Educate patient and family regarding the need to alter social atmosphere to promote wellness.
13. Educate patient and family regarding lifelong eating habits.
14. Monitor electrolyte levels.
15. Monitor for symptoms of complications.
16. Monitor for symptoms of dehydration, e.g. decreased urine output, hypotension, concentrated urine, weight loss, constipation, dry skin, dry mouth, tenting of skin, and confusion.
17. Monitor vital signs. (See Appendix D.)
18. Encourage communication on the part of the patient and family.
19. Educate patient regarding importance of follow-up care.
20. Calm, relaxed, social environment for meals.
21. Educate patient, family, and staff regarding behavior modification techniques that will be used to promote patient compliance while allowing control over choices.
22. Consider the use of a signed contract between the patient and staff regarding amounts to be eaten, weight gain goals, and behavior.

23. Allow the patient to ventilate feelings. Take threats of suicide seriously; threats of suicide should be dealt with promptly with referrals to counselors, physicians, and therapists. Protect patient from harm.

24. Develop a trusting relationship with the patient and family by establishing open and honest communication, responding to requests as soon as possible, and following through with requests.

25. Assist the patient to make mealtime pleasant, food attractive, and eating and tasting the food enjoyable.

26. Assist to identify strengths and build on these strengths.

27. Help patient develop methods to deal with conflict in positive ways.

FOR MORE INFORMATION

Center for the Study of Anorexia and Bulimia
1 West 91st Street
New York, NY 10024
(212) 595-3449

American Anorexia and Bulimia Association
418 East 76th Street
New York, NY 10021
(212) 734-1114

Anorexia Nervosa and Related Eating Disorders (ANRED)
1255 Hiliard
P.O. Box 5102
Eugene, OR 97405
(503) 344-1144

National Association of Anorexia Nervosa and Associated Disorders (ANAD)
P.O. Box 7
Highland Park, IL 60035
(708) 831-3438

ASSIGNMENT SHEET: ANOREXIA NERVOSA

Short Answer

1. Write a brief definition for the terms listed throughout the chapter.

2. Write a brief definition for anorexia nervosa.

3. Describe the incidence of anorexia nervosa.

4. List thirteen (13) risk factors for anorexia nervosa.

5. List thirty-four (34) signs and symptoms of anorexia nervosa.

6. Describe six (6) specific causes for the physical symptoms associated with anorexia nervosa.

7. Describe eight (8) possible complications of anorexia nervosa. Describe the rationale and associated care for each of the complications.

8. List six (6) specific methods used to aid in the diagnosis of anorexia nervosa.

9. List ten (10) specific methods used in the treatment of anorexia nervosa.

10. List six (6) specific requirements for the successful treatment of anorexia nervosa.

11. List twenty-seven (27) considerations for caring for a patient with anorexia nervosa.

12. Write the normal ranges for each of the following laboratory tests.
    a. Electrolytes
       • Sodium
       • Potassium
       • Chloride
    b. BUN
    c. SGOT
    d. SGPT
    e. Bilirubin
    f. Albumin
    g. Alkaline phosphatase
    h. Prothrombin time
    i. Amylase
    j. Calcium
    k. Glucose
    l. Urinalysis
    m. Creatinine

13. Describe how an EKG is used in the diagnosis and care of anorexia nervosa.

14. List three (3) foods that are a rich source of calcium.

15. List six (6) possible symptoms of pancreatitis.

16. List six (6) possible symptoms of renal insufficiency.

17. List thirteen (13) possible symptoms of an infection.

18. List nine (9) possible symptoms of dehydration.

19. Write the normal range for each of the following vital signs. (See Appendix D.)
    a. Blood pressure
       • Systolic
       • Diastolic
    b. Temperature
    c. Pulse
    d. Respiration

KNOWLEDGE INTO ACTION

1. Karen Wright, a 19-year-old, has been admitted to the hospital with a history of anorexia and now has syncope due to an electrolyte imbalance. What three elements make up electrolytes?

2. Due to her electrolyte imbalance, Karen Wright is on I and O. Cross out the items that would *not* be included on I and O.
    a. jello
    b. toast
    c. milk
    d. urine
    e. constipated bowel movement
    f. apple
    g. chocolate shake

3. Gregory King, a 21-year-old college student, is admitted with a history of anorexia. He also has symptoms of abdominal pain, nausea, vomiting, fever, and decreased bowel sounds. His serum amylase level is 422 U/L. Would you suspect an

initial diagnosis of acute dehydration, renal failure, pancreatitis, or osteoporosis?

4. Due to her anorexia, Angela Demarco has had increased frequency of infections. Currently, she is in your facility with a cough and sore throat. Describe precautions that should be taken to protect Angela. Describe precautions that should be taken to protect the staff from possible infection.

5. Meredith Johnson, a 36-year-old with a history of anorexia, is admitted to your facility. Her serum albumin is taken on admission with a result of 2.9 g/dL. What symptoms would you expect to see with this albumin level? (Choose the best answer.)

   a. Increased energy level and possible tremor

   b. Decreased energy level and possible confusion
   c. Weight gain and edema
   d. Weight loss and syncope

6. Once Meredith Johnson's condition becomes stabilized, she requests to go home for a weekend to see her family. At this point, she is 5' 6" tall and weighs 94 lbs. Her blood pressure is 86/50. She has refused to participate in group therapy sessions. Give an example of positive behavior modification that could be used with Meredith.

7. John and Mary Brand are taking their daughter, 15-year-old Sheila, home today. She has been diagnosed with anorexia. They are concerned about what they should be alert for. What will be your advice to them?

UNIT 3

MUSCULOSKELETAL DISORDERS

Myasthenia Gravis

KEY TERMS

Exacerbated – the severity of the symptoms of a specific disease are increased

Anticholinesterase – blocks cholinesterase in the body

Spontaneous – voluntary occurrence

Neuromuscular junction– place at which nerves and muscles meet or connect

Synapse – junction between the axon of one neuron and the dendrite of another neuron in the nervous system pathway; nerve impulse travels across this junction to continue the impulse along the nervous system pathway

Axon – transfers neurological impulses away from the neuron, across the synapse, and on to the dendrite of the next neuron

Acetylcholine – compound found in organs and tissues throughout the body; necessary for nerve

INTRODUCTION AND PHYSIOLOGY

Myasthenia gravis is characterized by progressive muscle weakness and fatigability of the skeletal muscles. The weakness and fatigability are **exacerbated** by exercise and improve with rest and **anticholinesterase** drugs. The disease is also characterized by exacerbations and remissions. Approximately 12% of patients with myasthenia gravis will experience a **spontaneous** remission. Symptoms of the disease are due to failure of nerve impulse transmission at the **neuromuscular junction**, which is the space (**synapse**) between the motor **axon** and the fiber of the muscle. **Acetylcholine** is a neurotransmitter that transmits the impulse from the nerve to the muscle fiber at a neuromuscular junction. **Cholinesterase** is an enzyme also present in the body. It destroys acetylcholine. Myasthenia gravis is caused from a decreased amount of acetylcholine, an excess of cholinesterase, or a decreased sensitivity of the muscles to the acetylcholine. (See Figure 14-1.)

STATISTICS

Myasthenia gravis affects approximately 2 to 20 out of 100,000 people in the United States. There is an increased incidence between the ages of 20 and 40 and another sharp increase at later middle-age. Females are affected three times more often than males. Approximately 15% of patients with myasthenia gravis also have **thymomas**.

RISK FACTORS

1. **Autoimmune** response
2. Decreased release of acetylcholine
3. Defective muscle response to acetylcholine
4. Presence of thymoma (See Figure 14-2)

impulse transmission at the synapses and neuromuscular junctions

Cholinesterase – enzyme capable of breaking down acetylcholine

Thymoma – tumor of the thymus gland

Autoimmune – process by which antibodies within a person's body destroy normal cells within the body

Insidious – refers to a gradual onset of symptoms

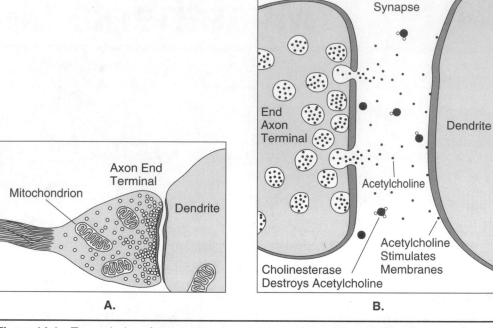

Figure 14-1   Transmission of a nerve impulse across a synapse (From Burke, *Human Anatomy and Physiology in Health and Disease, 3rd edition,* copyright © 1992, Delmar Publishers)

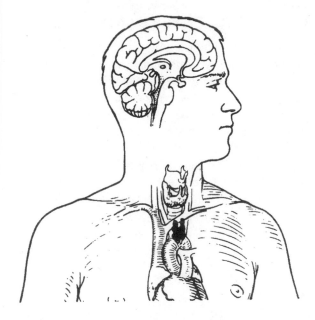

Figure 14-2   Location of the thymus gland (From Ehrlich, *Medical Terminology for Health Professions, 2nd edition,* copyright © 1993, Delmar Publishers)

SIGNS, SYMPTOMS, AND ASSOCIATED CARE

Symptoms for myasthenia gravis can be sudden or **insidious**.

1. Muscle weakness

    *   Allow plenty of time to do activities and procedures to avoid frustration or possible injury

    *   Encourage patient to do as much as possible for himself, even though it may take longer

    *   Assist patient with activities of daily living (ADLs) as necessary

    *   Encourage frequent rest periods as needed

Ptosis – drooping of a body part; frequently refers to the eyelid

Ophthalmologist – specialist (physician) whose main focus is diagnosing and treating diseases and disorders of the eye

Diplopia – double vision

Monotone – voice lacking character

- Schedule care, treatment, and activities around patient rest periods and periods of peak energy for patient
- Encourage patient not to overdo activity
- Assist with ambulation and transfer as needed to prevent injury

2. Muscle fatigability
   - Encourage frequent rest periods as needed
   - Schedule care, treatment, and activities around patient rest periods and periods of peak energy for patient
   - Assist patient with ADLs as necessary
   - Encourage patient not to overdo activity
   - Assist with ambulation and transfer as needed to prevent injury

3. **Ptosis**
   - Educate patient regarding head position to improve vision
   - Evaluate ability for patient to drive safely in presence of visual problems
   - Encourage alternate activities for patient who has difficulty with reading
   - Avoid eye strain
   - Provide large-print books or cassettes
   - Avoid injury to the patient due to visual disturbances
   - Evaluation by **ophthalmologist**
   - Provide adequate lighting when reading, watching TV, or doing other activities
   - Remove environmental hazards, such as throw rugs, cluttered hallways, and excessive furniture

4. **Diplopia**
   - Utilize an eyepatch over alternate eyes to correct diplopia
   - Evaluate ability for patient to drive safely in presence of diplopia
   - Encourage alternate activities for patient who has difficulty with reading due to diplopia

5. **Monotone** voice
   - Encourage to practice singing and reading aloud
   - Encourage to talk or read into a tape recorder and practice enunciation and expression
   - Encourage to practice making exaggerated facial expressions in the mirror
   - Be certain you correctly understand what the patient is saying
   - Allow time for the patient to respond to questions and comments
   - Maintain good eye contact when speaking with the patient
   - Concentrate on what the patient is saying
   - Avoid outside distractions, e.g. TV and radio
   - Avoid rooms that are congested with other people when visiting
   - Avoid finishing sentences for the patient
   - Encourage patient not to isolate himself
   - Provide alternative forms of communication, such as writing, word boards, and electronic devices (See Figure 14-3)
   - Encourage continued efforts at communication

6. Blank expression
   - Practice making exaggerated facial expressions in a mirror

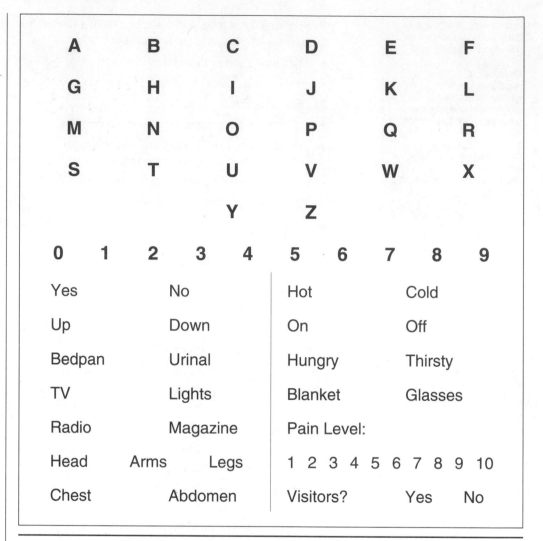

A	B	C	D	E	F
G	H	I	J	K	L
M	N	O	P	Q	R
S	T	U	V	W	X
	Y		Z		

0   1   2   3   4   5   6   7   8   9

Yes	No	Hot	Cold
Up	Down	On	Off
Bedpan	Urinal	Hungry	Thirsty
TV	Lights	Blanket	Glasses
Radio	Magazine	Pain Level:	

Head   Arms   Legs

1 2 3 4 5 6 7 8 9 10

Chest   Abdomen

Visitors?   Yes   No

Figure 14-3   Communication method for patient who needs alternative method of communication

7. Dysphagia
   - Offer foods that are easy to chew according to patient preference
   - Avoid fresh fruits and vegetables as these are often more difficult to chew
   - Alternate liquids and solids during meals
   - Monitor for choking
   - Instruct family members on the Heimlich maneuver should choking occur while they are with the patient and for when the patient returns home
   - Utilize suction equipment in the event of choking
   - Concentrate on chewing food thoroughly
   - Educate that food may need to be cut into smaller pieces, ground, or pureed
   - Provide method, such as a warming plate, to keep food warm during entire length of time needed for patient to eat
   - Obtain baseline weight and monitor on a routine basis
   - Encourage the patient to take as much time as necessary during meals
   - Avoid outside distractions during mealtime to avoid choking
   - Encourage the patient to sit upright to eat

Dysarthria – difficulty with speech due to impairment of the nerves or muscles that control speech

Tracheotomy – surgical creation of an opening between the trachea and the surface of the anterior neck

Thymectomy – surgical removal of the thymus gland

Plasmapheresis – separating the plasma from the cells in a specimen of blood by means of centrifuge; the red blood cells are then reinjected into the original donor or another person

- Be alert for symptoms of dehydration. Symptoms of dehydration include decreased urine output, hypotension, concentrated urine, weight loss, constipation, dry skin, dry mouth, tenting of skin, and confusion.
- Use a syringe to feed liquids in small amounts

8. Neck muscle weakness
   - Prevent injury to patient if unable to hold head up
   - Utilize assistive brace or neck support to hold head up
   - Provide neck support when in automobile to prevent injury during a sudden stop

9. **Dysarthria**
   - Be certain you heard the patient correctly
   - Maintain good eye contact when speaking
   - Concentrate on what the patient is saying
   - Avoid outside distractions, e.g. TV and radio
   - Avoid rooms that are congested with other people when visiting
   - Avoid finishing sentences for the patient

DIAGNOSIS

1. Symptoms
2. Physical examination
3. Muscle fatigability that improves with rest
4. *Electromyography* used to differentiate between muscle disorders versus nerve disorders
5. *Tensilon test* shows improvement of symptoms after administration of edrophonium or neostigmine
6. X-ray of mediastinum to rule out thymoma
7. Laboratory tests to rule out thyroid disease, e.g. *Thyroxin, T3,* and *TSH*
8. Serum analysis shows presence of *acetylcholine (ACh) receptor antibodies* in 90% of patients with myasthenia gravis
9. *CT scan* to determine presence of thymoma

TREATMENT

1. Anticholinesterase drugs are used to treat muscle weakness and fatigue by increasing neuromuscular transmission; prevent breakdown of acetylcholine, which is a neurotransmitter. Medications do not cure myasthenia gravis but help control symptoms by allowing increased availability of acetylcholine, e.g. Neostigmine and Pyridostigmine (Mestinon).
2. Corticosteroids are used to treat symptoms, e.g. Prednisone
3. **Tracheotomy** and ventilation therapy if respiratory muscle involvement is severe (See Figure 14-4)
4. **Thymectomy** is necessary for patients with thymomas, which results in remission in approximately 30 to 40% of patients with thymoma. Approximately 15% of patients with myasthenia gravis have thymomas.
5. **Plasmapheresis**—removal of plasma, which contains acetylcholine receptor antibodies, temporarily improves symptoms
6. Approximately 12% of people with myasthenia gravis will have a remission from symptoms for several years

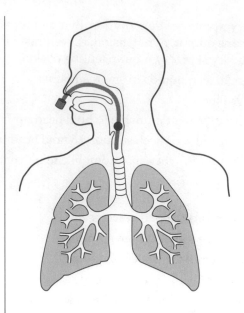

Figure 14-4 Placement of endotracheal tube

COMPLICATIONS

1. Myasthenic crises—sudden deterioration in the condition of the client with extreme exacerbation of the symptoms of the disease; often leads to cardiac or respiratory distress
2. Cholinergic crisis—excess acetylcholine at the neuromuscular junction resulting from an excess of anticholinergic medications
3. Brittle crisis—decreased sensitivity of the neuromuscular junction receptors to anticholinesterase medications
4. Respiratory distress due to myasthenia crisis or due to the normal progression of the disease
5. Eating and chewing difficulties due to myasthenia crisis or to the normal progression of the disease
6. Aspiration pneumonia caused from the drawing of foreign objects, by aspiration, into the lung or bronchi

CONSIDERATIONS FOR CARE

1. Educate patient and family regarding the disease process.
2. Educate patient and family regarding forms of treatment as well as side effects of medications.
3. Provide emotional support to patient and family.
4. Provide nonjudgmental acceptance of emotions and behavior of the patient and family.
5. Suggest a support group for patient and family.
6. Counseling may be necessary for patient and family to work through emotions associated with the disease.
7. Family members need to offer encouragement to the patient to do as much as possible for herself.
8. Family and friends should be available to help but should not encourage dependence.
9. Depression may develop as a result of the patient being unable to provide financially, contribute to responsibilities in the home, and address other responsibilities previously held by the patient.

Menses – menstruation

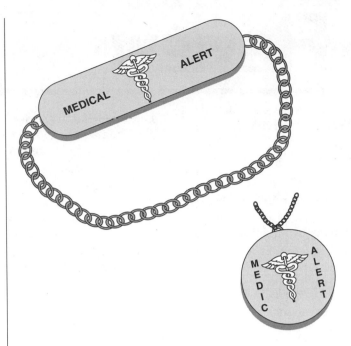

Figure 14-5 Medical alert bracelet and necklace

10. Educate patient and family regarding the importance of taking medications at the scheduled time.

11. Educate patient and family regarding the importance of follow-up care.

12. Educate patient regarding the importance of avoiding stress, infections, and excessive exposure to heat and cold as these tend to cause exacerbations; also exacerbations have a tendency to occur during **menses**.

13. Obtain baseline vital signs (See Appendix D) and respiratory status. Monitor on a frequent basis.

14. Obtain baseline neurologic function and muscle strength and monitor on a routine basis.

15. Encourage patient to perform activities around periods of peak energy.

16. Drug schedule should correlate with peak energy needs of the patient.

17. Avoid crowded areas and individuals infected with respiratory illness or other infections.

18. Instruct patient regarding the availability of self-help aids, such as long-handled devices, velcro closures, bath mitts, soap on a rope, large-handled utensils, devices for reaching, elastic shoe closures, electric razor, and handrails in hallways and bathroom.

19. Educate patient and family regarding the need to carry a medical alert card and wear a medical alert bracelet or necklace. (See Figure 14-5.)

20. If traveling, have medication with the patient rather than stored in luggage.

FOR MORE INFORMATION

Myasthenia Gravis Foundation Inc.
Suite 660
53 West Jackson Blvd.
Chicago, IL 60604
(312) 427-6252

ASSIGNMENT SHEET: MYASTHENIA GRAVIS

Short Answer

1. Write a brief definition for the terms listed throughout the chapter.

2. Write a brief definition for myasthenia gravis.

3. Describe four (4) risk factors associated with myasthenia gravis.

4. Describe the incidence of myasthenia gravis.

5. List nine (9) signs and symptoms associated with myasthenia gravis and associated care for each of these symptoms.

6. List nine (9) specific methods used to aid in the diagnosis of myasthenia gravis.

7. List six (6) specific methods used in the treatment of myasthenia gravis.

8. Describe six (6) complications associated with myasthenia gravis.

9. List twenty (20) considerations for caring for a patient with myasthenia gravis.

10. Write the normal range for each of the following laboratory thyroid tests.
    a. Thyroxine
    b. T3
    c. TSH

11. Describe the following procedures used in the diagnosis of myasthenia gravis.
    a. Electromyography
    b. CT scan
    c. Tensilon test

12. List the normal ranges for each of the following vital signs. (See Appendix D.)
    a. Blood pressure
       • Systolic
       • Diastolic
    b. Temperature
    c. Pulse
    d. Respirations

KNOWLEDGE INTO ACTION

1. A new nursing assistant has been hired at your facility. She is assigned to help Marcie Wheeler, a 53-year-old with a long history of myasthenia gravis, to eat her noon meal. She has read in the chart that Mrs. Wheeler has had a problem with dysphagia and is concerned about this. She asks you for suggestions. What suggestions could you provide?

2. Prior to Mrs. Wheeler's discharge, her husband talks to you about his wife's dysarthria. Visiting has gotten to be extremely difficult for them and he misses communication with his wife of 32 years. What suggestions could you give Mr. Wheeler regarding methods to improve their communication efforts? What alternate forms of communication could you suggest for Mrs. Wheeler's use?

3. David Lerner, a 39-year-old welder, has been admitted to your facility with weakness, dysarthria, and dysphagia. You are aware that the physician initially wants to rule out myasthenia gravis, due to Mr. Lerner's symptoms and a physical examination by the physician. What other tests might be done to make the diagnosis of myasthenia gravis? List three (3) and write a brief explanation for each.

4. Sandy Lerner, David's wife, stops you in the hall prior to David's discharge from your facility. She says they live in a two-story home with the bedrooms on the upper level. She asks you for suggestions for outside assistance and personal self-help aids that might make David's day-to-day life easier. What would your response be?

5. Amy Chang, a 38-year-old nurse, has been admitted to your facility to have some testing done to find out the cause of her increasing muscle weakness, fatigue, and visual problems. The physician is unsure whether the cause is from a thyroid gland disorder or possibly from myasthenia gravis. The physician orders thyroid tests to rule out a thyroid gland disorder. The results are back on her chart when you come to work today. For each thyroid test listed, tell if the level is low, normal, or high.
   a. _____ Thyroxine = 3.1 µg/dL
   b. _____ T3 = 82 ng/dL
   c. _____ TSH = 17 U/mL

6. As part of Amy Chang's initial examination, you were asked to take her vital signs. What would the normal ranges for each of the following vital signs be?
   a. Blood pressure
      • Systolic
      • Diastolic
   b. Temperature
   c. Pulse
   d. Respirations

CHAPTER 15

Multiple Sclerosis

OBJECTIVES

Upon completion of this chapter, the student should be able to:

- Define the key terms listed throughout the chapter
- State a specific definition for multiple sclerosis
- Describe the incidence of multiple sclerosis
- Describe the risk factors for multiple sclerosis
- List signs and symptoms often associated with multiple sclerosis and associated care for symptoms
- Identify specific methods for diagnosis of multiple sclerosis
- Identify specific methods for treatment of multiple sclerosis
- Describe specific considerations for caring for a patient with multiple sclerosis

KEY TERMS

Multiple sclerosis (MS) – disease of the nervous system caused by destruction of the myelin sheath

Myelin sheath – fatlike covering around the nerve fibers

Sclerosis – formation of scar tissue from normal, healthy tissue

INTRODUCTION AND PHYSIOLOGY

Multiple sclerosis (MS) is defined as a chronic central nervous system (CNS) disease caused by scar tissue, which is formed as a result of the destruction of the **myelin sheath**. The myelin sheath surrounds the nerve fibers of the brain and the spinal cord, allowing information and impulses to be relayed from the CNS to the body and back again. (See Figure 15-1.) When the myelin is destroyed, scar tissue replaces the myelin in these areas and the impulses are no longer able to get through. The name of the disease is very descriptive of what occurs: *multiple* refers to the many sites that are involved and *sclerosis* refers to the formation of scar tissue.

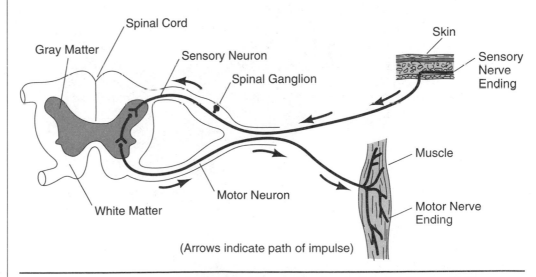

(Arrows indicate path of impulse)

Figure 15-1 The reflex arc (Adapted from Hegner, *Nursing Assistant: A Nursing Process Approach, 7th edition*, copyright © 1995, Delmar Publishers)

Immune system – system of the body that has the primary function of detecting pathogens in the body and removing or destroying the foreign pathogen; also known as the lymph system

STATISTICS

Multiple sclerosis most often occurs in people in their twenties and thirties accounting for approximately 75% of all cases. The disease occurs more often in females than in males (3:2 ratio). The disease also seems to be associated with people living in cold, damp climates, especially during the first 15 years of their lives. MS affects a total of 40 to 60 people per 10,000 in the United States. An average of 15% of patients with MS die due to complications of the disease.

RISK FACTORS

MS is believed to be caused by an autoimmune response, whereby the body's own T-cells, which are part of the **immune system**, attack the myelin sheath. (See Figure 15-2.)

1. Genetic factors increase the risk by fifteen times
2. Cold, damp climates
3. Trauma
4. Environmental toxins
5. Stress
6. Nutritional deficiencies
7. Viral infection
8. Pregnancy

SIGNS, SYMPTOMS, AND ASSOCIATED CARE

Multiple sclerosis is often difficult to diagnose due to the sporadic nature of the symptoms as well as the broad range of nonspecific symptoms (symptoms that could signify many other illnesses or diseases). The course of the disease is often marked by periods of exacerbation followed by periods of complete or partial remission. Following are some of the most common signs and symptoms associated with MS.

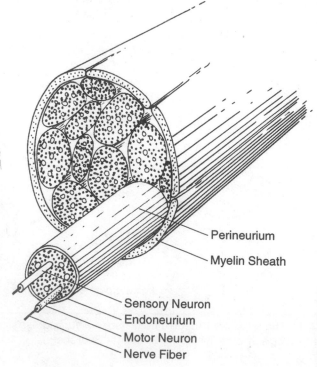

Perineurium
Myelin Sheath
Sensory Neuron
Endoneurium
Motor Neuron
Nerve Fiber

Figure 15-2 Cross section of a spinal nerve (From Burke, *Human Anatomy and Physiology in Health and Disease, 3rd edition,* copyright © 1992, Delmar Publishers)

Paresthesia – refers to a feeling of numbness or tingling

1. Muscle weakness
    - Encourage patient to do as much as possible for herself
    - Assist with activities of daily living (ADLs) as necessary
    - Prevent injury due to weakness
    - Assist with ambulation and transfer as needed
    - Encourage exercise to maintain muscle strength
    - Provide cane or walker to provide additional assistance for ambulation and transfer (See Figure 15-3)
    - Encourage patient to rest as needed

2. Blurred vision or diplopia
    - Educate patient regarding head position to improve vision
    - Evaluate ability for patient to drive safely in presence of visual problems
    - Encourage alternate activities for patient who has difficulty reading
    - Avoid eye strain
    - Provide large-print books or cassettes
    - Avoid injury to the patient due to visual disturbances
    - Provide evaluation by ophthalmologist
    - Provide adequate lighting when reading, watching TV, or doing other activities
    - Remove environmental hazards, such as throw rugs, cluttered hallways, and excessive furniture

3. **Paresthesia**
    - Assist with position for patient comfort
    - Prevent injury due to paresthesia from extreme heat, cold, or sharp instruments
    - Assist with ADLs as necessary

4. Decreased coordination
    - Provide wide base of support for standing and ambulating
    - Evaluate ability to drive and do activities that could cause injury due to decreased coordination

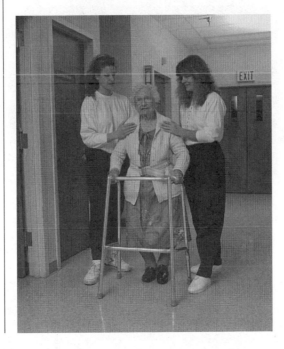

Figure 15-3   A walker is often needed to provide additional assistance for ambulation and transfer. (From Hegner, *Nursing Assistant: A Nursing Process Approach, 7th edition,* copyright © 1995, Delmar Publishers)

- Encourage use of assistive devices, such as large-handled utensils, bath mitts, velcro fasteners, long-handled shoehorns, soap on a rope, elevated toilet seat, and handrails (See Figure 15-4)
5. Fatigue
   - Assist patient with ADLs as necessary
   - Schedule care, activities, and treatment around patient's rest schedule
   - Monitor phone calls and visitors around patient's energy level and rest schedule
   - Encourage frequent rest periods
   - Encourage activity as able
   - Provide assistance as needed to prevent injury due to weakness
   - Provide method for patient to call for assistance
   - Encourage patient to set realistic goals of activities
   - Allow adequate time to do activities and procedures to avoid frustration or possible injury
   - Encourage exercise to maintain muscle strength
   - Provide cane or walker to provide additional assistance for ambulation and transfer
   - Provide private room for patient to promote rest periods

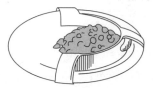

A Food bumper snaps over a dinner plate to keep the food on the plate

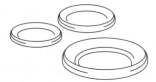

B Plates with inner lip to keep food on plate

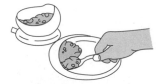

C Plate with high curved edge to help push food on fork or spoon

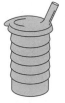

D Feeding cup

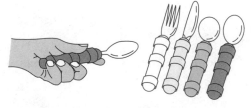

E Cutlery with built-in handles for easier gripping: movable grip rings adjust for comfort

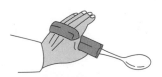

Hand clip for people who cannot grip handles

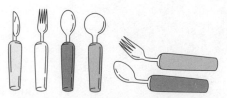

F Angled cutlery for people with limited arm and wrist movement

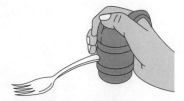

G Gripper for people who cannot grip standard or built-up handles

Figure 15-4   Adaptive equipment (Adapted from Hegner, *Nursing Assistant: A Nursing Process Approach, 7th edition,* copyright © 1995, Delmar Publishers)

Malodorous – refers to foul or unpleasant odor

Lability – instability; generally refers to the state of emotional well-being

6. Decreased bladder control
   - Assess for bladder control and observe for incontinence
   - Provide meticulous skin care especially in the presence of incontinence
   - Educate patient and family to observe for and report symptoms of urinary tract infection, e.g. burning with urination, frequency, urgency, pain, fever, cloudy urine, **malodorous** urine, and bloody urine
   - Encourage fluid intake
   - Encourage urination schedule
   - Be aware of nonverbal clues a patient may give to use the bathroom
   - Prevent odors in the room by changing linens as needed and washing off chairs and other items that become wet or soiled
   - Prevent embarrassment to the patient
   - Use a mild soap to cleanse the patient's skin and pat dry
   - Provide privacy for the patient when she is using the bathroom

7. Muscle spasms and cramps
   - Provide massage, relaxation techniques, imaging, and medications to control muscle spasms and cramps
   - Encourage activity as able
   - Encourage regular exercise program
   - Provide cane or walker to facilitate ambulation and transfer

8. Occasional forgetfulness or confusion
   - Encourage patient to make lists and write reminding notes as needed
   - Encourage patient to store items in the same place each time

9. Dysarthria
   - Encourage patient not to isolate herself
   - Provide alternative forms of communication, such as writing, word boards, and electronic devices
   - Practice singing or reading aloud
   - Practice making exaggerated facial expressions in the mirror
   - Be certain you correctly understand what the patient is saying
   - Maintain good eye contact when speaking with the patient
   - Concentrate on what the patient is saying
   - Avoid outside distractions, e.g. TV or radio
   - Avoid rooms that are congested with other people when visiting
   - Avoid finishing sentences for the patient
   - Encourage patient not to isolate herself
   - Encourage continued efforts at communication on the part of the patient
   - Allow time for the patient to respond to questions and comments

10. Emotional **lability**
    - Realize that the patient may not have complete control over emotions and this may be a normal part of the disease
    - Avoid embarrassment for the patient by refraining from drawing attention to emotions

11. Depression
    - Encourage communication between the patient and family
    - Provide professional counseling as necessary
    - Administer medications to help treat the depression

Gamma globulin – protein manufactured by the lymph system in response to toxins present in the system, e.g. bacteria or virus

- Help patient maintain as much control as possible over her life
- Observe for signs of severe depression or suicidal tendencies

12. Constipation

- Encourage fluids
- Encourage a high-fiber diet including fruits, vegetables, whole grains, prunes, and beans
- Increase exercise as tolerated
- Administer enemas, suppositories, stool softeners, and laxatives as prescribed by physician
- Monitor frequency, number, and consistency of stools
- Monitor for possible bowel obstruction. Symptoms of bowel obstruction include no stools or diarrhea, bloating, nausea, vomiting, abdominal pain, and fever
- Encourage fresh fruits and vegetables
- Establish regular bowel routine
- Provide privacy for bowel routine as able

13. Dysphagia

- Offer foods that are easy to chew according to patient preference
- Avoid fresh fruits and vegetables as these are often more difficult to chew
- Alternate liquids and solids during meals
- Monitor for choking
- Instruct family members on the Heimlich maneuver should choking occur while they are with the patient and for when the patient returns home
- Utilize suction equipment in the event of choking
- Concentrate on chewing food thoroughly
- Educate that food may need to be cut into smaller pieces, ground, or pureed
- Provide method, such as a warming plate, to keep food warm during entire length of time needed for patient to eat
- Obtain baseline weight and monitor on a routine basis
- Encourage the patient to take as much time as necessary during meals
- Avoid outside distractions during mealtime to avoid choking
- Have patient sit upright to eat
- Be alert for symptoms of dehydration
- Use a syringe to feed liquids in small amounts

DIAGNOSIS

For a diagnosis of MS to be made, there must be two factors present: (1) scar tissue must be present in the central nervous system, and (2) the patient must have had two separate attacks attributed to the disease. Methods of diagnosis include the following:

1. Symptoms
2. Physical examination
3. *Spinal tap* may show elevated WBC and elevated **gamma globulin**
4. *CT scan* will show evidence of scar tissue formation or swelling of myelin sheath and ventricular enlargement
5. Elevation of patient's body temperature will show increase of symptoms in many patients with MS
6. *MRI* used to show the number, location, and extent of scar tissue lesions

Immunosuppressives – medications that suppress the body's formation of antibodies in response to an antigen

Anticonvulsive – substance that prevents, reduces the frequency of, or treats convulsions (seizures)

Anticholinergic – blocking of cholinergic responses through the parasympathetic nervous system (cholinergic effect is that of acetylcholine)

Decubitus ulcer – ulcer or sore on the skin that results from long periods of pressure to an area of skin and the decreased circulation that results; also known as bedsore

7. Urological examination done in the presence of bladder dysfunction
8. *EEG* will be abnormal in 30% of patients with MS

TREATMENT

Treatment is based on caring for the symptoms of the disease, rather than the ability to cure the disease itself. Following are the most commonly used forms of treatment:

1. Corticosteroids may be used to speed recovery during exacerbations of the disease by decreasing the swelling around the myelin lesions, e.g. Prednisone, Dexamethasone
2. **Immunosuppressive** therapy may be used to speed recovery during exacerbations of the disease and to stabilize the disease, e.g. Cyclophosphamide, Azathioprine
3. Aspirin, acetaminophen, or other medications may be used to treat the muscle pain that often accompanies MS
4. **Anticonvulsive** medications may be used to treat the muscle spasms that often accompany MS, e.g. Diazepam, Dantrolene sodium
5. Medications to relax the bladder often are used to treat frequency and urgency of urination, e.g. Amitriptyline
6. Antispasmodic medications are used to treat the muscle spasm that often accompanies MS; e.g. Baclofen is available in oral form and also in an experimental form, which is transfused directly into the spinal canal
7. Medications to treat extreme fatigue, which often accompanies MS, e.g. Symmetrel
8. Antidepressant medications to treat depression, which often accompanies MS, e.g. Elavil
9. **Anticholinergic** medications used to treat bladder dysfunction, e.g. Pro-Banthine

CONSIDERATIONS FOR CARE

1. Educate patient and family regarding the disease process.
2. Educate patient and family regarding forms of treatment as well as side effects of treatment.
3. Provide emotional support to patient and family.
4. Provide nonjudgmental acceptance of emotions and behavior of patient and family.
5. Educate patient to avoid stressful situations, excessive fatigue, viral infections, and excessive heat or humidity as these have been shown to cause exacerbations of symptoms in patients with MS.
6. Encourage proper nutrition with high fiber to promote regularity.
7. Encourage patient to maintain appropriate weight.
8. Stress the importance of keeping the patient independent for as long as possible.
9. For patients with decreased mobility, stress the importance of monitoring for and preventing skin breakdown. (See Figure 15-5.)
   - Signs of skin breakdown (**decubitus ulcers**) include: redness, swelling, warm or hot to touch, open sores, cyanosis, pain, and blisters.
   - Prevention measures include: frequent repositioning (minimum of every 1 to 2 hours); meticulous skin care; massage areas at bony prominences;

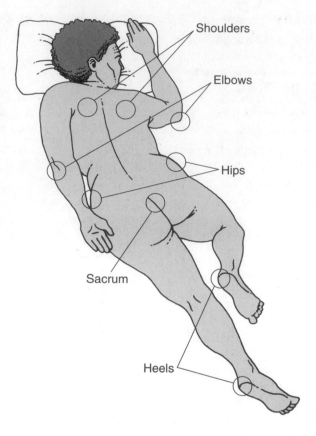

Figure 15-5 Body areas sensitive to skin breakdown (Adapted from Hegner, *Assisting in Long-Term Care, 2nd edition*, copyright © 1994, Delmar Publishers)

encourage activity as able; alternate pressure mattresses; prevent pressure from appliances or tubing; prevent friction when repositioning by using a lift sheet and adequate assistance; and linens must be clean, dry, and wrinkle-free. (See Table 15-1.)

10. Encourage patient and family to attend support groups.

11. Professional counseling may be necessary to deal with emotions they may be experiencing.

12. Promote patient self-esteem by encouraging them to be as active as possible, to take part in decision making, and to carry on a normal lifestyle.

13. Educate patient and family regarding financial assistance opportunities that may be available to them.

Table 15-1 Stages of Decubitus Ulcer Development

Bedsores (also known as decubitus ulcers or pressure sores) occur in stages and advance in seriousness according to the amount of pressure, the length of time the pressure is present, the size of the patient, the general health status of the patient, and the nutritional and fluid status of the patient.

- Bedsores begin at the area of pressure and will be reddened and tender to touch.

- If the pressure continues, the site may blister. Portions of the area may have broken skin integrity.

- As the bedsore progresses, subcutaneous tissue is involved and eventually, muscle, bone, and deep tissue are involved and exposed.

- In the advanced stages of bedsores, skin grafting and/or amputation may be needed to treat the bedsore.

During the course of the development of the bedsore, the area is painful and very vulnerable to infection.

14. Educate patient and family regarding the availability of community resources.

15. Educate patient and family regarding the need to carry a medical alert card and wear a medical alert bracelet or necklace.

16. Provide routine for ADLs to include rest periods.

17. Provide evaluation and treatment from the following therapy groups:
    - Physical therapy will assist the patient to walk better and increase and maintain strength
    - Speech therapy will assist with speech and swallowing difficulties
    - Occupational therapy will help to maintain hand coordination and dexterity

18. Avoid large crowds of people and people with respiratory or other infections.

FOR MORE INFORMATION

National Multiple Sclerosis Society (NMSS)
733 Third Avenue, 6th Floor
New York, NY 10017
1-800-624-8236

ASSIGNMENT SHEET: MULTIPLE SCLEROSIS

Short Answer

1. Write a brief definition for the terms listed throughout the chapter.

2. Write a brief definition for multiple sclerosis.

3. Describe the incidence of multiple sclerosis.

4. List eight (8) possible risk factors for multiple sclerosis.

5. List thirteen (13) signs and symptoms associated with multiple sclerosis and the associated care for each symptom.

6. List eight (8) specific methods used in the diagnosis of multiple sclerosis.

7. List nine (9) specific methods used in the treatment of multiple sclerosis.

8. List eighteen (18) considerations for caring for a patient with multiple sclerosis.

9. List seven (7) specific signs and symptoms of a decubitus ulcer.

10. Describe eight (8) specific measures to decrease the incidence of decubitus ulcers.

11. Describe the following procedures used in the diagnosis of multiple sclerosis.
    a. Spinal tap
    b. CT scan
    c. MRI
    d. EEG

KNOWLEDGE INTO ACTION

1. Maurice Lohman, a 43-year-old electrician, is admitted to your facility with a long history of multiple sclerosis. He has gotten weaker over the years to the point where he needs a great deal of assistance with ambulation. He has also developed incontinence, dysarthria, dysphagia, and severe constipation. You are responsible for developing a plan of care for Mr. Lohman while he is in the hospital that can also be used for him when he is discharged from the hospital to his own home. Describe what each of the symptoms means and describe four methods of associated care that could be utilized for Mr. Lohman in response to the apparent symptoms.

2. Mr. Lohman has been unable to be very active due to his weakness. You are concerned that he may develop decubitus ulcers. Describe four signs of a decubitus ulcer and four measures used in the prevention of the formation of decubitus ulcers.

3. Mrs. Lohman says to you, "Maurice has gotten so weak and just isn't able to take care of himself as well as he used to. I'm having a hard time doing it all myself anymore. Is there anyone who could suggest methods to help Maurice regain his strength or could show us ways he could do things for himself more easily?" What will your response be?

Parkinson's Disease

OBJECTIVES

Upon completion of this chapter, the student should be able to:

- Define the key terms listed throughout the chapter
- State a specific definition for Parkinson's disease
- Describe the incidence of Parkinson's disease
- List the risk factors associated with Parkinson's disease
- List signs and symptoms associated with Parkinson's disease and associated care
- Identify specific methods for diagnosis of Parkinson's disease
- Identify specific methods for treatment of Parkinson's disease
- Describe specific considerations for caring for a patient with Parkinson's disease

KEY TERMS

Substantia nigra – area of cells within the brain that produce dopamine

Dopamine – important for the process of neurotransmission in the central nervous system (CNS); produced by the adrenal glands

INTRODUCTION AND PHYSIOLOGY

Parkinson's disease is a chronic, progressive disease that affects muscle strength, coordination, and movement. The disease has an insidious onset. The **substantia nigra**, an area of cells in the brain that produces dopamine, is affected in Parkinson's disease. **Dopamine**, which is necessary for nerve transmission, is depleted at a very rapid rate or is deficient in the patient. Acetylcholine, which is also necessary for nerve transmission, must be in balance with the amount of dopamine available. As the amount of dopamine decreases, the dopamine/acetylcholine balance is disturbed, which enhances the symptoms. Symptoms associated with Parkinson's disease generally become evident when there is a 75 to 80% decrease in the amount of dopamine. The brain tries to compensate for the decrease in dopamine initially by increasing the amount of dopamine produced by the cells in the substantia nigra as well as making the nerve cells more sensitive to the remaining dopamine.

STATISTICS

An estimated 50,000 people in the United States are diagnosed annually with Parkinson's disease with a total of approximately 1,000,000 people affected. The disease affects men slightly more often than women with the average age at diagnosis of the disease being 65 years old. With medication and treatment, the patient with Parkinson's disease should be able to expect a normal life span. The incidence is increasing due to increased longevity in the United States. The age of diagnosis is equally divided between the under 50 age group, 50 to 60 age group, and over 60 age group with 10% of total new cases diagnosed being under the age of 40. Approximately 1% of the total population over the age of 60 in the United States are affected by the disease.

RISK FACTORS

The cause of Parkinson's disease currently is unknown, but the following several theories are being explored.

1. Trauma to the head or generalized severe trauma to the body

Anesthesia – decreased sensation generally accompanied by complete sedation, generally for the purpose of surgery

Gait belt – belt made of webbed fabric that is put around the waist of a person needing assistance with transfer or ambulation; added security by allowing the person who is assisting to have a firm hold on the belt

Bradykinesia – decreased or slowed movements

2. **Anesthesia**
3. Herbicides and pesticides used in certain occupations
4. Viral infections
5. Genetic predisposition
6. Carbon monoxide poisoning

SIGNS, SYMPTOMS, AND ASSOCIATED CARE

The onset of the symptoms is insidious with the early symptoms mimicking the normal aging process. Following are the more common, typical symptoms associated with Parkinson's disease.

1. Tremor during stress that disappears with purposeful movement and sleep; present in approximately 75% of cases
   - Allow plenty of time to do activities and procedures to avoid frustration or possible injury
   - Encourage patient to do as much as possible for himself, even though it may take longer
   - Assist with hot foods or liquids as needed to avoid burns from spills
   - Use large mugs with easy-to-grip handles
   - Fill mugs containing hot liquids only part-way full to avoid spills
   - Utilize straws to avoid spills when drinking liquids
   - Assist with activities of daily living (ADLs) as needed
   - Monitor intake and output (I and O) to ensure adequate patient hydration

2. Difficulty getting to a standing position after sitting
   - Provide a firm chair with armrests to assist with standing
   - Provide electric lift chair if necessary
   - Avoid lifting patient under the arms to prevent shoulder injury
   - Utilize **gait belt** around waist to assist to standing position (See Figure 16-1)
   - Provide raised toilet seat

3. **Bradykinesia**
   - Allow plenty of time to do activities and procedures to avoid frustration or possible injury

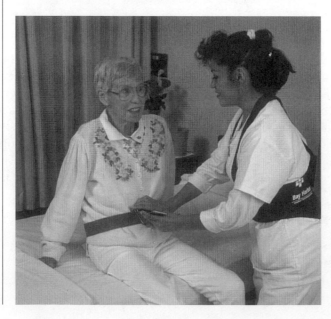

Figure 16-1   Gait belt (From Hegner, *Nursing Assistant: A Nursing Process Approach, 7th edition,* copyright © 1995, Delmar Publishers)

Rigidity – stiffness

Cogwheel – rigidity of movement that is jerky and uneven when the extremity is moved or manipulated

- Encourage patient to do as much as possible for himself even though it may take longer
- Avoid doing tasks for the patient that he can accomplish on his own

4. Masklike facial expression
   - Practice making exaggerated facial expressions in a mirror

5. Monotone speech, dysarthria
   - Practice singing or reading aloud
   - Practice making exaggerated facial expressions in the mirror
   - Be certain you correctly understand what the patient is saying
   - Maintain good eye contact when speaking with the patient
   - Concentrate on what the patient is saying
   - Avoid outside distractions, e.g. TV and radio
   - Avoid rooms that are congested with other people when visiting
   - Avoid finishing sentences for the patient
   - Encourage patient not to isolate himself
   - Provide alternative forms of communication, such as writing, word boards, and electronic devices
   - Encourage continued efforts at communication
   - Allow time for the patient to respond to questions and comments

6. Loss of volume of speech
   - Be certain you heard the patient correctly
   - Maintain good eye contact when speaking
   - Concentrate on what the patient is saying
   - Avoid outside distractions, e.g. TV and radio
   - Avoid rooms that are congested with other people when visiting
   - Avoid finishing sentences for the patient

7. **Rigidity** resulting in **cogwheel** movements
   - Maintain daily exercise routine
   - Provide warm baths, massage, and stretching, which may help reduce rigidity

8. Stooped posture with shoulders bent forward
   - Encourage broad base of support
   - Encourage to concentrate when walking to avoid injury
   - Encourage correct posture
   - Employ exercises to maintain correct posture

9. Drooling
   - Provide meticulous skin care to avoid skin breakdown around mouth
   - Educate regarding exercises to promote muscle control around mouth
   - Encourage patient to keep clean, dry cloth to wipe mouth as needed
   - Establish a signal for patient to wipe mouth to avoid embarrassment of drooling or the need to verbalize the need to wipe the mouth
   - Understand that patient may wish to wear protective bib or similar to protect clothing

10. Dysphagia
    - Offer foods that are easy to chew according to patient preference
    - Avoid fresh fruits and vegetables as these are often more difficult to chew

Seborrhea – increased secretions from the sebaceous (oil-producing) glands of the body; frequently refers to the sebaceous glands of the scalp; commonly called dandruff

Gait – pattern of movement or ambulation

- Alternate liquids and solids during meals
- Monitor for choking
- Instruct family members on the Heimlich maneuver should choking occur while they are with the patient and for when the patient returns home
- Utilize suction equipment in the event of choking
- Concentrate on chewing food thoroughly
- Educate that food may need to be cut into smaller pieces, ground, or pureed
- Provide a method, such as a warming plate, to keep food warm during entire length of time needed for patient to eat
- Obtain baseline weight and monitor on routine basis
- Encourage patient to take as much time as necessary during meals
- Avoid outside distractions during mealtime to avoid choking
- Have patient sit upright to eat
- Be alert for symptoms of dehydration, e.g. decreased urine output, constipation, dry skin, tenting of skin, dry mouth, dry eyes, concentrated urine, hypotension, and confusion
- Use a syringe to feed liquids in small amounts

11. **Seborrhea**
    - Avoid heavy soaps, lotions, cosmetics, or creams that increase oil production
    - Provide frequent bathing and hair washing
    - Provide meticulous skin care with mild, unscented soap
    - Avoid use of tapes and other adhesives on skin
    - Encourage fluid intake
    - Pat skin gently dry
    - Avoid harsh soaps or bleach in clothing and linens
    - Avoid clothing and bedding that is irritating
    - Assess skin redness and irritation on routine basis to monitor for infection. Symptoms of infection include redness, swelling, discharge, pain, hot to touch, and decreased ability to use.
    - Observe for open areas and signs of infection

12. Loss of balance control
    - Allow plenty of time to do activities and procedures to avoid frustration or possible injury
    - Encourage patient to do as much as possible for himself, even though it may take longer
    - Assist patient with ambulation and transfer as needed to avoid injury
    - Provide handrails in bathrooms and hallways

13. Shuffling **gait**
    - Educate that leather-soled shoes may be preferred as other shoes may "stick" to the floor and cause patient to stumble or fall
    - Maintain a wide base of support
    - Concentrate on taking large steps
    - Concentrate on lifting feet off ground completely for each step
    - Concentrate on swinging arms to maintain balance
    - Avoid use of throw rugs to prevent falls
    - Remove doorsills between rooms to avoid tripping

Orthostatic hypotension – results when a person moves from a recumbent to a standing position; also known as postural hypotension

Blood pressure – measurement of the pressure within the arteries of the body as it relates to the contraction (systole) and relaxation (diastole) of the heart

- Remove unnecessary furniture and decorations
- Install handrails for safety

14. Fine motor coordination impairment
    - Provide clothing that has zippers or velcro as opposed to small buttons
    - Avoid clothing that has the opening in the back
    - Encourage patient to do as much as possible for himself, even though it may take longer
    - Provide assistive devices for patient use, e.g. velcro fasteners, elastic shoe closures, long-handled reaching devices for reaching items, bath mitt, electric razor, large-handled eating and cooking utensils, oven mitts when cooking to avoid burns, and handrails in hallways and bathrooms

15. Intense emotions
    - Realize that the patient may not have control over emotions
    - Realize that emotions may be inappropriate for the situation
    - Avoid drawing attention to the patient's intense or inappropriate displays of emotions

16. Fatigue due to constant muscle activity
    - Assist patient with ADLs as necessary
    - Schedule care, activities, and treatment around patient's rest schedule
    - Monitor phone calls and visitors around patient's energy level and rest schedule
    - Encourage frequent rest periods
    - Provide assistance as needed to prevent injury due to weakness
    - Provide method for patient to call for assistance
    - Encourage patient to set realistic goals of activities
    - Allow adequate time to do activities and procedures to avoid frustration or injury
    - Encourage exercise to maintain muscle strength
    - Provide cane or walker for assistance in ambulation and transfer
    - Provide private room for patient to promote rest periods

17. Constipation due to the disease or medications
    - Exercise as able
    - Encourage a high-fiber diet. Foods high in fiber include fruits, vegetables, whole grains, prunes, and beans
    - Encourage fluids, fresh fruits, and vegetables
    - Establish regular bowel program
    - Increase exercise as tolerated
    - Administer enemas, suppositories, stool softeners, and laxatives as prescribed by physician
    - Monitor frequency, number, and consistency of stools
    - Monitor for possible bowel obstruction. Symptoms of bowel obstruction include no stools or diarrhea, bloating, nausea, vomiting, abdominal pain, and fever.
    - Provide privacy for bowel routine

18. **Orthostatic hypotension**
    - Educate patient to get up slowly from a lying position and sit on edge of bed for several minutes prior to standing
    - Monitor **blood pressure** (See Appendix D)

- Provide method for patient to call for assistance as needed
- Respond to call for assistance promptly

19. Insomnia is often related to depression associated with Parkinson's disease
    - Utilize relaxation techniques, music, or other methods to relax patient at bedtime
    - Avoid caffeine an other stimulants prior to bedtime
    - Encourage patient to establish a routine for bedtime to promote relaxation
    - Avoid distractions and noise once the patient is in bed
    - Schedule medications and treatment at times other than bedtime
    - Avoid large meals close to bedtime
    - Exercise at regular intervals throughout the day
    - Avoid sleeping throughout the day as able

20. Weight loss due to frequent movement, tremors, and dysphagia
    - Obtain baseline weight and monitor weight on routine basis
    - Encourage patient to participate in dietary choices
    - Offer nutritional supplements and vitamins
    - Encourage clothing that enhances patient appearance
    - Encourage family and friends to bring in food that is appealing to patient as dietary restrictions allow
    - Administer parenteral fluids as necessary
    - Monitor intake and output (I and O)
    - Encourage rest periods before and after meals
    - Avoid unpleasant sights and odors in room to make meals more appealing
    - Provide meticulous mouth care
    - Monitor for skin breakdown due to loss of body tissue
    - Monitor for symptoms of dehydration, e.g. decreased urine output, constipation, dry skin, tenting of skin, dry mouth, dry eyes, concentrated urine, hypotension, and confusion

21. Urinary difficulties due to rigidity of the bladder muscle
    - Provide the patient opportunity to use the restroom, urinal, or commode on frequent basis
    - Provide night light for patient who needs to urinate during the night
    - Watch for signals that the confused patient needs to urinate
    - Change bedding or briefs frequently and provide meticulous skin care for the patient who may be incontinent
    - Assist the patient to the bathroom as needed
    - Be aware of urinary difficulties when planning treatments or when traveling
    - Provide method for patient to contact staff if assistance is needed
    - Respond promptly to patient requests for assistance

22. Edema of lower extremities due to rigidity of muscles in the legs being unable to circulate fluid back to the heart
    - Avoid constrictive clothing or undergarments
    - Restricted salt diet as prescribed by physician
    - Provide elastic stockings or Jobst stockings to reduce swelling
    - Monitor edema on routine basis

Dementia – diminished or deterioration of mental functioning; confusion

Toxicity – refers to a state of overwhelming poisonous substances in the body

- Encourage patient to elevate edematous extremity above the level of the heart to reduce swelling
- Monitor for skin breakdown in edematous areas
- Monitor for symptoms of decreased circulation in edematous areas, e.g. skin cool to touch, cyanosis, and decreased sensation
- Obtain baseline weight and monitor on routine basis
- Monitor intake and output (I and O)

23. **Dementia** occurs in approximately 30% of patients with Parkinson's disease
    - Label cupboards, doors, and drawers. As the memory fades, resort to pictures if necessary.
    - Display labeled photos of family members
    - Keep a notebook of appointments
    - Place items frequently used in a consistent location
    - Display large calendars and large clocks. Clocks may need to be digital with AM and PM clearly marked.
    - Provide behavior cues to patient as appropriate
    - Avoid situations that could cause embarrassment to the patient while continuing to encourage socialization
    - Avoid situations, like driving, that could cause potential harm to the patient

DIAGNOSIS

1. Symptoms
2. Physical examination
3. Rule out other possible causes of symptoms, e.g. tumors, stroke, depression, and drug **toxicity**, with the use of *CT scans* and *MRI*
4. *Urinalysis* may show decreased dopamine levels

TREATMENT

1. Medications
   - Carbidopa/levodopa (dopamine replacement therapy) is used to treat symptoms; Levodopa is converted to dopamine in the brain; Carbidopa enhances the action of Levodopa as well as decreasing side effects of Levodopa; does not cure the disease, e.g. Sinemet
   - Anticholinergics may be given to counteract the action of acetylcholine in the patient's CNS. Cholinergic pathways are thought to be oversensitive in the presence of dopamine deficiency, e.g. Cogentin, Pagitane, Kemadrin.
   - Antihistamine compounds may be helpful in treating tremors, e.g. Benadryl
   - Antidepressants may be helpful in treating depression, e.g. Elavil
   - Antiviral medications may increase the release of dopamine in the brain while decreasing production of acetylcholine, e.g. Symmetrel
2. Exercise—continue exercise program on a daily basis
3. Therapy
   - Physical therapy will assist the patient with ambulation and maintain strength
   - Speech therapy to assist with speech and swallowing difficulties
   - Occupational therapy will help to maintain hand coordination and dexterity

Thalamotomy – surgical removal or destruction of all or part of the thalamus

Thalamus – the portion of the brain that receives sensory input

Ultrasound – sound-wave visualization of organs and tissues of the body as the sound waves "bounce off" the various tissues and organs of the body and are recorded

4. Surgical intervention

- Fetal cell transplants by replacing the diseased dopamine-releasing cells in the striatum of the patient with cells obtained from 6- to 11-week-old fetuses. These cells are injected into the brain of the patient in a liquid suspension.

- Transplantation of dopamine-secreting cells from patient's own adrenal glands into the brain

- **Thalamotomy**—ventrolateral nucleus of the **thalamus** is destroyed with the use of **ultrasound**, freezing, or *radiation*, which prevents involuntary movements. The function of the thalamus is to receive and react to sensory stimuli.

CONSIDERATIONS FOR CARE

1. Educate patient and family regarding the disease process.

2. Educate patient and family regarding forms of treatment as well as side effects of medications.

3. Provide emotional support to patient and family.

4. Provide nonjudgmental acceptance of emotions and behavior of patient and family.

5. Encourage proper nutrition. Educate that protein interferes with the absorption of Sinemet and may be reduced in the diet according to physician recommendations.

6. Family members need to offer encouragement to the patient to do as much as possible for himself.

7. Patient may be more apt to exercise if family and friends exercise with him.

8. Educate family that they may experience normal feelings of anger, resentment, or fear.

9. Recommend a support group for patient and family.

10. Counseling may be necessary for patient and family to work through emotions associated with the disease.

11. Weigh patient on a routine basis and encourage to maintain as there is a tendency for patients to lose weight due to constant muscle movement.

12. Family and friends should be available to help but should not encourage dependence.

13. Depression may develop as a result of the patient being unable to provide financially, contribute to responsibilities in the home, and other responsibilities previously held by the patient.

14. Educate patient and family that even though the patient has muscle involvement, the mental capacity generally remains unimpaired.

15. Educate patient and family regarding the importance of taking medications at the scheduled time.

16. Educate patient and family regarding importance of follow-up care with physician.

17. For patients with decreased mobility, stress the importance of observing for and preventing skin breakdown.

- Signs of skin breakdown (decubitus ulcers) include: redness, swelling, warm or hot to touch, open sores, cyanosis, pain, and blisters.

- Prevention measures include: frequent repositioning (minimum of every 1 to 2 hours); meticulous skin care; massaging areas at bony prominences;

encouraging activity as able; alternating pressure mattresses; preventing pressure from appliances or tubing; prevent friction when repositioning by using a lift sheet and adequate assistance; and linens must be clean, dry, and wrinkle-free.

18. Medical alert card and medical bracelet or necklace should be obtained and worn or carried at all times.

19. Stress that approximately 90% of all clients with Parkinson's disease are able to continue living in their own home.

20. Meticulous mouth and dental care are required due to saliva pooling in the mouth and difficulty of self-care.

21. Soap-on-a-rope may be used for bathing to reduce the need to stoop to pick up dropped soap or the need to retrieve after placing in the soap dish.

FOR MORE INFORMATION

National Parkinson Foundation Hotline
1-800-327-4545

American Parkinson Disease Association
Suite 401
60 Bay Street
Staten Island, NY 10301

National Parkinson Foundation, Inc.
1501 NW Ninth Avenue
Bob Hope Road
Miami, FL 33136
(305) 547-6666

Parkinson's Disease Foundation
William Black Medical Research Building
650 West 168th Street
New York, NY 10032
(800) 457-6676

Institute of Rehabilitation Medicine
New York University
(212) 340-7300*

---

* Call to obtain catalog containing garments for clients with disabilities.

ASSIGNMENT SHEET: PARKINSON'S DISEASE

Short Answer

1. Write a brief definition for the terms listed throughout the chapter.

2. Write a brief definition for Parkinson's disease.

3. Describe the incidence of Parkinson's disease.

4. List six (6) possible risk factors of Parkinson's disease.

5. List twenty-three (23) symptoms associated with Parkinson's disease and associated care for each symptom.

6. List and describe four (4) specific methods used in the diagnosis of Parkinson's disease.

7. List and describe four (4) specific methods used in the treatment of Parkinson's disease.

8. List twenty-one (21) considerations for caring for a patient with Parkinson's disease.

9. Describe the following procedures used in the diagnosis or treatment of Parkinson's disease.
   a. CT scan
   b. MRI
   c. Urinalysis
   d. Fetal cell transplant
   e. Ultrasound
   f. Radiation therapy

KNOWLEDGE INTO ACTION

1. Peter Danning, a 72-year-old with a history of Parkinson's disease, comes to your clinic with complaints of "skin problems." The physician diagnoses Mr. Danning as having seborrhea. How could the physician describe the cause of seborrhea to Mr. Danning? What are methods of associated care for the seborrhea?

2. As a home health nurse, you are assigned to Mr. Danning. Mr. Danning has a shuffling gait. What suggestions could you make to Mr. Danning regarding precautions to take to prevent injury in the home due to his shuffling gait?

3. While you are in Mr. Danning's home, he says to you, "Things aren't as easy as they used to be. I can't get dressed like I used to. I'm all thumbs when I do anything in the kitchen." What will your response be regarding assistive devices Mr. Danning could use?

4. Angie Preston, a 66-year-old with a history of Parkinson's disease, is in your facility. She says to you, "I get so dizzy when I stand up." What will your response be regarding the possible cause of her dizziness? Which of her vital signs could you check to help determine the cause of her dizziness?

5. Erika Belez, a 71-year-old with a history of Parkinson's disease, is a resident in your long-term care facility. She has lost 25 pounds over the past year. What methods of associated care could be utilized to help her gain or maintain her weight?

6. Eloise Lunde, a 61-year-old female, comes to your clinic with tremor, cogwheel movements, fatigue, and constipation. Her physician suspects Parkinson's disease. What methods of diagnosis could be used to rule out other diseases and also help to determine an accurate diagnosis of Parkinson's disease?

7. Mrs. Lunde's physician determines that she does have Parkinson's disease. List and describe two types of medications that could be used in the treatment of Mrs. Lunde's Parkinson's disease. List and describe two forms of treatment, other than medications, that could be used to treat Mrs. Lunde's Parkinson's disease.

8. Ronald McCrain, a 68-year-old male with a history of Parkinson's disease, is in your facility. During morning report, the night shift nurse reports that Mr. McCrain is developing a decubitus ulcer. What symptoms could Mr. McCrain have that would lead the nurse to report this? What methods of associated care could be used to treat the decubitus ulcer and prevent it from becoming worse?

Rheumatoid Arthritis

OBJECTIVES

Upon completion of this chapter, the student should be able to:

- Define the key terms listed throughout the chapter
- Describe the physiology of a joint
- State a specific definition for rheumatoid arthritis
- Describe the incidence of rheumatoid arthritis
- List the risk factors for rheumatoid arthritis
- Describe the signs and symptoms of rheumatoid arthritis and associated care
- Identify specific methods for diagnosis of rheumatoid arthritis
- Identify specific methods for treatment of rheumatoid arthritis
- Describe considerations for caring for a patient with rheumatoid arthritis

KEY TERMS

Inflammation – localized response to injury; symptoms may include redness, swelling, pain, or increased local temperature

Bilateral – refers to both sides, generally of the body

Synovium – synovial membrane

Synovitis – inflammation of the synovial membrane

Pannus – tissue covering a surface of the body

Joint – the place where two bones meet

Cartilage – fibrous connective tissues that make up the nasal septum, external portion of the ear, eustachian tube, trachea, cushion between the vertebrae, and portions of the ribs

Synovial membrane – lining of the synovial (joint) capsule

INTRODUCTION

Arthritis refers to the more than 100 diseases that involve **inflammation** of one or more joints. Rheumatoid arthritis is characterized by inflammation of the joints, commonly in the hands, feet, and other connective tissues in the body. Other joints of the body that are commonly involved are the hips, shoulders, knees, elbows, neck, jaw, and ankles. There is usually **bilateral** involvement of the joints. The joint lining (**synovium**) becomes inflamed (**synovitis**). The inflammation then spreads to the other tissues of the joints. The inflamed tissue eventually causes damage which may change the shape of the joints. The disease is also characterized by the formation of **pannus**, which are inflammatory cells that form a growth at the joint, eroding the cartilage surface of the joint and eventually eroding the bone itself. Movement becomes painful and limited due to the involvement of the ligaments and tendons. Any organ or system of the body can be involved by this disease. Rheumatoid arthritis is a chronic disease, which is characterized by exacerbations and remissions.

PHYSIOLOGY OF JOINTS

A **joint** is a place in the body where two bones meet. The ends of the bones are covered by **cartilage**. Cartilage is a tough, elastic tissue that protects the ends of the bones by absorbing shocks and preventing the bones from rubbing together. The joints are enclosed in a capsule called the **synovial membrane**, which releases **synovial fluid** into the space between the bones. The synovial fluid lubricates the joint for smooth, easy movement and also provides nourishment to the cartilage.

Outside the joint space are muscles, **tendons**, and **ligaments**. Tendons "tie" muscles to bone, and ligaments "link" bones together. These help to support the joints as well as assist in skeletal movement. **Bursae** are fluid-filled sacs that are located near the joints and help to keep the muscles, bones, ligaments and tendons moving smoothly against each other. (See Figure 17-1.)

Synovial fluid – fluid that is secreted by the synovial membrane; located in bursae and cavities of joints; functions to protect and lubricate joints

Tendon – fibrous tissue that connects muscles to bones

Ligament – connective tissue that connects bones to one another

Bursa (plural: **bursae**) – fluid-filled sac located at the joints of the body; purpose is to reduce the friction at the site of the joint

Pathogen – disease-producing substance

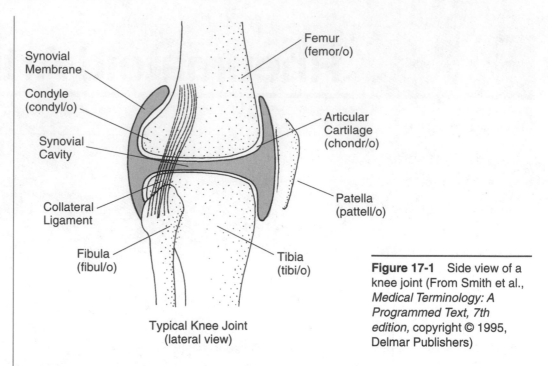

Synovial Membrane

Condyle (condyl/o)

Synovial Cavity

Collateral Ligament

Fibula (fibul/o)

Femur (femor/o)

Articular Cartilage (chondr/o)

Patella (pattell/o)

Tibia (tibi/o)

Typical Knee Joint
(lateral view)

Figure 17-1 Side view of a knee joint (From Smith et al., *Medical Terminology: A Programmed Text, 7th edition,* copyright © 1995, Delmar Publishers)

STATISTICS

More than 2,500,000 people in the United States are affected by rheumatoid arthritis, with women affected 2.5 to 3 times more often than men. Approximately 1 to 3% of the adult population in the United States has rheumatoid arthritis. The total cost for health care for all forms of arthritis is in excess of $35 billion annually in the United States.

RISK FACTORS

The exact cause of rheumatoid arthritis is unknown. The following are several of the risk factors.

1. A genetic susceptibility has been shown. A genetic marker called HLA-DR4 has been associated with rheumatoid arthritis. This genetic marker occurs in approximately 25% of the total population but is present in 75% of people with rheumatoid arthritis.

2. An autoimmune reaction has been suggested as part of the cause of rheumatoid arthritis. The immune system is necessary to protect the body from disease. However, instead of fighting disease, the immune system may attack the body, especially the joints.

3. Emotional stress has been shown to cause exacerbations of the symptoms of rheumatoid arthritis. In most patients, when stress decreases, the symptoms decrease as well.

4. Infection in the joint may be caused by virus or other **pathogens**.

SIGNS, SYMPTOMS, AND ASSOCIATED CARE

Symptoms may exacerbate due to physical injury, emotional stress, physical stress, or injury to a joint.

1. Joint pain, swelling, warmth, and tenderness due to inflammation of the synovium

- Offer heat or other methods of pain control, such as massage, relaxation, and imaging
- Administer medications as prescribed by physician for pain control
- Monitor level of comfort
- Protect and immobilize joints and decrease weight bearing
- Assist with activities of daily living (ADLs) as necessary due to pain
- Assist with position for patient comfort
- Encourage patient to keep as active as possible
- Facilitate frequent rest periods to provide joint rest and pain relief
- Offer warm, moist packs for the relief of pain
- Allow adequate time to do as much as possible for themselves, even though it may take longer
- Use pillows to support extremities

2. Fatigue
   - Assist patient with ADLs as necessary
   - Schedule care, activities, and treatment around patient's rest schedule
   - Monitor phone calls and visitors around patient's energy level and rest schedule
   - Encourage frequent rest periods
   - Provide assistance as needed to prevent injury due to weakness
   - Provide method for patient to call for assistance
   - Encourage patient to set realistic goals of activities
   - Allow adequate time to do activities and procedures to avoid frustration or possible injury
   - Encourage exercise to maintain muscle strength
   - Provide cane or walker for ambulation and transfer
   - Provide private room to promote rest periods

3. Weight loss
   - Obtain baseline weight and routinely monitor weight
   - Encourage patient to participate in dietary choices
   - Offer nutritional supplements and vitamins
   - Encourage clothing that enhances patient appearance
   - Encourage family and friends to bring in food that is appealing to patient as dietary restrictions allow
   - Administer parenteral fluids as necessary
   - Monitor intake and output (I and O)
   - Encourage rest periods before and after meals
   - Avoid unpleasant sights and odors in room to make meals more appealing
   - Provide meticulous mouth care
   - Monitor for skin breakdown due to loss of body tissue
   - Monitor for symptoms of dehydration, e.g. decreased urine output, constipation, dry skin, tenting of skin, dry mouth, dry eyes, concentrated urine, hypotension, and confusion

4. Loss of appetite (anorexia)
   - Obtain baseline weight and routinely monitor
   - Offer small, frequent meals as tolerated
   - Encourage patient to participate in dietary choices

Nodule – refers to a node or a swelling of a specific location on the body

Immobility – inability or a decrease in the ability to be mobile (movement)

- Provide nutritional supplements and vitamins
- Monitor for signs of dehydration, such as decreased urine output, concentrated urine, dry skin, tenting of skin, dry mucous membranes, dry mouth, dry eyes, confusion, and constipation
- Encourage family and friends to bring in food that is appealing to patient as dietary restrictions allow
- Administer parenteral fluids as necessary
- Monitor intake and output (I and O)
- Encourage fluids to prevent dehydration
- Avoid unpleasant sights and odors in the room to make meals more appealing
- Provide meticulous mouth care
- Maintain social atmosphere for mealtimes to encourage the patient to eat
- Encourage clothing that enhances patient appearance
- Encourage exercise program as tolerated to increase appetite

5. Anemia
   - Administer blood transfusions and iron supplements as necessary to treat anemia
   - Monitor *hemoglobin* and *hematocrit*
   - Monitor for weakness associated with anemia, assist with ADLs as necessary due to weakness, and protect from possible injury due to weakness
   - Monitor for physical symptoms of anemia, such as pallor, weakness, and vertigo

6. Lumps (**nodules**) under the skin, especially on the backs of the elbows
   - Provide meticulous skin care
   - Prevent skin breakdown. Signs of skin breakdown (decubitus ulcers) include redness, swelling, warm or hot to touch, open sores, cyanosis, pain, and blisters. Prevention measures include frequent repositioning (minimum of every 1 to 2 hours); meticulous skin care; massage areas at bony prominences; encourage activity as able; alternating pressure mattresses; prevent pressure from appliances or tubing; prevent friction when repositioning by using a lift sheet and adequate assistance; and linens must be clean, dry, and wrinkle-free.

7. Muscle stiffness after **immobility** that eases with activity
   - Encourage exercise at routine intervals throughout the day
   - Avoid long periods of immobility throughout the day
   - Encourage frequent stretch breaks if traveling long distances
   - Avoid injury to muscles by overexertion after rest periods
   - Avoid injury due to muscles stiffness after immobility

8. Low-grade fever
   - Monitor temperature at routine intervals
   - Provide comfort measures for patient with elevated temperature, such as cool cloth to forehead, partial or complete bath as needed, clothing and bedding changed frequently due to diaphoresis, and encourage fluids to prevent dehydration
   - Avoid exposing patient to a draft
   - Cover with blankets as necessary
   - Monitor intake and output (I and O)

Pleura – membrane that encloses the lung

Scleritis – inflammation of the sclera (fibrous tissue that covers the "white of the eye")

Arteritis – Inflammation of an artery of the body

Range of motion (ROM)– exercises during which each of the joints of the body is put through its entire range of movements; generally done when a patient is immobile to prevent the formation of contractures, decubitus ulcers, and other complications that may occur as a result of immobility

- Maintain comfortable room temperature for patient
- Avoid plastic mattresses and plastic bed protectors that increase perspiration
- Use antiperspirant or deodorant to minimize sweating and odor

9. Reddened palms
   - Protect hands from injury in the presence of decreased sensation
   - Avoid irritating the palms of the hands with scented soaps and lotions

10. Pleurisy due to inflammation of the **pleura**
    - Monitor for signs of hypoxia, e.g. cyanosis, diaphoresis, decreased level of consciousness, and confusion
    - Administer medications as directed for pain relief
    - Offer heating pad or other form of heat treatment as directed for pain relief
    - Observe for complications relating to pain, such as insomnia, decreased appetite, and mood changes
    - Offer alternative methods of pain relief, such as relaxation techniques, imaging, and massage
    - Facilitate rest periods as necessary
    - Monitor for increased respiratory distress

11. **Scleritis** due to inflammation of the tear glands
    - Prevent further irritation by refraining from wearing eye makeup and rubbing eyes
    - Encourage alternate activities for patient who has difficulty with reading
    - Avoid eye strain
    - Avoid injury to the client due to visual disturbances
    - Facilitate evaluation by an ophthalmologist
    - Provide adequate lighting when reading, watching TV, or other activities

12. **Arteritis**
    - Monitor for symptoms of arteritis, e.g. headache, decreased vision, and pain over the area of the affected artery

13. Ankle edema
    - Avoid constrictive clothing or undergarments
    - Restrict salt in diet as prescribed by physician. Foods that are high in sodium and should be avoided include processed foods, cured meats, salted chips and crackers, pickles, and table salt.
    - Utilize elastic stockings or Jobst stockings to reduce swelling
    - Monitor edema on a routine basis
    - Encourage patient to elevate edematous extremity above the level of the heart to reduce swelling
    - Monitor for skin breakdown and decreased circulation in edematous areas, e.g. skin cool to touch, cyanosis, and decreased sensation
    - Obtain baseline weight and monitor on routine basis
    - Monitor intake and output (I and O)

14. Muscle spasms
    - Provide **range of motion (ROM)** and exercise as directed by the physician and physical therapist
    - Provide proper alignment

Pericarditis –
inflammation of the sac
around the heart

Neuropathy – refers to a
disease of the nerves

Carpal tunnel syndrome
– pain, numbness, and
loss of function of the
thumb and first two or
three fingers of the hand
due to pressure or injury
to the nerve in the wrist;
often caused by frequent,
repetitive movements

- Change patient position at least every 2 hours with proper support of joints and extremities. Patient should be on the unaffected side when in the side-lying position.
- Provide relaxation techniques
- Offer heat or other methods of pain control, such as massage, relaxation, and imaging
- Administer medications as prescribed by physician for pain control
- Monitor level of comfort

15. **Pericarditis**
   - Monitor for symptoms of pericarditis, e.g. fever, chest pain, dyspnea, irregular or rapid pulse, and presence of murmur
   - Monitor vital signs (See Appendix D)
   - Monitor heart rate and rhythm through the use of a heart monitor

16. Lymphadenopathy
   - Monitor for lymphadenopathy
   - Comfort measures as necessary due to lymphadenopathy

17. Splenomegaly
   - Monitor for splenomegaly
   - Avoid abdominal injury in the presence of splenomegaly
   - Monitor for signs of internal bleeding in the presence of splenomegaly, such as abdominal pain, tachycardia, hypotension, and abdominal distention
   - Monitor hemoglobin and hematocrit

18. **Neuropathy**
   - Facilitate rest to decrease strain
   - Decrease weight-bearing to painful extremities
   - Provide heat or other methods of pain control, such as massage, relaxation techniques, distraction, and medications
   - Encourage patient to request pain control methods prior to having pain become too severe

19. Fingers become spindle-shaped due to edema in the joints
   - Facilitate alternative methods of doing activities if difficulty due to finger shape

20. **Carpal tunnel syndrome** due to synovial pressure
   - Educate client regarding the use of a splint and assist in applying as necessary
   - Avoid repetitive movements with the hands and arms

DIAGNOSIS

1. Symptoms
2. Physical examination
3. *Rheumatoid factor* is present in 75 to 80% of people with rheumatoid arthritis
4. *Antinuclear antibodies* are present in 25% of people with rheumatoid arthritis
5. Elevated *ESR* is present in 85 to 90% of patients
6. Joint x-ray may appear normal in the early stages of the disease
7. *Bone scan* to show joint inflammation
8. Decreased *RBC*, elevated *WBC*

Gout – disease that causes inflammation of the joint(s) due to an accumulation of uric acid

Salicylate – salt of salicylic acid, which, in the form of acetylsalicylic acid, is used as an analgesic (aspirin)

Nonsteroidal anti-inflammatory drugs (NSAID) – medications that decrease inflammation, relieve pain, and reduce fever

Diabetes mellitus – disease in which the body is unable to break down and use carbohydrates for energy due to the lack of insulin or the inability of the body to use insulin adequately

Cataract – visual impairment caused by an opacity (cloudiness) of the lens of the eye

Orally – taken by mouth

Analgesic – substance taken to reduce or relieve pain

9. *Biopsy* of rheumatoid nodule to distinguish between rheumatoid arthritis and **gout**

10. *Joint aspiration* to rule out other diseases

11. *Arthroscopy* to examine the lining of the joint

TREATMENT

The goals of treatment are to reduce inflammation, relieve pain, prevent damage to the joints, prevent joint deformity, and keep joints functioning properly. Specific examples of treatment include the following.

1. Rest; too much exercise can lead to inflammation and pain while too much rest may lead to poorly moving joints and stiffness. It is generally recommended to increase rest periods during periods of increased symptoms and exercise during periods when symptoms subside.

2. Medications

   • Aspirin relieves pain and reduces inflammation. Aspirin is a **salicylate**, and a patient who takes large doses of aspirin for rheumatoid arthritis should have periodic *serum salicylate levels* drawn.

   • **Nonsteroidal anti-inflammatory drugs (NSAID)** are used to reduce joint swelling, reduce inflammation, and reduce pain and stiffness. NSAID are usually more expensive than aspirin but tend to produce fewer side effects, e.g. Ibuprofen, Naprosyn, Nalfon, Indocin, Clinoril.

   • Corticosteroids reduce joint inflammation. These medications are used if the symptoms of rheumatoid arthritis cannot be controlled with aspirin or other drugs. Corticosteroids can cause serious side effects, such as thinning of bones (osteoporosis), weight gain, **diabetes mellitus**, emotional problems, decreased resistance to disease, hypertension, and **cataracts**, e.g. Hydrocortisone, Prednisone, Methylprednisolone.

   • Corticosteroid injections are injected directly into the joints and are used to relieve pain. They have less side effects than corticosteroids taken orally.

   • Gold treatments are used when traditional medications have failed to control symptoms of rheumatoid arthritis. Gold can be given **orally** or in the form of an injection. It may take several months of medication before the effects can be noticed.

   • Penicillamine is also reserved for people who have not responded well to other forms of treatment. It may take several months of medications before the effects can be noticed.

   • Antimalarial drugs can also be used to reduce the symptoms of rheumatoid arthritis when other methods have failed. Use of this medication can lead to serious eye damage, and regular eye examinations are necessary.

   • Immunosuppressive drugs have been used to decrease the inflammatory process caused by the body's immune system. In addition to serious side effects, these medications can also increase the risk of certain types of cancer, e.g. Imuran, Cytoxan.

   • Medications may also be taken for treatment of anemia, e.g. iron, which may accompany rheumatoid arthritis

   • **Analgesic** medications in conjunction with medications to control the symptoms of arthritis

Transcutaneous electrical nerve stimulation (TENS) – transmission of an electrical stimulus over the body to the area of pain that interferes with pain sensation and transmission

Synovectomy – surgical removal of synovial membrane

Arthroplasty – surgical repair or reconstruction of a joint

3. Pain control methods that include visualization techniques, relaxation techniques, hypnosis or self-hypnosis, **transcutaneous electrical nerve stimulation (TENS)** units, and massage

4. Exercise is important to keep joints flexible, build muscle strength, improve circulation, and protect joints from further stresses

5. Joint protection

- Canes, walkers, and crutches are used to decrease the amount of weight-bearing on individual joints
- Splints are used primarily at night but may also be used during the day to rest joints and hold them in proper position
- Use more than one joint/muscle group to do work when able. Examples of this include using your body or whole arm to open a door rather than just one hand or using both arms to lift an object rather than carrying it in just one hand.
- Maintain weight within normal limits to decrease stress on joints
- Braces and splints are used to protect joints from overuse and injury, as well as to provide rest, immobilization, and correct alignment for joints
- Use large muscle groups for lifting
- Use alternative methods for ADLs that cause less joint strain
- Avoid activities that cause impact to joints
- Maintain correct posture

6. Surgery (See Figure 17-2)

- Surgery may be done to remove the damaged tissue which reduces pain and increases joint mobility (*synovectomy*)
- Replace or repair damaged joints with man-made joints (*arthroplasty*)

7. Heat and/or cold applications

- Heat is used to relax muscles and decrease pain due to joint inflammation. Examples include heat pads, heat lamps, warm moist compresses, and paraffin wax dips.
- Cold treatments are used to relieve pain in some people. Examples include ice packs or cold compresses.

8. Self-help aids include long-handled combs, shoehorns, and kitchen utensils; heightened chairs and toilet seats, clothing with velcro, mittens instead of gloves, hand-held shower nozzle, and palm-held brush

CONSIDERATIONS FOR CARE

1. Educate patient and family on the disease process and forms of treatment.
2. Instruct patient on the importance of weight control to decrease stress on joints.
3. Emotional support for the patient and family.
4. Coping strategies may be necessary to address changes in appearance due to weight loss or joint deformity.
5. Offer options for alternative leisuretime activities due to physical limitations.
6. Counseling may be necessary for the emotional stresses placed upon the patient.
7. Be aware that the patient may experience stress and depression due to pain; offer emotional support and counseling options.

Prone – positioned on the abdomen

Flexion – bending

Contracture – permanent shortening of a muscle often related to immobility

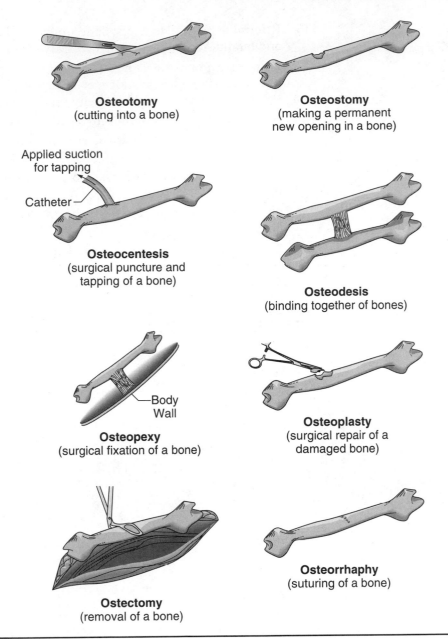

Figure 17-2   Surgical procedures involving bones (From Layman, *The Medical Language*, copyright © 1995, Delmar Publishers)

8. Vocational changes may need to be made due to limitations placed upon the person by the symptoms of the disease.

9. Offer resources that would assist the person due to financial burdens placed upon the patient and family due to medical expenses, job difficulties, or home changes.

10. Assist with ADLs due to limitations from stiffness, pain, deformity, and fatigue.

11. Schedule care, treatment, and activities around rest periods.

12. Monitor visitors to promote rest.

13. Patient should lie in a **prone** position twice daily to prevent hip **flexion** and knee **contractures**.

14. Specially designed shoes or shoe inserts may be needed to decrease stress on feet and ankle joints.

15. Encourage correct posture and instruct regarding body mechanics.

16. Referral to physical therapist or occupational therapist to assist with exercises and modifications that may be necessary.

17. Encourage proper nutrition, especially foods high in protein and calcium. Foods high in protein include meats, fish, milk, cheese, soybeans, and eggs. Foods high in calcium include dairy products and green leafy vegetables.

18. A positive but realistic approach to patient care is encouraged.

19. Allow patient as much control as possible while in the hospital as well as at home.

20. Assess level of pain and offer comfort measures as available.

21. Physical therapy and occupational therapy consults to assist client in planning an exercise program, using splints, and variations and adaptations for performing ADLs.

22. Alcohol should be consumed in limited amounts only in conjunction with aspirin and NSAIDs. Alcohol should *not* be consumed by clients taking methotrexate due to possible liver damage.

FOR MORE INFORMATION

Arthritis Foundation
1314 Spring Street, NW
Atlanta, GA 30309
(404) 872-7100

CHAPTER 17 REVIEW

ASSIGNMENT SHEET: RHEUMATOID ARTHRITIS

Short Answer

1. Write a brief definition for the terms listed throughout the chapter.

2. Describe the physiology of joints.

3. Write a brief definition for rheumatoid arthritis.

4. Describe four (4) risk factors for rheumatoid arthritis.

5. Describe the incidence of rheumatoid arthritis.

6. List twenty (20) signs and symptoms of rheumatoid arthritis and associated care.

7. Describe eleven (11) specific methods used to diagnose rheumatoid arthritis.

8. Describe the following diagnostic tests used in the diagnosis of rheumatoid arthritis.
   a. Bone scan
   b. Biopsy
   c. Joint aspiration
   d. Arthroscopy
   e. Synovectomy
   f. Arthroplasty

9. Describe the five (5) goals for treatment of rheumatoid arthritis.

10. Describe eight (8) specific methods for treatment of rheumatoid arthritis.

11. Describe the specific benefits from each of the following medications used for the treatment of rheumatoid arthritis.
    a. Aspirin
    b. NSAID
    c. Corticosteroids
    d. Corticosteroid injections
    e. Gold treatment
    f. Penicillamine
    g. Antimalarial
    h. Immunosuppressive

12. List twenty-two (22) considerations for caring for a patient with rheumatoid arthritis.

13. Write the normal ranges for each of the following laboratory tests.
    a. ESR
    b. Hemoglobin
    c. Hematocrit
    d. Rheumatoid factor
    e. Antinuclear antibodies
    f. Red blood cell count (RBC)
    g. White blood cell count (WBC)
    h. Salicylate level

KNOWLEDGE INTO ACTION

1. Natasha Kanaranze, a 57-year-old production worker, comes to your clinic to check her rheumatoid arthritis. You notice that her weight has increased 8 pounds since her visit 3 months ago and her ankles are swollen. What is the medical term for this accumulation of fluid in Ms. Kanaranze's ankles? What methods of associated care could be utilized to decrease the swelling and prevent complications?

2. Charles Lanning is a 58-year-old mine worker with a history of rheumatoid arthritis. He is admitted to your facility to regulate his medications due to an increase in joint pain and muscle spasms. Mr. Lanning's physician writes an order that states, "Range of motion to be performed by physical therapy twice daily." As the physical therapist, briefly describe what you would do in response to this order.

3. Alfred Johanson, a 36-year-old meat cutter, comes to your clinic. He has a history of rheumatoid arthritis. Today, he complains of increased pain and numbness to his right hand, especially his thumb and first two fingers. The pain also shoots up into his right arm. Keeping in mind the repetitive movements often associated with Mr. Johanson's occupation, as well as his symptoms, what could an initial diagnosis be that would explain the symptoms? Circle the best answer.
   a. Synovectomy
   b. Carpal tunnel syndrome
   c. Lymphadenopathy
   d. Pleuritis

4. You are studying with a friend for your test on rheumatoid arthritis. Your friend asks you to list five possible methods of diagnosis for rheumatoid arthritis and describe each of the methods. What will your response be?

5. Joyce Benfield, a 48-year-old day-care provider, comes to your clinic to have a checkup for her rheumatoid arthritis. She has been on aspirin for the past 2 years to control her joint pain. She states that recently the aspirin does not control her pain effectively and has begun to cause stomach upset. What are some other medications that could be used to control the symptoms associated with rheumatoid arthritis other than the aspirin?

6. Mrs. Benfield's physician tells her she needs to increase her intake of protein and calcium. She asks you for suggestions of foods high in protein and calcium. What will your response be?

Osteoarthritis

OBJECTIVES

Upon completion of this chapter, the student should be able to:

■ Define the key terms listed throughout the chapter

■ Describe the physiology of joints

■ State a specific definition for osteoarthritis

■ Describe the incidence of osteoarthritis

■ List the risk factors for osteoarthritis

■ List the signs and symptoms of osteoarthritis and associated care for these symptoms

■ Identify specific methods for diagnosis of osteoarthritis

■ Identify specific methods for treatment of osteoarthritis

■ Describe specific considerations for caring for a person with osteoarthritis

KEY TERMS

Spur – hard, bonelike growth located on the bone at the joint; common in arthritis

INTRODUCTION

Osteoarthritis is a chronic form of arthritis that causes pain, stiffness, and loss of joint mobility. It is thought to develop primarily from the general wear and tear on the joints. The joints most often affected are the weight-bearing joints of the hands, feet, hips, spine, and knees. The cartilage responsible for protecting the bones of the joints from rubbing together becomes worn away, allowing the bones to rub together. In addition to cartilage being worn away, the bone ends form growths called **spurs**.

PHYSIOLOGY OF JOINTS

A joint is a place in the body where two bones meet. The ends of the bones are covered by cartilage. Cartilage is a tough, elastic tissue that protects the ends of the bones by absorbing shocks and preventing the bones from rubbing together. The joints are enclosed in a capsule called the synovial membrane, which releases synovial fluid into the space between the bones. The synovial fluid lubricates the joint for smooth, easy movement and provides nourishment to the cartilage. (See Figure 18-1.)

Outside the joint space are muscles, tendons, and ligaments. Note that tendons "tie" muscles to bone, and ligaments "link" bones together. These help support the joints and assist in skeletal movement. Bursae are fluid-filled sacs that are located near the joints and help keep the muscles, bones, ligaments, and tendons moving smoothly against each other.

STATISTICS

Osteoarthritis is the most common form of arthritis with 16 million people in the United States affected, of which 11.7 million are female. The disease mainly affects people 25 to 75 years old. The symptoms are generally apparent after the age of 40. (See Table 18-1.)

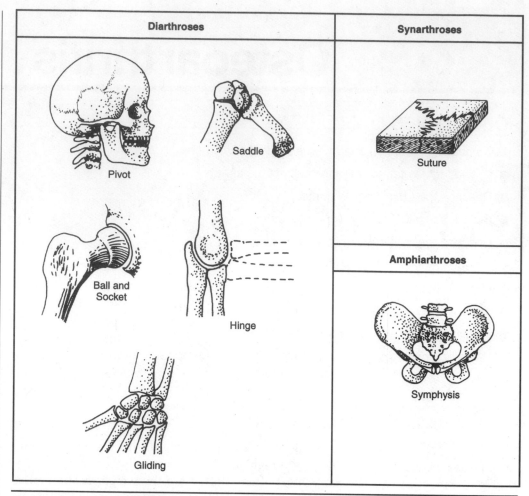

Figure 18-1 Types of joints (From Burke, *Human Anatomy and Physiology in Health and Disease, 3rd edition,* copyright © 1992, Delmar Publishers)

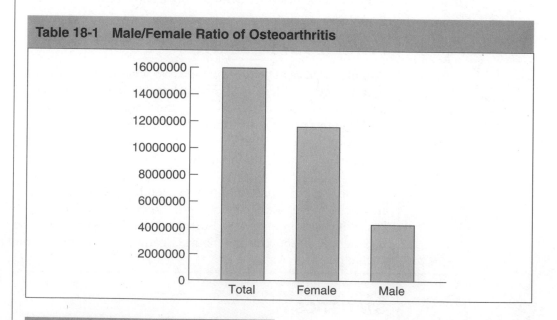

Table 18-1 Male/Female Ratio of Osteoarthritis

RISK FACTORS

1. Heredity
2. Joint trauma
3. Obesity

Malalignment – displaced alignment; refers frequently to the bones or teeth

Crepitus – grating sound heard with the movement of a joint

4. Aging
5. **Malalignment** of joints
6. Excessive stress on joints

SIGNS, SYMPTOMS, AND ASSOCIATED CARE

The symptoms of osteoarthritis increase with obesity, poor posture, and mechanical stress on the body.

1. Arthralgia
   - Offer heat or other methods of pain control, such as massage, relaxation, and imaging
   - Administer medications as prescribed by physician for pain control
   - Protect joints, immobilize joints, and decrease weight-bearing as able
   - Assist with activities of daily living (ADLs) as necessary due to pain
   - Assist with position for patient comfort
   - Encourage patient to keep as active as possible
   - Facilitate frequent rest periods to provide joint rest and pain relief
   - Offer warm, moist packs for the relief of pain
   - Allow adequate time to do as much as possible for themselves, even though it may take longer
   - Use pillows to support extremities
2. Joint stiffness in mornings and after exercise
   - Encourage to do stretching exercises and increase activity gradually in the mornings
   - Encourage frequent rest periods throughout the day and especially after exercise
   - Schedule activities, care, and treatment around periods when patient's stiffness is at a minimum
3. Enlargement of joints
   - Prevent pressure, which could result in skin breakdown, on enlarged joints
4. Joint pain caused by changes in the weather
   - Administer pain control methods and medications as prescribed by a physician
   - Protect joints, immobilize joints, and decrease weight-bearing
   - Assess for level of comfort and offer pain control methods
5. Grating joints (**crepitus**)
   - Reassure patient that this is a normal symptom of the disease
6. Decreased mobility
   - Encourage exercise and activity as able
   - Assist with ADLs as needed due to decreased mobility
   - Offer self-help aids as desired by patient
   - Encourage patient to develop compensatory measures for activities
   - Prevent skin breakdown for patients with decreased mobility. Signs of skin breakdown (decubitus ulcers) include redness, swelling, warm or hot to touch, open sores, cyanosis, pain, and blisters. Prevention measures include frequent repositioning (minimum of every 1 to 2 hours); meticulous skin care; massage areas at bony prominences; encourage activity as able; alternating pressure mattresses; prevent pressure from appliances or tubing; prevent friction when repositioning by using a lift sheet and adequate assistance; and linens must be clean, dry, and wrinkle-free.

Heberden's nodes – nodules located on the joints of the fingers; present with osteoarthritis

Bouchard's nodes – nodes that appear in the middle joints of the fingers, which are characteristic of osteoarthritis

Fusion – join or grow together

Joint aspiration – removal of fluid from the space around a joint

Arthrodesis – surgical fusion of a joint causing immobilization of that joint

Osteoplasty – surgical repair of a bone

Osteotomy – refers to surgically cutting into a bone

7. **Heberden's nodes** (spurs) and **Bouchard's nodes** on finger joints
   - Administer pain control methods and medications as prescribed by physician

DIAGNOSIS

1. Symptoms
2. Physical examination
3. *X-ray* shows joint deformity, narrowed joint spaces, spur formation, and eventually **fusion** of the joint
4. Blood tests and *joint aspiration* are useful in ruling out other disorders

TREATMENT

The goal of treatment is to reduce joint destruction, relieve pain, decrease inflammation, and improve joint mobility.

1. Medications
   - Aspirin is used to relieve pain and reduce inflammation. Aspirin is a salicylate and periodic *salicylate levels* should be determined for a patient taking large doses of aspirin.
   - Nonsteroidal anti-inflammatory drugs (NSAID) relieve pain and reduce inflammation, e.g. Ibuprofen, Naprosyn, Nalfon, Indocin, and Clinoril
   - Corticosteroids reduce inflammation, e.g. Hydrocortisone, Prednisone, and Methylprednisolone
   - Cortisone injection into the joint spaces
2. Physical therapy
   - Retain joint flexibility, maintain muscle strength, protect joints from further destruction
3. Heat or cold treatments are used to relieve pain
   - Warm baths; heating pads; paraffin dips; and warm, moist packs
   - Cold compresses or ice packs
4. Occupational therapy
   - To assist in maintaining mobility in arms and hands
   - Educate regarding compensatory methods of doing things
5. Surgery
   - *Arthroplasty*—surgical replacement of a diseased joint
   - *Arthrodesis*—fusion of a joint to diminish or relieve pain
   - *Osteoplasty*—surgically removing the diseased portion of the joint
   - *Osteotomy*—correcting alignment of a joint to reduce pressure
6. Self-help aids
   - Canes, walkers, and crutches are used to provide support and reduce weight-bearing with ambulation and transfer
7. Protection of joints
   - Braces and splints are used to protect joints from overuse and injury, as well as to provide rest, immobilization, and correct alignment for joints
   - Use large muscle groups for lifting
   - Use alternative methods for ADLs that cause less joint strain
   - Avoid activities that cause impact to joints

- Ambulatory aids, e.g. walker, crutch, or cane to decrease weight-bearing to joints
- Lose weight to decrease weight-bearing to joints
- Maintain correct posture

8. Rest
- Stress and increased exercise promote joint inflammation, which is reduced with rest
- Especially important after exercise or exertion

9. Pain control methods
- Visualization techniques, relaxation techniques, hypnosis, or self-hypnosis, Transcutaneous electrical nerve stimulation (TENS), and massage

10. Weight control
- To decrease weight-bearing on joints

CONSIDERATIONS FOR CARE

1. Educate patient and family regarding the disease process.
2. Educate patient and family regarding forms of treatment as well as side effects of treatment.
3. Encourage patient to rest as needed.
4. Encourage proper nutrition and maintenance of correct weight.
5. Encourage moderation.
6. Provide emotional support to patient and family.
7. Provide firm mattress and correct alignment for patient.
8. Encourage patient to wear shoes that provide correct alignment and support.
9. Educate regarding safety devices and self-help aids in the home, such as hand-rails, elevated toilet seats, no throw rugs, avoid clutter, avoid stairs as needed and able, large-handled utensils, long-handled combs, clothing with velcro, hand-held shower nozzles, bath mitts, and soap-on-a-rope.
10. Avoid activities that aggravate or initiate pain.
11. Encourage correct posture and body mechanics.
12. Develop coping strategies for the patient due to joint deformity and physical appearance.
13. Offer alternative leisure time activities due to physical limitations.
14. Counseling may be necessary for the emotional stresses placed upon the patient due to the disease.
15. Be aware that the patient may experience stress and depression due to pain and other factors; offer emotional support and counseling options.
16. Vocational changes may need to be made due to limitations placed upon the person.
17. Offer resources that would assist the person due to financial burdens placed upon the patient and family due to medical expense, job difficulties, or home changes.
18. Assist with ADLs due to limitations from stiffness, pain, or fatigue.
19. Referral to physical therapist or occupational therapist as needed.
20. A positive but realistic approach to patient care is encouraged.
21. Allow patient as much control as possible while in the hospital as well as at home.

22. Assess level of pain and offer comfort measures as available.

23. Dietary consult to promote weight control.

FOR MORE INFORMATION

Arthritis Foundation
1314 Spring Street, NW
Atlanta, GA 30309
(404) 872-7100

Arthritis Foundation
P.O. Box 19000
Atlanta, GA 30326

ASSIGNMENT SHEET: OSTEOARTHRITIS

Short Answer

1. Write a brief definition for the terms listed throughout the chapter.

2. Describe the physiology of joints.

3. Write a brief definition for osteoarthritis.

4. Describe the incidence of osteoarthritis.

5. List six (6) possible risk factors for osteoarthritis.

6. List seven (7) signs and symptoms of osteoarthritis and associated care.

7. Identify four (4) specific methods of diagnosis for osteoarthritis.

8. Identify four (4) specific goals of treatment used for osteoarthritis.

9. Identify ten (10) specific methods of treatment used for osteoarthritis.

10. List twenty-three (23) considerations for caring for a patient with osteoarthritis.

11. Write the normal range for a serum salicylate level.

12. Describe the following procedures used in the diagnosis or treatment of osteoarthritis.
    a. X-ray
    b. Joint aspiration
    c. Arthroplasty
    d. Arthrodesis
    e. Osteoplasty
    f. Osteotomy
    g. Transcutaneous electrical nerve stimulation (TENS)

KNOWLEDGE INTO ACTION

1. Due to the large amount of aspirin Mr. Jong is taking, the doctor wants Mr. Jong to have a blood level checked periodically. Mr. Jong asks you what the name of the blood level is that checks the aspirin to see if it is in a therapeutic range. What will your response be regarding the name of this blood test? What is the normal range for this test?

2. Six weeks later, Mr. Jong returns to the clinic. He tells you he has been taking the aspirin and using the other methods of pain control the physician had suggested. He reports there has been minimal control of his pain. What other medications could the physician prescribe for Mr. Jong?

3. You are a home health aid and are going on a home visit to help Fred Charles, an 81-year-old who has recently had surgery. Mr. Charles's wife, Hanna, has a history of osteoarthritis. She says to you, "Fred used to be such a help around the house before his surgery. Since he's been down, I've had to do more housework. I'm having a hard time taking care of my personal needs and the housework the way this arthritis is acting up. Do you have any good suggestions for me?" What will your response be?

4. Marion Bernstein is your supervisor at the hospital where you work. She generally is very energetic and enthusiastic, even though she has a history of osteoarthritis. The past few days, you notice Marion is moving more slowly and has been very quiet. Today, she snaps at you for not responding quickly enough to a patient call light, even though she knows you were helping a physician with a procedure at the time. You suspect she snapped at you only because her osteoarthritis is making her uncomfortable. What will your response be?

5. You are at a family reunion. Your 6-year-old niece comes up to you and says, "I'm worried about Grandma. She said, 'This arthritis and these old knees of mine are sure giving me fits.' What does she mean by arthritis? Does it make her knees hurt?" What will your response be?

UNIT 4

NEUROLOGICAL DISORDERS

OBJECTIVES

Upon completion of this chapter, the student should be able to:

- Define the key terms listed throughout the chapter
- State a specific definition for stroke
- Describe the physiology of the brain
- Describe the incidence of stroke
- Describe the specific causes of stroke
- List the risk factors for stroke
- Describe the signs and symptoms of stroke and the associated care for these symptoms
- Identify specific methods for diagnosis of stroke
- Identify specific methods for treatment of stroke
- List complications of stroke and the associated care
- Describe specific considerations for caring for a patient with a stroke
- State a specific definition for transient ischemic attack (TIA)
- List the cranial nerves, the function of each and a method of testing the function of each
- Describe the process involve in a neurological examination
- List assistive devices available for individuals with physical impairments due to a stroke

KEY TERMS

Cerebrovascular – refers to the blood vessels of the brain

Necrosis – tissue death

Cranium – the bones of the skull excluding the jawbone and facial bones

Cerebrospinal fluid (CSF) – fluid that surrounds the brain and spinal cord and protects from injury by acting as a cushion

Membrane – external or internal covering of an organ

Meninges – membranes covering the brain and spinal cord (dura mater, arachnoid, and pia mater); *singular,* meninx

Cerebrum – largest portion of the brain;

INTRODUCTION

Cerebrovascular accident (CVA) or stroke is defined as interruption of blood supply to the brain or bleeding into the brain, which disrupts the oxygen supply to the brain and causes tissue death, called **necrosis**.

The symptoms from a stroke depend on the region of the brain tissue that has the oxygen and blood supply cut off as well as the amount of tissue involved. (See Figure 19-1.)

PHYSIOLOGY OF THE BRAIN

The brain is located in the **cranium** and is covered and protected by **cerebrospinal fluid (CSF)**, **membranes (meninges)**, and the skull. The meninges of the brain include the dura mater, arachnoid, and pia mater. The brain is divided into three areas: the cerebrum, cerebellum, and the brain stem. (See Figure 19-2.)

1. The **cerebrum** is the largest portion of the brain. The surface of the cerebrum is covered with grooves (**fissures**) and ridges (**convolutions**). The cerebrum is divided into left and right **hemispheres** and functions as a control for voluntary movement, emotion, thought processes, sensation, and consciousness. The right hemisphere of the brain controls spatial relations and perception, creativity, fantasy, and concrete thinking. The left hemisphere of the brain controls communication, abstract thinking, language skills, and auditory memory.

responsible for voluntary movement and thought processes

Fissure – formation of a groove or crack

Convolution – surface that has many folds or coils

Hemisphere – refers to half of the cerebrum or cerebellum

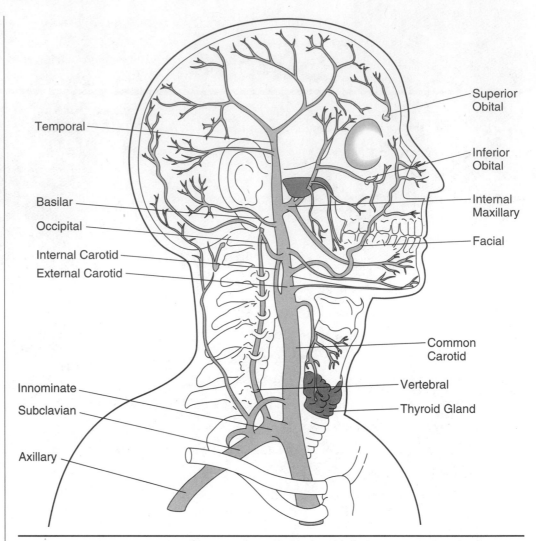

Figure 19-1   Arterial circulation to the head (Adapted from Burke, *Human Anatomy and Physiology in Health and Disease, 3rd edition,* copyright © 1992, Delmar Publishers)

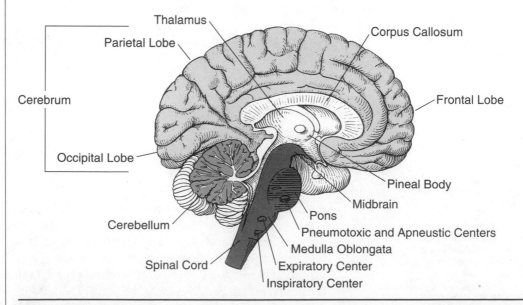

Figure 19-2   Cross section of the brain (From Fong et al., *Body Structures and Functions, 8th edition,* copyright © 1993, Delmar Publishers)

Lobe – specific portion of an organ

Frontal lobe – anterior portion of the cerebrum of the brain

Parietal lobe – sections of the cerebrum located at the side

Temporal lobe – lobe of the brain necessary for hearing and smelling

Auditory – in reference to hearing; eighth cranial nerve

Olfactory – the first of the twelve cranial nerves; responsible for the sense of smell

Occipital lobe – lobe of the cerebrum located directly above the cerebellum in the posterior of the brain

Cerebellum – portion of the brain located directly under the cerebrum; responsible for coordination of balance and muscle tone

Equilibrium – state of being equal or balanced; refers to chemical or physical balance within the body

Brain stem – the portion of the brain that connects the brain with the spinal cord; the parts of the brain stem are the medulla, pons, and midbrain

Anterior – front

Midbrain – uppermost section of the brain stem

Pons – portion of the brain anterior to the cerebellum and between the medulla and the midbrain

Medulla – lowest section of the brain stem

Cerebral – refers to the cerebrum, the largest portion of the brain

Thrombosis – blood clot formation within the blood vessels

Embolism – substance or blood clot that travels through the vascular system of the body often causing obstruction by lodging in the lumen of a vessel

Each hemisphere of the brain is further divided into four sections or **lobes**:

- **Frontal lobe**—contains the motor area; the left side of the brain controls the right side of the body and the right side of the brain controls the left side of the body. The frontal lobe also contains the speech center of the brain (Broca's area) and controls emotions and intellect.
- **Parietal lobe**—contains the sensory area, which is responsible for touch, temperature, pain, pressure, and recognition of size, shape, location, and intensity of stimuli. The parietal lobe is also necessary for awareness of body parts.
- **Temporal lobe**—contains the **auditory** area, which is responsible for receiving and interpreting sound as well as the **olfactory** area, which is responsible for the sense of smell.
- **Occipital lobe**—contains the visual area, which is responsible for images that arise from the retina of the eye.

2. The **cerebellum** is the second largest part of the brain and lies directly under the occipital lobe of the cerebrum. The function of the cerebellum is to control the coordination of movement, **equilibrium**, muscle tone, and posture.

3. The **brain stem** is the smallest portion of the brain and is located directly **anterior** to the cerebellum. The brain stem is further divided into the **midbrain**, **pons**, and **medulla**. The function of the brain stem is to provide a pathway between the body and the brain as well as to control respirations, heartbeat, and blood vessel diameter.

STATISTICS

There are approximately 500,000 strokes that occur annually in the United States with more than 150,000 of these ending in death. Stroke is the third leading cause of death in the United States following heart disease as first and cancer as second. An average of 30% of stroke victims are under the age of 65.

More than $25 billion is spent annually in the United Sates as a result of direct and indirect costs associated with strokes. Nearly 85% of strokes could be prevented by reducing or deleting risk factors. Rehabilitation helps 65% of clients regain all their abilities. In the United States, 20% of all people will be affected by a stroke in their lifetime.

CAUSES

A stroke follows one of the following events.

1. **Cerebral thrombosis.** The most common cause of stroke is a blood clot that originates in the brain and blocks the blood flow in an artery that supplies blood and oxygen to a specific portion of the brain. The event is called cerebral thrombosis and it accounts for approximately 60% of all strokes; it is common in the elderly.

2. Cerebral **embolism.** When a blood clot originates in a distant area of the body (often in the heart) and travels to the brain through the bloodstream and lodges in an artery in the brain, the event is called a cerebral embolism. The clot then blocks blood and oxygen to that specific portion of the brain. Cerebral embolism accounts for approximately 20% of all strokes and is also common in the elderly.

3. Cerebral hemorrhage. When bleeding from an artery in the brain, caused by head injury or **aneurysm**, leads to a blood and oxygen shortage in the brain, it is a cerebral hemorrhage. Not only is blood supply and oxygen cut off from

Aneurysm – blood-filled sac formed by tearing and separation of the walls of blood vessels, allowing blood to escape into the layers of the vessel

Subarachnoid – located below the arachnoid (middle membrane or meninx that covers the brain and spinal cord)

Skull – the bones that form the head

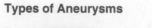

Types of Aneurysms

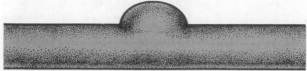

Saccular–Unilateral Pouchlike Bulge

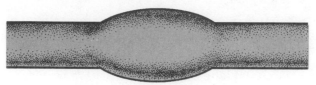

Fusiform–A Spindle-shaped Bulge of the Entire Artery Wall

Figure 19-3 Aneurysms in blood vessel walls (From Keir et al., *Medical Assisting: Administrative and Clinical Competencies, 3rd edition*, copyright © 1993, Delmar Publishers)

the specific portion of the brain, but temporary or permanent damage may occur due to the pressure of the accumulated blood in the tissue. Cerebral hemorrhage accounts for approximately 20% of all strokes and is common is younger clients. (See Figure 19-3.)

4. **Subarachnoid** hemorrhage. The most rare event leading to a stroke is when bleeding from a blood vessel on the surface of the brain accumulates blood between the brain and the **skull**. Damage may occur due to pressure of accumulated blood and lack of blood and oxygen to brain tissue. (See Figure 19-4.)

RISK FACTORS

1. Hypertension in 40 to 70% of clients indicates an increased risk factor of 4 to 6 times that of an average person.

   - Check blood pressure on a routine basis
   - Control elevated blood pressure with low-salt diet, weight loss, regular exercise program, smoking cessation, and stress reduction as instructed by physician. If these methods fail, the physician may prescribe medications to control hypertension.

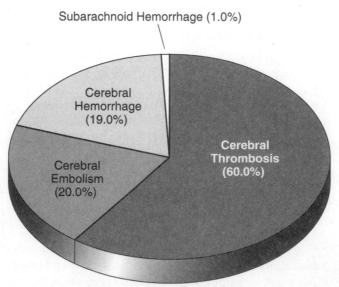

Figure 19-4 Causes of stroke

Atrial fibrillation – irregular beating and contractions of the atria of the heart

Cholesterol – substance found normally in many foods including animal fats and egg yolks

Nicotine – poisonous substance found in tobacco

Saturated fat – fats from animal sources that are solid at room temperature

Polycythemia – increased number of red blood cells in the blood

Transient ischemic attack (TIA) – "mini-stroke"; caused by the temporary lack of blood supply to a specific portion of the brain

2. Heart disease. The general population of people with heart disease are six times more likely to have a stroke. Approximately 15% of stroke patients have a history of **atrial fibrillation.**
   - Control heart disease by blood pressure control, blood **cholesterol** control, and smoking cessation

3. Cigarette smoking doubles the risk of having a stroke
   - Cease smoking due to **nicotine** causing an elevation in blood pressure as well as reducing the amount of oxygen in the blood due to carbon monoxide in the blood. Smoking also causes blood to thicken, which increases the chance of blood clots forming in the brain or travelling to the brain.

4. Diabetes mellitus
   - Schedule regular examinations by physician
   - Control blood sugar levels with diet, exercise, weight loss, and medications as prescribed by physician
   - Monitor blood sugar levels

5. Alcohol
   - Consume alcohol in moderation, if at all

6. High blood cholesterol
   - Monitor blood cholesterol on regular basis as advised by physician
   - Consume foods low in **saturated fats** and cholesterol
   - Exercise and weight maintenance as prescribed by physician
   - Utilize medications to control blood cholesterol levels as prescribed by physician

7. **Polycythemia**
   - The increase in the amount of RBCs cause blood to thicken and increase the chance of clot formation; therefore: (1) administer blood thinners as directed by physician and (2) periodically donate blood as a control

8. Age
   - Schedule regular physical exams and control other risk factors. Note that greater than 70% of strokes occur in people over the age of 65.

9. Gender
   - Schedule regular physical exams and control other risk factors. Note that the majority of strokes occur in males.

10. Heredity
    - Schedule regular physical exams and control other risk factors.

11. Race
    - Schedule regular physical exams and control other risk factors. Note that African-Americans are at a greater risk for stroke due to their increased risk of hypertension.

12. Geographic location
    - Schedule regular physical exams and control other risk factors. Note that strokes are most common in the Southeastern states and least common in Southwestern states.

13. Oral contraceptives
    - Utilize alternate form of birth control
    - Cease smoking due to stroke risk increasing considerably in the combination of smoking and oral contraceptives

14. History of **Transient Ischemic Attack (TIA)**
    - Schedule regular physical exams and control other risk factors based on the observation that TIAs precede approximately 10% of all strokes

Carotid – carotid arteries located in the neck that supply blood to the head

Bruit – abnormal sound present when auscultating a vein or artery

Endarterectomy – surgical removal of plaque and fat buildup from the lumen of an artery

15. Obesity
    - Reduce weight due to the increase in heart disease, hypertension, and related stroke with the presence of obesity
16. **Carotid bruit**
    - Schedule regular physical exams and control other risk factors. Note that carotid bruit increases the risk for stroke.
    - Possible need for *carotid* **endarterectomy**

SIGNS, SYMPTOMS, AND ASSOCIATED CARE

Signs and symptoms of a stroke depend on the area of the brain involved and the extent of the involvement. (See Figure 19-5.)

1. Weakness or numbness, generally on only one side of the body
   - Obtain baseline neurological function and monitor on routine basis
   - Prevent injury to patient due to weakness and numbness
   - Provide assistance with activities of daily living (ADLs) as needed
   - Provide assistance with ambulation and transfer as needed
   - Provide range of motion (ROM) exercises if immobile to decrease the risk of decubitus ulcers, pneumonia, muscle wasting, and contractures
   - Consultation and therapy provided by physical therapy and occupational therapy
   - Prevent skin breakdown for patients with decreased mobility. Signs of skin breakdown (decubitus ulcers) include redness, swelling, warm or hot to touch, open sores, cyanosis, pain, and blisters. Prevention measures include frequent repositioning (minimum of every 1 to 2 hours); meticulous skin care; massage areas at bony prominences; encourage activity as able; alternating pressure mattresses; prevent pressure from appliances or tubing; prevent friction when repositioning by using a lift sheet and adequate assistance; and linens must be clean, dry, and wrinkle-free.
   - Encourage use of assistive devices, such as large-handled utensils, bath mitts, velcro fasteners, long-handled shoehorns, soap-on-a-rope, elevated toilet seat, and handrails
2. Visual disturbance, generally in only one eye
   - Educate patient regarding head position to improve vision

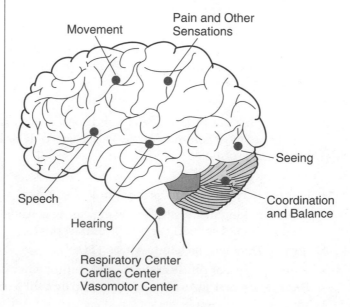

Figure 19-5 Functional areas of the brain (From Hegner, *Nursing Assistant: A Nursing Process Approach,* 7th edition, copyright © 1995, Delmar Publishers)

- Evaluate ability of patient to drive safely in presence of visual problems
- Encourage alternate activities for patient who has difficulty with reading
- Avoid eye strain
- Provide large print books or cassettes
- Avoid injury to the patient due to visual disturbances
- Facilitate evaluation by ophthalmologist
- Provide adequate lighting when reading, watching TV, or other activities
- Remove environmental hazards, such as throw rugs, cluttered hallways, and excessive furniture

3. Dysphagia
   - Offer foods that are easy to chew according to patient preference
   - Avoid fresh fruits and vegetables as these are often more difficult to chew
   - Alternate liquids and solids during meals
   - Monitor for choking
   - Instruct family members on the Heimlich maneuver should choking occur while they are with the patient and for when the patient returns home
   - Educate that food may need to be chopped or pureed
   - Utilize suction equipment in the event of choking
   - Concentrate on chewing food thoroughly
   - Provide method such as a warming plate to keep food warm during entire length of time needed for patient to eat
   - Obtain baseline weight and monitor on routine basis
   - Encourage patient to take as much time as necessary during meals
   - Avoid outside distractions during mealtime to avoid choking
   - Encourage patient to sit upright to eat
   - Be alert for symptoms of dehydration. Symptoms include constipation, decreased amounts of urine, concentrated urine, dry skin, tenting of skin, dry mouth, dry eyes, hypotension, and confusion.
   - Use a syringe to feed liquids in small amounts

4. Severe headaches
   - Provide dim lights in the event of photophobia
   - Administer medications or other methods of pain relief, such as relaxation techniques, imaging, and massage
   - Assist with position for patient comfort
   - Provide calm, quiet environment for the patient
   - Administer pain control methods such as relaxation techniques, massage, imaging, and pain medications as prescribed by physician
   - Encourage patient to avoid eye strain during periods of headache
   - Encourage frequent rest periods as necessary
   - Monitor phone calls and visitors to promote rest periods

5. Dizziness, balance disturbance, or falls
   - Monitor for vertigo
   - Monitor vital signs (See Appendix D)
   - Assist with ambulation and transfer to prevent injury in the presence of vertigo
   - Educate patient to ask for assistance when out of bed in presence of syncope
   - Provide method for patient to call for assistance

Seizure – episode affecting the nervous system that is characterized by symptoms ranging from alteration in consciousness to severe tremors involving the entire body, which can be accompanied by a temporary loss of consciousness

Hemianopia – loss of vision of half of the visual field of an eye or eyes

6. Dysarthria
   - Practice singing or reading aloud
   - Practice making exaggerated facial expressions in the mirror
   - Be certain you correctly understand what the patient is saying
   - Maintain good eye contact when speaking with the patient
   - Concentrate on what the patient is saying
   - Avoid outside distractions (TV, radio)
   - Avoid rooms that are congested with other people when visiting
   - Avoid finishing sentences for the patient
   - Encourage patient not to isolate themselves
   - Provide alternative forms of communication that may need to be used, such as writing, word boards, and electronic devices
   - Encourage continued efforts at communication on the part of the patient
   - Allow time for the patient to respond to questions and comments

7. **Seizures**
   - Protect patient from injury during a seizure
   - Monitor patient for seizures and administer medications as prescribed by physician
   - Offer reassurance to patient and family during and after a seizure
   - Note behavior prior to seizure to determine presence of an aura
   - Monitor duration and intensity of seizure as well as body involvement
   - Monitor airway and breathing following a seizure
   - Provide privacy for the patient during and after a seizure
   - Turn patient to their side after a seizure if they begin to choke or vomit

8. Impaired mental activity
   - Provide calm, quiet environment for patient
   - Avoid startling patient
   - Avoid approaching patient from behind
   - Reorient patient as necessary
   - Allow family members or friends to stay with patient as much as needed if this is reassuring to the patient

9. Loss of consciousness
   - Reposition patient frequently to prevent skin breakdown
   - Prevent skin breakdown for patients with decreased mobility. Signs of skin breakdown (decubitus ulcers) include redness, swelling, warm or hot to touch, open sores, cyanosis, pain, and blisters. Prevention measures include frequent repositioning (minimum of every 1 to 2 hours); meticulous skin care; massage areas at bony prominences; encourage activity as able; alternating pressure mattresses; prevent pressure from appliances or tubing; prevent friction when repositioning by using a lift sheet and adequate assistance; and linens must be clean, dry, and wrinkle-free.
   - Complete neurological examination on routine basis
   - Provide adequate hydration
   - Continue to explain care and treatment to patient even though unresponsive
   - Offer comfort and reassurance to patient and family

10. **Hemianopia**
    - Prevent injury to the patient due to visual field cut
    - Facilitate evaluation by ophthalmologist

Palpate – to examine or feel with the fingers or hand

Auscultate – process of listening to sounds within the body, generally with a stethoscope, as the organs within the body carry out their specific functions

Cranial nerves – twelve pairs of nerves that originate in the brain and control various functions of the body

Plaque – abnormal accumulation of a substance; generally refers to the lumen of the blood vessel or to the teeth

Anticoagulant – substance that prevents or delays blood from clotting

Vasodilation – refers to dilation of the vessels of the body

DIAGNOSIS

1. Presence of symptoms
2. Physical examination including:
   - **Palpate** and **auscultate** all major blood vessels
   - Vital signs (See Appendix D)
3. Neurological examination
   - **Cranial nerves** (see section on cranial nerves)
   - Mental status and level of consciousness
   - Reflex testing
   - Sensation to touch, pain, and temperature
   - Muscle strength and tone
   - Hearing check
   - Vision check
4. *CT scan* used to differentiate between hemorrhage and clots
5. *MRI* used to evaluate the size and location of the lesion or hemorrhage
6. *Dopplar ultrasound test* is used to detect blockages in the carotid artery
7. *Radionuclide angiography* is used to show the function of the brain and can detect blocked blood vessels as well as the area of damage
8. *EEG* is used to detect specific areas of the brain that have reduced electrical activity
9. *Lumbar puncture* used to rule out infection and subdural hematoma as evidenced by bloody spinal fluid and increased intracranial pressure
10. *Digital subtraction angiography* is used to show an image of blood vessels in the brain and detect blood vessel abnormalities
11. *Positron emission tomography* is used to detect changes in the cerebral vascular blood flow

TREATMENT

Treatment is aimed at helping the patient to regain independence and improve physical ability. Specific methods of treatment include:

1. Surgery may be needed for the following:
   - *Carotid endarterectomy* to remove **plaque** from the carotid artery
   - Relieve pressure in the brain caused by hemorrhage
   - Remove a tumor or blood clot that may have caused the stroke
   - Repair aneurysm if present
2. Medication may be needed for the following:
   - **Anticoagulants** in the event of blood clot to the brain to prevent further clots from forming
   - Medications to reduce the swelling in the brain accompanied by brain tissue injury, e.g. Corticosteroids, Mannitol
   - **Vasodilators** to treat arterial spasm in the brain
   - Anticonvulsants for the control of seizures, e.g. Dilantin, Phenobarbital
   - Pain medications to control the headaches, which often accompany a stroke
3. Rehabilitation to regain independence and improve physical ability

Spasticity – increased muscular tone that makes movement or stretching of the muscles difficult

Plantar – refers to the sole of the foot

Pulmonary embolism – obstruction of a portion of the arterial circulation of the lungs due to a blood clot that travels from another part of the body and lodges in the arterial circulation

COMPLICATIONS OF STROKE AND ASSOCIATED CARE

1. **Spasticity** and joint contracture
   - Provide range of motion (ROM) as directed by the physician and physical therapist
   - Provide proper alignment
   - Splints and braces to maintain joints in proper alignment
   - Utilize foot board to prevent **plantar** flexion of feet. Note that high-top tennis shoes also work well for this.
   - Change patient position at least every 2 hours with proper support of joints and extremities. Patient should be on the unaffected side when in the side-lying position.

2. Pneumonia
   - Prevent aspiration by the following methods: Assess patient's ability to swallow, sit patient up when eating, small bites of food, don't rush, and suction as necessary
   - Be alert for symptoms of pneumonia, e.g. cough, phlegm, chest pain, fever, dyspnea, chills, and diaphoresis
   - Encourage coughing and deep breathing
   - Educate patient and family to report symptoms of respiratory infection to physician
   - Educate patient regarding importance of completing medication prescribed for respiratory infection
   - Encourage fluids to thin secretions and make them easier to expel
   - Prevent transmission of infection by hand washing, correctly disposing of tissues and phlegm
   - Avoid people with respiratory infections
   - Maintain optimal health to fight off infections
   - Administer influenza and pneumonia vaccinations as directed by physician
   - Avoid crowded areas which increase the likelihood of contracting a respiratory infection

3. Depression
   - Encourage communication between the patient and family
   - Provide professional counseling as necessary
   - Administer medications to help treat the depression
   - Help patient maintain as much control as possible over his life
   - Observe for signs of severe depression or suicidal tendencies

4. **Pulmonary embolism** or deep vein thrombosis
   - Encourage exercise or range of motion to decrease pooling of blood in the extremities
   - Provide antiembolism stockings (TED hose) for patient use
   - Educate patient to refrain from crossing the legs

5. Skin breakdown
   - Prevent skin breakdown for patients with decreased mobility. Signs of skin breakdown (decubitus ulcers) include redness, swelling, warm or hot to touch, open sores, cyanosis, pain, and blisters. Prevention measures include frequent repositioning (minimum of every 1 to 2 hours); meticulous skin care; massage areas at bony prominences; encourage activity as able; alternating pressure mattresses; prevent pressure from appliances or tubing; prevent friction when repositioning by using a lift sheet and adequate assistance; and linens must be clean, dry, and wrinkle-free.

CONSIDERATIONS FOR CARE

1. Educate patient and family regarding:
   - Exercises and therapy
   - Nutrition
   - Follow-up care at home
   - Assistive devices that can be used
2. Maintain bowel and bladder program through the following:
   - Take to the bathroom or offer the bedpan/commode/urinal at regular intervals
   - Promote bowel regularity by fluids, fiber, exercise, and stool softeners
   - Laxatives, enemas, or suppositories as prescribed by the physician
   - Provide privacy for the patient during elimination
   - Encourage fluids
   - If incontinence is a problem, provide for proper skin care as well as initiation of a bowel or bladder retraining program
   - Watch for signs of bladder infection
3. Encourage patient to complete ADLs with adaptive equipment if necessary.
4. Watch for complications associated with stroke.
5. Involve family and friends in patient care as willing and able.
6. Encourage communication and verbalization of feelings.
7. Provide information for support groups.
8. Expect some degree of emotional lability and possible depression.
9. Encourage patient to do as much for himself as possible and avoid doing those things for the patient that he can do for himself.
10. Safety devices need to be used in the hospital and may need to be installed at home, e.g. handrails, wheelchair ramps, nonskid strips on bathtub, shower or tub chair, and elevated toilet seats and chairs.
11. Help the patient set realistic goals and offer encouragement in attaining these goals.
12. Understand that the patient and family are going through a grieving process in addition to worrying about long-term care, financial burdens, and changes in previous level of responsibility.
13. Provide adequate rest and relaxing environment.
14. Allow patient control over as many aspects of care as possible.
15. Observe patient for visual complications associated with the stroke.
16. Support extremities that may be flaccid following the stroke with slings or other forms of support.
17. Obtain baseline vital signs and monitor on routine basis.
18. Transfer patient to the unaffected side, which allows her to lead with the stronger leg as well as improving visualization of the bed or chair.
19. Avoid lifting patient by the affected shoulder or putting tension on the affected arm or leg.
20. Teach patient to do things one-handed.
21. Involve physical therapy, occupational therapy, and speech therapy as indicated.
22. Be aware that patient may avoid affected side.
23. Prevent injury to affected side due to visual loss and loss of sensation.
24. Approach the patient from the unaffected side.
25. Place call bell, water, and other necessary items on the unaffected side.

Cardiac output – amount of blood that is pumped from the heart via the left ventricle per minute

26. Be aware that the patient may be more easily fatigued and compensate for this.

27. When dressing the patient, put clothes on the affected side first; when undressing, remove from the unaffected side first.

28. Educate patient and family regarding need to carry a medical alert card and wear a medical alert bracelet or necklace.

29. Elevate the head of the bed (HOB) approximately 30 degrees to decrease cerebral swelling.

30. Obtain baseline neurological status and monitor on routine basis.

31. Monitor intake and output (I and O).

32. Provide quiet, relaxed environment for the patient; dim lights in the room.

33. Bedrest as directed by physician.

34. Avoid straining with bowel movements or other forms of exertion.

35. Have suction equipment available at the bedside.

36. Develop method of communication for the patient who has decreased ability to communicate verbally.

TRANSIENT ISCHEMIC ATTACK (TIA)

Transient ischemic attacks, nicknamed "mini strokes," are caused by the temporary lack of blood supply to a specific portion of the brain. TIAs generally only last several minutes with symptoms normally completely disappearing within 24 hours. Causes of TIAs include the following:

1. Small emboli, which attack a small vessel in the brain

2. Hypotension, which decreases the amount of blood flow to the brain

3. Compression of neck veins from turning the head, constrictive clothing, or possibly from pressure when shaving the neck

4. Decreased **cardiac output** caused from dysrhythmias

5. Spasm of the vessels of the brain

Symptoms of TIAs are similar to those of stroke and include:

1. Temporary weakness or numbness generally on only one side of the body

2. Temporary visual disturbances

3. Temporary speech disturbances

4. Temporary dizziness or loss of balance

CRANIAL NERVES

A mnemonic that can be used to memorize the cranial nerves is to remember that the first letter of each of the cranial nerves is also the first letter of each of the words of the following sentence: "On old Olympus's towering tops a Finn and German viewed some hops." (See Table 19-1 and Figure 19-6.)

NEUROLOGICAL EXAMINATION

A baseline neurological examination should be completed on admission to the hospital and monitored on a routine basis. Basic areas of the neurological examination include the following:

1. Check patient level of consciousness (LOC)

2. Cranial nerve check

Table 19-1 Cranial Nerves

Nerve	Function	Test
I — Olfactory	Sense of smell	Test each nostril individually for smell recognition
II — Optic	Vision	Check vision and visual field cuts
III — Oculomotor	Eyelid movements	Check ability to open and close eyes
	Pupil constriction	Check pupil constriction
IV — Trochlear	Eye movements	Check for ability to move eyes downward/inward
V — Trigeminal (trifacial)	Chewing	Open and close mouth; clench jaw
	Sensory impulses of the face	Check face for sensation and ability to distinguish between pain, touch, and temperature
VI — Abducens	Eye movement	Check for ability to move eyes in all directions
VII — Facial	Facial expression	Check for ability to raise eyebrows, puff cheeks, and movement of mouth
	Taste	Test for ability to taste foods and ability to distinguish between various foods
VIII — Acoustic (Vestibulocochlear)	Balance; hearing	Check for balance and ability to hear
IX — Glossopharyngeal	Saliva secretion	Check for gag reflex and ability to swallow
	Sensory impulses of the tongue and throat	Test for ability to taste foods and ability to distinguish between various foods
X — Vagus	Control of most organs in abdominal and thorasic cavities; voice production	Check for ability to speak and swallow
	Slows heartbeat	Monitor rhythm and rate of heartbeat
XI — Spinal accessory	Shoulder and head movement	Check for ability to shrug shoulders actively and against resistance
XII — Hypoglossal	Tongue movement	Check various tongue movements as well as ability to stick out tongue

3. Check patient orientation to time, place, and person with questions to determine the presence of short-term and long-term memory
4. Check muscle strength, movement, and coordination as well as tendon reflexes
5. Check sensations to heat, cold, touch, and pain

ASSISTIVE DEVICES

Examples of assistive devices that can assist a patient who has loss of function in a specific part of the body include the following:

1. Cane, walker, wheelchair, or other methods to assist ambulation and transfer

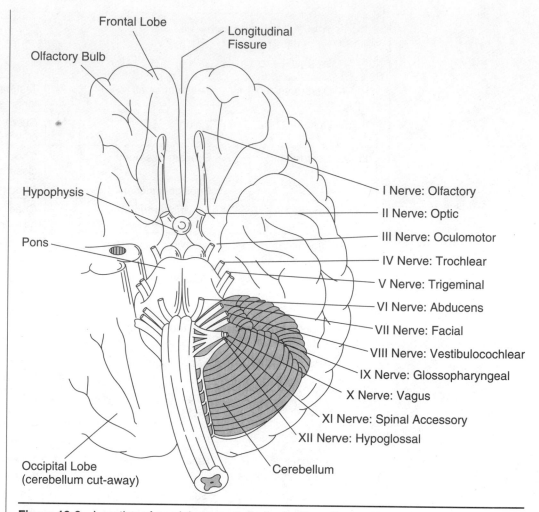

Frontal Lobe

Longitudinal Fissure

Olfactory Bulb

Hypophysis

Pons

I Nerve: Olfactory
II Nerve: Optic
III Nerve: Oculomotor
IV Nerve: Trochlear
V Nerve: Trigeminal
VI Nerve: Abducens
VII Nerve: Facial
VIII Nerve: Vestibulocochlear
IX Nerve: Glossopharyngeal
X Nerve: Vagus
XI Nerve: Spinal Accessory
XII Nerve: Hypoglossal

Occipital Lobe
(cerebellum cut-away)

Cerebellum

Figure 19-6   Location of cranial nerves in the brain (From Burke, *Human Anatomy and Physiology in Health and Disease*, *3rd edition*, copyright © 1992, Delmar Publishers)

2. Large-handled appliances: silverware, toothbrush, hairbrush, pens, and pencils
3. Clothing and shoes with elastic or velcro closures
4. Long-handled shoe horns or devices for grasping hard-to-reach items

FOR MORE INFORMATION

National Stroke Association
Suite 1000
8480 East Orchard Drive
Englewood, CO 80111-5015
(303) 771-1700

National Easter Seal Society
2023 West Ogden Avenue
Chicago, IL 60612

American Heart Association
7320 Greenville Avenue
Dallas, TX 75231

ASSIGNMENT SHEET: STROKE

Short Answer

1. Write a brief definition for the terms listed throughout the chapter.

2. Describe the physiology of each of the following parts of the brain.
    a. Cerebrum
    b. Cerebellum
    c. Brain stem

3. Describe the function of each of the four (4) lobes of the hemispheres of the brain.
    a. Frontal lobe
    b. Parietal lobe
    c. Temporal lobe
    d. Occipital lobe

4. Describe items that could be considered indirect costs associated with stroke.

5. List the three (3) membranes (meninges) that surround the brain.

6. Describe the following procedures used in the diagnosis of stroke.
    a. Digital subtraction angiography
    b. Endarterectomy
    c. CT scan
    d. Lumbar puncture (spinal tap)
    e. MRI
    f. Dopplar ultrasound test
    g. Radionuclide angiography
    h. EEG

7. Describe the incidence of stroke.

8. Describe the four (4) specific causes of stroke.

9. Describe the sixteen (16) risk factors associated with stroke and methods to reduce the risk factors.

10. Describe ten (10) signs and symptoms of a stroke and associated care.

11. Describe specific problems that could be associated with the symptom of hemianopia.

12. Describe specific problems that could be associated with the symptoms of "hemiparesis."

13. Describe what is meant by "neglect" as associated with stroke.

14. List seven (7) symptoms of pneumonia.

15. Describe eleven (11) specific methods used to diagnose a stroke.

16. Describe three (3) areas of treatment associated with a diagnosis of stroke.

17. Describe the care associated with each of the following complications of stroke.
    a. Contractures
    b. Pneumonia
    c. Depression
    d. Pulmonary embolism or deep vein thrombosis.
    e. Skin breakdown

18. List three (3) specific questions a physician may ask to determine whether a patient is having a stroke.

19. List three (3) home health care considerations that would need to be considered prior to discharging the patient home.

20. Describe what is meant by transient ischemic attack (TIA).

21. List the normal ranges for the following laboratory tests.
    a. Cholesterol
    b. Blood sugar (glucose)

KNOWLEDGE INTO ACTION

1. Dallas White Chief, a 72-year-old with a history of a stroke and right-sided paralysis, is being transferred from the hospital to your long-term care facility. You are aware that complications of strokes can include contractures, thrombosis formation, and decubitus ulcers. List three (3) methods of associated care that could reduce the risk for Mr. White Chief from developing the listed complications.

2. As you are writing Mr. White Chief's plan of care, you are asked to list ten (10) considerations for care that would help to make his stay in your long-term care facility better and less stressful for

him, while also helping to improve his ability to care for himself. List ten (10) methods of associated care that could be included in the plan of care that would meet those objectives.

3. After 7 weeks in your long-term care facility, Mr. White Chief is preparing to go home with his wife. Mrs. White Chief is anxious to give the best care possible to her husband. She asks you to make a list of "a dozen or so" things she needs to do or be aware of regarding her husband's care. What will your response be?

4. Mavis Creighton, an 81-year-old retired teacher, is admitted to your facility with dizziness, numbness to the right side of her body, and visual loss. Her blood pressure is 168/104. By the next morning, her symptoms are completely gone and her blood pressure is 148/84. Her physician tells her she has had a "mini stroke." She asks you, "The doctor was called to the emergency room before he had a chance to tell me what that 'mini stroke' thing was and what caused it. Can you tell me, please?" What will your response be?

Meningitis

Upon completion of this chapter, the student should be able to:

■ Define the key terms listed throughout the chapter

■ Describe the physiology of the meninges of the brain and spinal cord

■ State a specific definition for meningitis

■ Describe the incidence of meningitis

■ List the primary causes of meningitis

■ Describe the mode of transmission for meningitis

■ Identify risk factors for meningitis

■ List signs and symptoms associated with meningitis and associated care for these symptoms

■ Describe the steps of a neurological examination

■ List the cranial nerves, the function of each, and a specific method of testing each cranial nerve

■ Identify specific methods for diagnosis of meningitis

■ Identify specific methods for treatment of meningitis

■ Describe specific complications associated with meningitis

■ Describe specific considerations for caring for a patient with meningitis

KEY TERMS

Dura mater – the outer meninx (membrane) that covers the brain and spinal cord

Arachnoid – the middle meninx (membrane) that covers the brain and spinal cord

Pia mater – innermost meninx (membrane) covering the brain and spinal cord

Mortality – refers to the state of being subject to death

INTRODUCTION

Meningitis is defined as inflammation of the meninges of the brain and spinal cord, generally caused by bacterial infection. All three layers of the meninges may be involved.

PHYSIOLOGY OF THE MENINGES

The meninges surround the brain within the cranium. There are three layers of meninges: the **dura mater**, **arachnoid**, and **pia mater**. The function of the meninges is to protect and cushion the brain. (See Figure 20-1.)

STATISTICS

Meningitis is a very serious disease, especially in the very young patient or in the elderly. There is a **mortality** rate of 70 to 100% if left untreated.

CAUSATIVE AGENTS

Meningitis can be caused by several agents and can be transmitted to the person in a variety of methods. The most common causes are as follows:

1. *Neisseria meningitidis*
2. *Haemophilus influenzae*

Sinusitis – inflammation of the sinus cavity

Bacteremia – accumulation of bacteria in the blood

Otitis media – inflammation of the middle ear

Encephalitis – inflammation of the brain and the meninges

Immune – resistant to disease either by natural defenses in the body (antibodies) or through the use of a vaccine

Sickle cell anemia – disease in which the red blood cells are elongated rather than biconcave and increase the thickness or viscosity of the blood

Pneumonia – inflammation or infection of the lungs

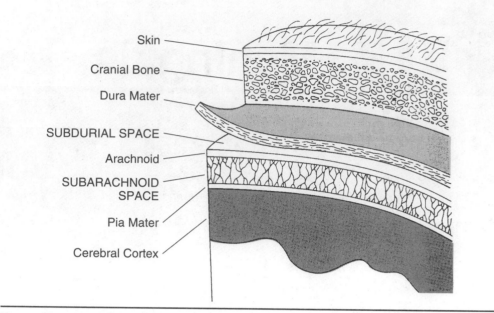

Figure 20-1   Location of subdural and subarachnoid bleeding (From Whitaker, *Comprehensive Perinatal and Pediatric Respiratory Care,* copyright © 1992, Delmar Publishers)

3. *Escherichia coli*

4. *Streptococcus pneumoniae*

5. Viral meningitis secondary to viral infections elsewhere in the body

The mode of transmission is generally one of the following methods.

1. Direct transmission from **sinusitis**

2. **Bacteremia**

3. Direct transmission from **otitis media**

4. Spread via **encephalitis**

5. Following skull fracture

6. Penetrating head wound

7. Human carriers—respiratory droplets

8. Direct contact with respiratory secretions or mucous

RISK FACTORS

1. **Immune** disorders

2. Alcoholism

3. Traumatic head injury

4. Neurosurgical procedures

5. Neoplastic disease

6. **Sickle cell anemia**

7. **Pneumonia**

8. Kidney disease

9. Splenectomy

10. Crowded living quarters

Nuchal – refers to the neck

Delirium – extreme mental confusion or agitation

Brudzinski's sign – in a supine position when the neck is flexed, flexing of the hips automatically occurs; presence of this sign is a positive indicator of meningitis

Kernig's sign – inability to straighten the leg while in a sitting position without extreme pain to the hamstring area; frequent symptom of meningitis

Intracranial – refers to the area within the cranium

Aura – sensation that is often perceived by an individual prior to the onset of an epileptic seizure or migraine headache; perceived by the individual as a sensation in hearing, smell, taste, or vision

SIGNS, SYMPTOMS, AND ASSOCIATED CARE

1. **Nuchal** rigidity
   - Assist with position for patient comfort
   - Move patient slowly and carefully to prevent discomfort
   - Provide pain management with relaxation techniques, warm packs, imaging, massage, and pain medications as prescribed by physician
   - Utilize pillows to support head and neck

2. Irritability
   - Employ nonjudgmental acceptance of patient's behavior
   - Encourage to rest as much as possible
   - Encourage patient to take part in decision making as possible
   - Provide comfort and reassurance to patient
   - Provide reassurance to friends and family that irritability is a normal symptom
   - Refrain from taking emotional outbursts personally
   - Provide a calm, quiet environment for patient
   - Give patient advance notice prior to care and treatment

3. **Delirium**
   - Provide calm, quiet environment for patient
   - Avoid startling patient
   - Avoid approaching patient from behind
   - Reorient patient as necessary
   - Allow family members or friends to stay with patient as much as needed if this is reassuring to the patient

4. Positive **Brudzinski's sign**
   - Obtain baseline on admission to hospital and monitor routinely

5. Positive **Kernig's sign**
   - Obtain baseline on admission to hospital and monitor routinely

6. Seizures due to increased **intracranial** pressure
   - Protect patient from injury during a seizure
   - Monitor patient for seizures and administer medications as prescribed by physician
   - Offer reassurance to patient and family during and after a seizure
   - Note behavior prior to seizure to determine presence of an **aura**
   - Monitor duration and intensity of seizure as well as body involvement
   - Monitor airway and breathing following a seizure
   - Provide privacy for the patient during and after a seizure
   - Turn patient on his side after a seizure if he begins to choke or vomit

7. Headache due to infection and increased intracranial pressure
   - Provide dim lights or indirect lighting in event of photophobia and accompanying headache
   - Assist with position for patient comfort
   - Provide calm, quiet environment for the patient
   - Administer pain control methods such as relaxation techniques, massage, imaging, and pain medications as prescribed by physician
   - Encourage patient to avoid eye strain during periods of headache

- Encourage frequent rest periods as necessary
- Monitor phone calls and visitors to promote rest periods

8. Vomiting due to increased intracranial pressure
   - Administer antiemetics before meals as prescribed by physician
   - Offer dietary choices according to patient preference
   - Control odors and unpleasant sights in room
   - Offer fluids frequently to prevent dehydration
   - Monitor intake and output (I and O) to avoid dehydration. Symptoms of dehydration include decreased urine output, concentrated urine, dry skin, tenting of skin, dry mucous membranes, dry mouth, dry eyes, confusion, hypotension, and constipation.
   - Monitor serum electrolytes (*Sodium*, *potassium*, and *chloride*)
   - Encourage rest periods after meals
   - Avoid foods that are spicy, rich, or previously disagreeable to patient
   - Provide receptacle for patient to vomit into as needed; this should be cleaned whenever used and changed on a frequent basis
   - Provide meticulous mouth care
   - Prevent aspiration of vomit
   - Utilize universal precautions at all times when coming in contact with blood or body fluids (See Appendix C)
   - Avoid greasy foods as they tend to stay in the stomach for a long period of time
   - Avoid cooking food if possible due to increased nausea with odors of foods
   - Avoid hot foods as necessary due to the increased odors of hot foods
   - Eat in well-ventilated area to decrease the accumulation of odors of foods while eating

9. Fever due to presence of infection
   - Monitor temperature at routine intervals
   - Provide comfort measures for patient with elevated temperature, such as cool cloth to forehead, partial or complete bath as needed, clothing and bedding changed frequently due to diaphoresis, and encourage fluids to prevent dehydration
   - Avoid exposing patient to a draft
   - Cover with blankets as necessary
   - Monitor intake and output (I and O)
   - Maintain comfortable room temperature for patient
   - Avoid plastic mattresses and plastic bed protectors as they increase perspiration
   - Use antiperspirant or deodorant to minimize sweating and odor

10. Malaise due to presence of infection
    - Assist patient with activities of daily living (ADLs) as necessary
    - Schedule care, activities, and treatment around patient's rest schedule
    - Monitor phone calls and visitors around patient's energy level and rest schedule
    - Encourage frequent rest periods
    - Provide assistance as needed to prevent injury due to weakness
    - Provide method for patient to call for assistance
    - Encourage patient to set realistic goals of activities

Coma – stupor or unconsciousness from which a person cannot be aroused

Opisthotonos – spasm involving the entire body in which the back is arched backward; seen as a symptom of meningitis, tetanus, and poisoning

Arrhythmia – abnormal rhythm of the beat of the heart

Vagal nerve – tenth cranial nerve; responsible for swallowing and speaking as well as functioning of the aorta, stomach, and esophagus

- Allow adequate time to do activities and procedures to avoid frustration or possible injury
- Encourage exercise and activity to maintain muscle strength
- Utilize cane or walker for ambulation and transfer
- Provide private room as able for patient to promote rest periods

11. Photophobia
    - Avoid eye strain
    - Dim lights in room
    - Provide sunglasses per patient preference
    - Pull curtains in patient room
    - Encourage to get fresh air in the evening when sunlight diminished
    - Provide indirect lighting in patient room

12. Diplopia
    - Educate patient regarding head position to improve vision
    - Evaluate ability for patient to drive safely in presence of visual problems
    - Encourage alternate activities for patient who has difficulty with reading due to visual problems
    - Avoid eye strain
    - Provide large print books or cassettes
    - Avoid injury to the patient due to visual disturbances
    - Facilitate evaluation by ophthalmologist
    - Provide adequate lighting when reading, watching TV, or other activities
    - Remove environmental hazards, such as throw rugs, cluttered hallways, and excessive furniture

13. **Coma**
    - Reposition patient frequently to prevent skin breakdown
    - Prevent skin breakdown for patients with decreased mobility. Signs of skin breakdown (decubitus ulcers) include redness, swelling, warm or hot to touch, open sores, cyanosis, pain, and blisters. Prevention measures include frequent repositioning (minimum of every 1 to 2 hours); meticulous skin care; massage areas at bony prominences; encourage activity as able; alternating pressure mattresses; prevent pressure from appliances or tubing; prevent friction when repositioning by using a lift sheet and adequate assistance; and linens must be clean, dry, and wrinkle-free.
    - Complete neurological examination on routine basis
    - Provide adequate hydration
    - Continue to explain care and treatment to patient even though unresponsive
    - Offer comfort and reassurance to patient and family

14. **Opisthotonos**
    - Assist with position for patient comfort
    - Reposition patient frequently to prevent skin breakdown
    - Monitor patient for skin breakdown

15. Sinus **arrhythmia** due to **vagal nerve** involvement
    - Monitor vital signs (See Appendix D)
    - Monitor heart rate and rhythm
    - Instruct patient to report symptoms of vertigo, palpitations, chest pain, dyspnea, or diaphoresis

Fontanel – soft spot or open space between the skull bones in a fetus or infant

Apnea – absence of respirations

Arterial blood gases (ABGs) – test done to determine the amount of oxygen, carbon dioxide, and other gases present in the arterial blood

16. Altered level of consciousness
    - Complete neurological examination on routine basis
    - Monitor level of consciousness
    - Protect from injury due to altered level of consciousness

17. Hyperactive reflexes
    - Obtain baseline reflex check and monitor routinely while in the hospital

18. Bulging **fontanel** in infants
    - Obtain baseline on admission to hospital and monitor routinely while in the hospital

19. **Apnea**
    - Monitor respiratory status routinely while in the hospital
    - Utilize apnea monitor as necessary
    - Utilize ventilatory support as necessary
    - Monitor *arterial blood gases (ABGs)*
    - Monitor for cyanosis, diaphoresis, and decreased level of consciousness

20. Back and shoulder pain due to inflammation
    - Assist with position for patient comfort
    - Administer pain control methods such as massage, relaxation techniques, imaging, and pain medications as prescribed by physician
    - Use pillows to support head, neck, and back
    - Avoid constrictive garments
    - Encourage patient to report pain before it gets too severe
    - Monitor appetite due to pain
    - Encourage activity as able
    - Assist with ADLs as needed due to pain

21. Anorexia
    - Obtain baseline weight and monitor on routine basis
    - Offer small, frequent meals as tolerated
    - Provide nutritional supplements and vitamins
    - Monitor for signs of dehydration, such as decreased urine output, concentrated urine, dry skin, tenting of skin, dry mucous membranes, dry mouth, dry eyes, confusion, and constipation
    - Encourage family and friends to bring in food that is appealing to patient as dietary restrictions allow
    - Offer menu choices according to patient preference
    - Administer parenteral fluids as necessary
    - Monitor intake and output (I and O)
    - Encourage fluids to prevent dehydration
    - Avoid unpleasant sights and odors in room to make meals more appealing
    - Provide meticulous mouth care
    - Maintain social atmosphere for mealtimes to encourage the patient to eat
    - Encourage clothing that enhances patient appearance
    - Facilitate exercise program as tolerated to increase appetite

Nasopharyngeal – nose and throat

Antipyretic – substance used to decrease a fever

CRANIAL NERVES

A mnemonic that can be used to memorize the cranial nerves is to remember that the first letter of each of the cranial nerves is also the first letter of each of the words of the following sentence: "On old Olympus's towering tops, a Finn and German viewed some hops." (Refer to Table 19-1, page 193.)

NEUROLOGICAL EXAMINATION

A baseline neurological examination should be completed on admission to the hospital and monitored on a routine basis. Basic areas of the neurological examination include the following.

1. Check patient level of consciousness (LOC)
2. Cranial nerve check
3. Check client orientation to time, place, and person with questions to determine the presence of short-term and long-term memory
4. Check muscle strength, movement, coordination, and tendon reflexes
5. Check sensations to heat, cold, touch, and pain

DIAGNOSIS

1. Symptoms
2. Physical examination
3. *Lumbar puncture*
   - Increased cerebrospinal fluid (CSF) pressure
   - Fluid may be cloudy or blood-tinged
   - Culture CSF
   - Presence of elevated WBCs, decreased glucose, and elevated protein
4. Positive Brudzinski's sign
5. Positive Kernig's sign
6. *CT scan to rule out tumor or hemorrhage*
7. *CBC indicates elevated WBC*
8. *Platelet count*
9. *Urinalysis*
10. Cultures of urine, blood, and **nasopharyngeal** fluid to determine origin of infection
11. *Chest x-ray (CXR)*

TREATMENT

1. Antibiotics for the specific antigen; IV antibiotics are generally recommended for a 2-week period followed by oral antibiotics, e.g. Penicillin G, ampicillin, Ceftriaxone
2. Bedrest
3. Isolation is recommended for a minimum of 24 hours after starting antibiotics
4. Fluids orally or intravenously (IV)
5. Mannitol used to decrease cerebral edema
6. Analgesics administered for relief of pain
7. **Antipyretics** administered for reduction of fever

Disseminated intravascular coagulation – accumulation of platelets in the small vessels in the body causing clots to form, while at the same time the platelets are depleted in other areas of the body and hemorrhaging occurs

Shock – condition in which the heart and circulatory system fail to provide adequate oxygenated blood to all the organs and tissues of the body

Hydrocephalus – accumulation of cerebrospinal fluid within the cranium; the excess fluid may cause an enlargement of the skull in infants and causes extreme pressure on the brain; accumulation of fluid caused from overproduction of cerebrospinal fluid or inadequate drainage of the cerebrospinal fluid

COMPLICATIONS

1. Permanent cranial nerve damage
2. **Disseminated intravascular coagulation**
3. Brain stem herniation due to increased intracranial pressure
4. **Shock**
5. Seizures
6. Cerebral edema
7. **Hydrocephalus**

CONSIDERATIONS FOR CARE

1. Educate patient and family regarding the disease process.
2. Educate patient and family regarding forms of treatment as well as side effects of medications.
3. Provide emotional support for the patient and family.
4. Provide respiratory isolation for the first 24 hours after beginning antibiotic therapy.
5. Monitor family and friends and anyone who had been in close contact with the patient for signs of meningitis.
6. Monitor for complications.
7. Monitor intake and output (I and O).
8. Encourage fluids.
9. Follow medication regimen as ordered with doses at correct times.
10. Monitor for side effects of medications.
11. Monitor level of comfort and offer comfort measures: relaxation techniques, positioning, massage, imaging, and medications as prescribed by physician.
12. Meticulous handwashing on the part of the patient, staff, family, and visitors.
13. Proper disposal of nasopharyngeal discharge and tissues.
14. Obtain baseline vital signs and monitor routinely throughout hospital stay.
15. Obtain baseline neurological examination and monitor routinely throughout hospital stay.
16. For infants, obtain baseline head circumference and monitor routinely throughout hospital stay.
17. Precautions should be taken to prevent the client from injury in the presence of seizures; monitor for seizure activity.
18. Provide quiet, darkened environment for the patient.
19. Monitor for skin breakdown due to inactivity.
20. Prevent constipation due to inactivity, e.g. fluids, fiber, and range of motion exercises (ROM).
21. Monitor for symptoms of increased intracranial pressure which include decreased level of consciousness (LOC), elevated blood pressure (BP), decreased pulse rate, irregular or difficult respirations, and diminished or unequal pupil response to light.
22. Educate client to lie flat 4 to 6 hours after a *spinal tap* (*lumbar puncture*).
23. Elevate head of bed (HOB) approximately 30 degrees to decrease intracranial swelling.
24. Suction equipment available at bedside.
25. Avoid straining with a bowel movement or other forms of exertion.
26. Provide quiet, relaxed environment for the client.

ASSIGNMENT SHEET: MENINGITIS

Short Answer

1. Write a brief definition for the terms listed throughout the chapter.
2. Describe the physiology of the meninges.
3. Write a brief definition for meningitis.
4. Describe the incidence of meningitis.
5. List five (5) primary causes for meningitis.
6. Describe eight (8) common modes of transmission of meningitis.
7. List ten (10) risk factors which could make a person more susceptible to meningitis.
8. List twenty-two (22) signs and symptoms associated with meningitis and associated care.
9. Describe what is included in a neurological examination.
10. Identify eleven (11) specific methods used in the diagnosis of meningitis.
11. Identify seven (7) specific methods used in the treatment of meningitis.
12. Describe the following procedures used in the diagnosis of meningitis.
    a. Lumbar puncture
    b. CT scan
    c. Chest x-ray (CXR)
13. Write the normal range for each of the following laboratory tests.
    a. Electrolytes
       - Sodium
       - Potassium
       - Chloride
    b. Arterial blood gases (ABGs)
       - pCO_2
       - pH
       - pO_2
       - HCO_3
    c. CBC
       - Hematocrit
       - Hemoglobin
       - Platelet count
       - Red blood cell count (RBC)
       - White blood cell count (WBC)
    d. Urinalysis
       - Color
       - Specific gravity
       - pH

14. Describe seven (7) complications associated with meningitis.
15. List twenty-six (26) considerations for caring for a patient with meningitis.
16. List the twelve (12) cranial nerves and describe a specific problem/complication associated with decreased function of each.

KNOWLEDGE INTO ACTION

1. Marian Gouter, a 19-year-old college student, tells you that she is concerned about her 16-month-old baby, Serina. She says for the past few days the child has been irritable, vomiting, less responsive, has a poor appetite, and has a fever of 102.4° rectally. The child frequently has ear infections. You are concerned that the child could have meningitis and tell the mother the child should be seen by a physician immediately. The mother says to you, "We don't have insurance, and with both of us in college, we don't have enough money the way it is. We'll have to wait and see how things go and hope Serina is better in a few days." What will your response be?

2. A 6-month-old child is admitted to the hospital to rule out meningitis. A physical finding that could be an indication of meningitis in an infant would be: (Choose the best answer.)
   a. Hyperactivity
   b. Increased appetite
   c. Blue discoloration of the skin around the mouth
   d. Bulging fontanels

3. The 6-month-old child is admitted to the hospital due to an initial diagnosis of probable meningitis. A lumbar puncture is done, as well as a CBC, platelet count, and urinalysis. Which of the following laboratory results would be the best indicator that the child has meningitis? (Choose the best answer.)
   a. Spinal fluid is clear, WBC is 7200 mm^3, and platelet count is 300,000 mm^3.
   b. Urine is clear with a specific gravity of 1.012, RBC is 4.9 $10^6/mm^3$.
   c. Spinal fluid is cloudy, WBC is 16,100 mm^3
   d. CT scan is normal, platelet count is 174,000 mm^3.

Alzheimer's Disease

OBJECTIVES

Upon completion of this chapter, the student should be able to:

- Define the key terms listed throughout the chapter
- State a specific definition for Alzheimer's disease
- Describe the incidence of Alzheimer's disease
- List the risk factors for Alzheimer's disease
- Discuss the care that is associated to specific symptoms for a patient with Alzheimer's disease
- Identify specific methods for diagnosis of Alzheimer's disease
- Identify specific methods for treatment of Alzheimer's disease
- Describe the process involved with a neurological examination
- Explain considerations for caring for a patient with Alzheimer's disease

KEY TERMS

Alzheimer's disease – disease characterized by gradually worsening dementia; generally affects individuals over the age of 60

Stroke – nerve and brain damage resulting from diminished blood flow or cessation of blood flow to a specific portion of the brain

Parkinson's disease – disease of the nervous system characterized by weakness, muscle rigidity, and tremor

INTRODUCTION AND PHYSIOLOGY

Alzheimer's disease is characterized by progressive, irreversible dementia. Approximately 55% of dementia noted in elderly in the United States is caused by Alzheimer's disease. This dementia impairs the individual's ability to think, remember, speak, reason, and care for personal, physical, social, and nutritional needs. Other causes of dementia in the United States include **stroke**, **Parkinson's disease**, and injury or trauma to the brain.

The physiology of the brain leads to several theories of the onset of Alzheimer's disease. Several of these theories, along with the associated risk factors, are provided in the following section.

STATISTICS

Alzheimer's disease is the most common form of dementia and the main cause of institutionalization of the elderly, affecting more than 4 million people in the United States. An estimated 10% of the population in the United States over the age of 65 is affected, and by age 90, more than 45 to 50% will be affected. More than 100,000 to 120,000 people die from the disease annually in the United States, which makes it the fourth leading cause of death among adults, following heart disease, cancer, and stroke. The time span from onset of symptoms until death occurs can range from 3 years to more than 20 years. The cost of total care for patients with Alzheimer's disease in the United States is estimated at more than $80 to $90 billion annually. This cost includes long-term care, hospital care, lost wages, use of community services, and early death.

RISK FACTORS

The cause of Alzheimer's disease is unknown although there have been many theories. Several of these theories include:

Amyloid – a protein similar to starch

Basal ganglia – areas of gray matter located in the brain that assist in coordination of the muscles

Ventricle – refers to a cavity within the body; generally refers to either the ventricles within the brain or the ventricles in the lower chambers of the heart

Cortical – cortex or outer membrane of an organ

Herpes simplex virus – virus that causes vesicles on the skin, generally in the facial area

Terminal – pertaining to the end of life; often refers to a disease or illness that is expected to hasten death or be the direct cause of death

1. A decrease in the amount of acetylcholine in the brain. Acetylcholine, a neurotransmitter, is necessary for the transmission of information between the 100 billion nerve cells in the brain.

2. A development of plaque on the cells of the brain known as senile plaques. The plaques are caused from deposits of a form of protein called **amyloid**.

3. Physical factors, which include wasting of the **basal ganglia**, **ventricle** enlargement, and **cortical** atrophy.

4. A structural and functional impairment of the neurotransmitters of the brain associated with the aging process or chemical imbalance.

5. Chromosomal defect to chromosomes 14 and 19 have been shown to occur in hereditary Alzheimer's disease, especially in the clients who are 40 to 55 years old.

6. An increase in the amount of Alzheimer's disease in certain families, which suggests a genetic cause. An estimated 50% of patients with Alzheimer's disease also has a close relative with the disease.

7. A connection has been shown between Alzheimer's disease and Trisomy 21, the primary cause of Down syndrome. Patients with Down syndrome are three times more likely to get Alzheimer's disease.

8. A possible link has been suggested between the **Herpes simplex virus** and Alzheimer's disease.

9. A correlation has been shown between individuals who have head trauma and later develop Alzheimer's disease.

10. Aluminum and silicon deposits have been found in the brains of patients with Alzheimer's disease.

SIGNS, SYMPTOMS, AND ASSOCIATED CARE

The onset of Alzheimer's disease is insidious. The patient generally goes through several stages of the disease, which are as follows:

Stage 1—During this stage, the patient experiences mild memory lapses and a shortened attention span. The patient also has a decreased interest in personal and social affairs.

Stage 2—During this stage, the memory lapses become much more obvious. The patient experiences short-term memory loss while retaining long-term memory. The patient begins to forget appointments, birthdays, and other important information. Personal items may be frequently lost or misplaced. In an effort to cover up their memory loss, the patient may begin to make things up.

Stage 3—During this stage, the patient may become completely disoriented to people, places, and time. Due to extreme memory loss, the patient will have difficulty carrying on a conversation. In addition, the patient will exhibit deficits in motor coordination and may tend to wander off.

Stage 4—Stage 4 is the **terminal** stage of the disease. The patient completely loses the ability to communicate, has complete loss of recognition of family and friends, loses bowel and bladder control and has a decreased gag reflex. Death often occurs due to aspiration pneumonia or other types of infection. From the onset of symptoms to the time of death is an average of 8 to 20 years.

The symptoms of Alzheimer's disease come on gradually and worsen with time.

1. Forgetfulness
   - Label cupboards, doors, and drawers. As the memory fades, you may need to resort to pictures to label these.

- Display labeled photos of family members
- Keep a notebook of appointments
- Place items frequently used in a location that is consistent
- Display calendars and large clocks. Clocks may need to be digital with AM and PM clearly marked.

2. Recent memory loss
- Retain familiar surroundings as much as possible.
- Follow routines daily that are consistent so the patient knows what to expect. Have the routine marked on a visual spot so the patient is aware of the routine. A checklist of the day's activities may help.
- Keep a calendar of events that have occurred and what will be happening for the patient to refer to. (See Figure 21-1.)

3. Aphasia
- Provide alternate methods of communication to be used as the aphasia worsens. Word boards and symbol boards are examples. (See Figure 21-2.)
- Encourage communication efforts on the part of the patient
- Use brief, clear instructions for the patient to more easily understand
- Allow time for the patient to respond to directions or questions
- Avoid directions that can be taken too literally, such as "Jump up on the scale"
- Practice singing and reading aloud
- Practice making exaggerated facial expressions in the mirror
- Be certain you correctly understand what the patient is saying
- Maintain good eye contact when speaking with the patient
- Concentrate on what the patient is saying
- Avoid outside distractions (TV, radio)
- Avoid rooms that are congested with other people when visiting
- Avoid finishing sentences for the patient
- Encourage patient not to isolate themselves
- Encourage continued efforts at communication on the part of the patient
- Allow time for the patient to respond to questions and comments

4. Apraxia
- Provide frequent verbal, nonverbal, and written cues as necessary
- Provide short, concise explanations as needed

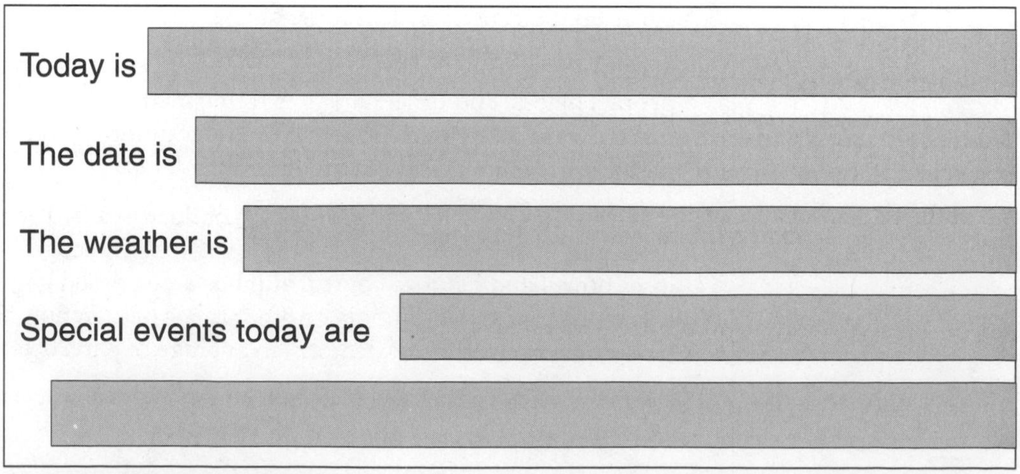

Today is

The date is

The weather is

Special events today are

Figure 21-1   Memory board

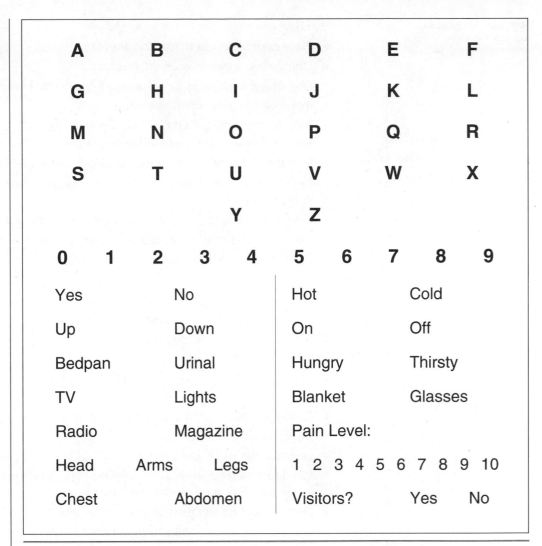

Figure 21-2   Word boards may be used as a method of communication.

5. Judgment impairment
   - Provide behavior cues to patient as appropriate
   - Avoid situations that could cause embarrassment to the patient while continuing to encourage socialization
   - Avoid situations that could cause potential harm to the patient, such as driving
6. Behavior changes
   - Recognize that these behavior changes are among the symptoms of the disease
   - Respond positively to appropriate behavior
   - Refocus patient's attention elsewhere if inappropriate behavior
7. Personal hygiene deterioration
   - Prevent skin breakdown by keeping skin clean and dry; linens clean, dry, and free of wrinkles; and change patient position at least every 2 hours
   - Substitute zippers for buttons, velcro for shoelaces, and elastic waste and slip-on clothing when available
   - Remove out-of-season and unnecessary clothing from closets and drawers
   - Offer warm, wet washcloth before and after meals, before bedtime and after using the bathroom
   - Offer clean articles of clothing as necessary.

Agnosia – inability to understand sensory input (seeing, hearing, and feeling)

8. Wandering
   - Place door locks out of the line of vision
   - Double bolt locks on each outside exit
   - Encourage exercise as daily routine to use stored energy
   - Install safety gate across steps and doors
   - Install security alarms on outside doors and exits
   - Provide patient with an identification bracelet
   - Install night lights throughout the house, especially in bathroom
   - Remove breakable items from shelves where they could easily be bumped off
   - Keep medications and cleaning supplies out of reach in a locked cabinet
   - Keep cigarettes and matches out of reach in a locked cabinet
   - Block access to kitchen and appliances when not in use

9. Dysphagia
   - Offer foods that are easy to chew according to patient preference
   - Avoid fresh fruits and vegetables as these are often more difficult to chew
   - Alternate liquids and solids during meals
   - Monitor for choking
   - Instruct family members on the Heimlich maneuver should choking occur while they are with the patient and for when the patient returns home
   - Utilize suction equipment in the event of choking
   - Concentrate on chewing food thoroughly
   - Educate that food may need to be cut into smaller pieces, ground, or pureed
   - Provide a method, such as a warming plate, to keep food warm during the entire length of time needed for patient to eat
   - Obtain baseline weight and monitor on routine basis
   - Encourage patient to take as much time as necessary during meals
   - Avoid outside distractions during mealtime to avoid choking
   - Have patient sit upright to eat
   - Be alert for symptoms of dehydration. Symptoms of dehydration include constipation, decreased amounts of urine, concentrated urine, dry skin, tenting of skin, dry mouth, dry eyes, hypotension, and confusion.
   - Use a syringe to feed liquids in small amounts

10. **Agnosia**
    - Protect from harm due to inability to recognize possibly harmful outside stimuli
    - Provide verbal, nonverbal, and written cues to orient patient to outside stimuli

11. Short attention span
    - Encourage eye contact with the patient when talking to him
    - Avoid outside distractions as much as possible

12. Mood changes
    - Recognize that these mood changes may be part of the disease
    - Maintain quiet, calm atmosphere as much as possible

13. Inappropriate affect
    - Avoid situations that could be potentially embarrassing to the patient
    - Remove patient from situations if the behavior is causing them embarrassment

Paranoia – mental disturbance characterized by delusions of persecution or illusions of grandeur

Delusion – false thought or belief that is not consistent with the actual external stimuli or with the truth

Hallucination – sensory perception that is not based on actual external stimuli; may relate to the sense of taste, smell, sight, sound, or touch

Confabulation – a person who has experienced memory loss may imagine or make up events to fill in the gaps of the loss of memory

14. Restlessness
   - Provide activities that the patient enjoys throughout the day
   - Offer regular exercise routines for the patient

15. Gait disturbance
   - Install hand rails and grab bars
   - Remove unnecessary throw rugs
   - Remove excess furniture and knick-knacks
   - Provide adequate lighting
   - Refrain from the use of restraints if possible

16. **Paranoia**
   - Reorient as needed
   - Avoid arguing with the patient when trying to reorient or explain
   - Remind patient frequently who you are and what your role is
   - Explain to patient what will be happening in clear, concise sentences
   - Offer patient as much control over his situation as possible
   - Remain consistent when answering questions

17. **Delusions** or **hallucinations**
   - Don't confront patient when trying to explain reality
   - Refocus attention to a different area

18. **Confabulation**
   - Do not go along with a confabulation when you know it to be untrue
   - Refrain from teasing or belittling the patient
   - Use consistency in explanations for the patient

19. Depression
   - Offer choices in care and routine as available
   - Continue to treat the patient as an adult
   - Offer frequent reassurance as needed by the patient
   - Avoid situations that have been known to cause depression in the patient
   - Administer medications as needed to treat the depression

20. Incontinence
   - Keep a written record of the patient's toileting schedule and adhere to it as much as possible
   - Be aware of nonverbal cues the patient may exhibit when needing to use the bathroom
   - Keep the patient's skin clean and dry to avoid skin breakdown and odor
   - Prevent odors in the room by changing linens as needed and washing off furniture that becomes wet or soiled
   - Prevent embarrassment to the patient
   - Do not tease or belittle the patient
   - Respond to the patient request to go to the bathroom as soon as possible
   - Use a mild soap to cleanse the patient skin and pat dry
   - Massage pressure points to prevent skin breakdown
   - Provide privacy for the patient when he is using the bathroom
   - Assess for bladder control and observe for incontinence
   - Observe for and educate family to observe for and report symptoms of urinary tract infection, e.g. burning with urination, frequency, urgency, pain, fever, cloudy urine, malodorous urine, and bloody urine
   - Encourage fluid intake

Autopsy – surgical examination of the body and tissues of the body after death; often done to determine the cause of death

21. Insomnia
    - Avoid caffeine and other stimulants late in the day
    - Utilize relaxation techniques, music, or other methods to relax patient at bedtime
    - Encourage patient to establish a ritual for bedtime to promote relaxation
    - Avoid distractions and noise once the patient is in bed
    - Avoid large meals close to bedtime
    - Schedule medications and treatments at times other than bedtime
    - Encourage exercise at regular intervals throughout the day
    - Avoid sleeping throughout the day if possible

22. Violent outbursts
    - Always tell the patient what will be happening in concise terms
    - Remain calm and supportive for the patient
    - Never approach the patient from behind
    - Speak to the patient when entering the room
    - Diminish noise and distractions as much as possible
    - Move slowly so as not to frighten the patient
    - Be aware of situations that cause problems and avoid them

23. Seizures in advanced stages
    - Protect patient from injury during a seizure
    - Be aware of any aura the patient may experience prior to a seizure
    - Turn patient on his side after a seizure if he begins to choke or vomit
    - Call an ambulance if needed
    - Monitor patient for seizures and administer medications as prescribed by physician
    - Offer reassurance to patient and family during and after a seizure
    - Monitor duration and intensity of seizure as well as body involvement
    - Monitor airway and breathing following a seizure
    - Provide privacy for the patient during and after a seizure

DIAGNOSIS

Early diagnosis of Alzheimer's disease is difficult due to the insidious onset of the symptoms. The absence of other diseases or disorders needs to be ruled out, as well as ruling out reversible causes of dementia. Diagnosis has been 80 to 90% accurate when compared with the results of an **autopsy**.

Forms of diagnosis include the following.

1. Patient history
2. Physical examination
3. Psychological testing
4. *Computed tomography scan*
5. *Liver* and *thyroid function studies*
6. Analysis of diet
7. *Magnetic resonance imaging (MRI)*
8. Family history of Alzheimer's
9. Family interview
10. Neurological examination (See section entitled Neurological Examination)

Neurofibrillary tangles –
nerve fibers twisted in
tangles that are located in
the neuron of the cell;
present in Alzheimer's
disease

Vasodilator – medication
or substance that causes
dilation of the vessels of
the body

Hyperbaric – increased
pressure and increased
amounts of oxygen

11. *Electroencephalogram*

12. *Lumbar puncture*

13. *EKG*

14. History of medication

15. *Positron emission transaxial tomography scan*, measures metabolic activity of the cerebral cortex

16. Onset of symptoms between 40 to 90 years old

Positive diagnosis of the disease can only be made postmortem during which time the findings will be senile plaques and **neurofibrillary tangles**. Neurofibrillary tangles are nerve fibers twisted in tangles that are located in the neuron of the cell.

NEUROLOGICAL EXAMINATION

A baseline neurological examination should be completed on admission to the hospital and monitored on a routine basis. Basic areas of the neurological examination include the following:

1. Check patient level of consciousness (LOC)

2. Cranial nerve check

3. Check client orientation to time, place, and person with questions to determine the presence of short-term and long-term memory

4. Check muscle strength, movement, coordination, and tendon reflexes

5. Check sensations to heat, cold, touch, and pain

TREATMENT

Most treatment for Alzheimer's disease consists of palliative rather than curative measures. Some of the treatments currently used are as follows.

1. Cerebral **vasodilators** are used to increase the vascular circulation in the brain.

2. Antidepressants are used to treat the symptoms of depression that may accompany Alzheimer's disease.

3. **Hyperbaric** oxygen is used in the attempt to increase the oxygen available to the brain for consumption.

4. Avoid use of products that contain aluminum such as antacids, aluminum-containing deodorant, and aluminum cooking utensils.

5. Several drugs are being used in an attempt to slow the disease process. Examples of these drugs include lecithin, naloxone, and choline salts.

6. Tetradroaminoacridine (THA) has been shown to improve memory function in some patients with Alzheimer's disease.

7. Physostigmine increases the level of acetylcholine by blocking its breakdown.

CONSIDERATIONS FOR CARE

The prime concern when caring for a patient with Alzheimer's disease, in addition to patient safety, is to promote the patient's remaining abilities and provide compensation for the patient's lost abilities. Other considerations for care are listed.

1. Offer support to the patient and family. Allow them to verbalize feelings and concerns. Family members are often the primary caregivers and suffer from financial burdens of care as well as exhaustion, isolation, and physical health problems.

2. Constitute a communication system with the patient and the patient's family that allows him to freely verbalize thoughts and feelings.

3. Instruct the patient and family about available community resources.

4. Put the patient and family in touch with an Alzheimer's support group if one is available.

5. Keep the patient as active as possible to promote physical mobility.

6. Establish a routine of care for the patient and adhere to it as strictly as possible, both in the hospital or long-term care facility as well as in the home.

7. Install safety devices such as grab bars, ramps, and nonskid flooring.

8. Involve the family in all aspects of the patient's care, treatment, and planning.

9. Monitor nutrition, weight, and intake and output (I and O).

10. Retain a calm, soothing atmosphere with a minimum of stress and distractions.

11. Assess the patient's sleeping pattern. Work around this pattern as needed when carrying out the activities of daily living.

12. Test the temperature of the food for the patient to prevent burns.

13. Provide cues for the patient that will aid in reality orientation, such as clocks, calendars, photos, and bulletin boards with recent information.

14. When offering the patient choices, limit these choices to two or three items.

15. Assess for need of bowel or bladder retraining program and instruct the patient and family as necessary.

16. Give instructions to the patient that are clear, simple, and concise.

17. Ensure that personal hygiene needs are met to include mouth, hair, and skin care.

18. With input from the patient and family, set realistic goals for the patient.

19. Promote independence when possible on the part of the patient.

20. Talk to the patient about things that are familiar to him, remembering that long-term memory is often the best.

21. Continue to accept the patient as a human being and demonstrate this in your care.

22. Realize the importance of nonverbal communication, such as smiling, touching, and hugging as appropriate.

23. Explain routines and procedures to the patient to gain compliance.

24. Educate patient and family regarding need to carry a medical alert card and wear a medical alert bracelet or necklace.

FOR MORE INFORMATION

Alzheimer's Disease and Related Disorders Association
70 East Lake Street
Chicago, IL 60601
1-800-621-0379 or 1-800-572-6037 (in Illinois)

Alzheimer's Disease Education and Referral Center
P.O. Box 8250
Silver Spring, MD 20907-8250
1-800-438-4380

Alzheimer's Association
Suite 1000
919 North Michigan Avenue
Chicago, IL 60611
1-800-272-3900

ASSIGNMENT SHEET: ALZHEIMER'S DISEASE

Short Answer

1. Write a brief definition for the terms listed throughout the chapter.

2. Write a brief definition for Alzheimer's disease.

3. Describe the incidence of Alzheimer's disease.

4. Briefly describe ten (10) risk factors for Alzheimer's disease.

5. Briefly describe the four (4) stages of Alzheimer's disease.

6. Describe the associated care for each of the following symptoms.
   a. Forgetfulness
   b. Recent memory loss
   c. Aphasia
   d. Apraxia
   e. Judgment impairment
   f. Behavior changes
   g. Personal hygiene deterioration
   h. Wandering
   i. Dysphagia
   j. Agnosia
   k. Short attention span
   l. Mood changes
   m. Inappropriate affect
   n. Restlessness
   o. Gait disturbance
   p. Paranoia
   q. Delusions or hallucinations
   r. Confabulation
   s. Depression
   t. Incontinence
   u. Insomnia
   v. Violent outbursts
   w. Seizures in advanced stages

7. Describe what is meant by each of the following methods of diagnosis.
   a. Computerized tomography scan (CT Scan)
   b. Electroencephalogram
   c. Lumbar puncture
   d. Electrocardiogram
   e. Magnetic resonance imaging (MRI)
   f. Positron emission transaxial tomography scan

8. Describe seven (7) specific forms of treatment for Alzheimer's disease.

9. Describe twenty-four (24) considerations for caring for a patient with Alzheimer's disease or to assist the family of a patient with Alzheimer's disease.

10. Write the normal range for each of the following serum laboratory tests.
    a. Thyroxine
    b. T3
    c. TSH
    d. SGOT
    e. SGPT
    f. Bilirubin
    g. Albumin
    h. Alkaline phosphatase
    i. Prothrombin time

KNOWLEDGE INTO ACTION

1. Lester Two Hawks, a 78-year-old retired social worker, is in your long-term care facility. He has a 15-year history of Alzheimer's disease and is no longer able to care for himself in his own home. List three methods of associated care relating to patient safety due to the symptoms of wandering, dysphagia, impaired judgment, gait disturbance, and seizures.

2. Veronica Languin, a 71-year-old retired concert pianist, is in your long-term care facility due to her inability to care for herself due to her Alzheimer's disease. Her symptoms include, among other symptoms, incontinence and insomnia. List four methods of associated care that should be included in Mrs. Languin's plan of care that should be done on a daily basis, or more frequently, due to her incontinence and insomnia.

3. Your neighbor tells you she is concerned about her 76-year-old father who is becoming more forgetful, withdrawn, has been losing things, and whose personal hygiene has deteriorated. She says to you, "I'm concerned that Dad might have

Alzheimer's disease, and I am trying to get him to go to the doctor. What would they do to diagnose Alzheimer's disease? I don't want him to go through a lot of painful tests." What will your response be?

4.   After you have talked to your neighbor about how Alzheimer's disease is diagnosed, she asks, "If it is Alzheimer's disease, how do they treat it?" What will your response be?

5.   Two weeks later, you receive a phone call from your neighbor. She states that her father has been diagnosed with Alzheimer's disease and has chosen to live with his daughter, your neighbor. She is concerned about being able to care adequately for her father and asks you to make a list of suggestions that would better help her care for her father. Make a list of fifteen (15) items that could make the care of your neighbor's father easier and safer for your neighbor.

UNIT 5

CARDIOVASCULAR DISORDERS

Hypertension

OBJECTIVES

Upon completion of this chapter, the student should be able to:

- Define the key terms listed throughout the chapter
- State a specific definition for hypertension
- Describe normal blood pressure
- Describe the incidence of hypertension
- List risk factors associated with essential hypertension
- List risk factors associated with secondary hypertension
- Describe the signs and symptoms associated with hypertension
- List specific methods used to diagnose essential hypertension
- List specific methods used to diagnose the causes of secondary hypertension
- Identify specific methods of treatment for hypertension
- Describe complications associated with hypertension as they relate to specific organs of the body
- Write a specific definition for hypertensive crisis
- Describe specific considerations for caring for a patient with hypertension

KEY TERMS

Systolic – refers to the first or top number in blood pressure; maximum blood pressure during contraction of the ventricles of the heart

Diastolic – refers to the lower or bottom number of the blood pressure; the amount of pressure needed to keep the arteries open during relaxation of the ventricles of the heart

Renal – refers to the kidney

Systole – refers to the period of contraction of the ventricles of the heart

Arterial – pertains to artery

Aorta – normally the largest vessel in the body; artery that transports blood to the systemic circulatory system from the left ventricle

Diastole – period of relaxation of the heartbeat that alternates with contraction, or systole, of the heart muscle

INTRODUCTION

Hypertension is defined as high blood pressure, with an elevation in either the **systolic** reading or the **diastolic** reading. Hypertension can be classified as either essential hypertension, for which the cause is unknown, or secondary hypertension, which is caused by an identifiable cause, such as **renal** disease, endocrine imbalance, pregnancy, or blood vessel disease.

PHYSIOLOGY

Blood pressure is the reading obtained by measuring the pressure exerted on arterial walls during left ventricular **systole**. Systole is the amount of pressure exerted on the **arterial** walls during contraction of the left ventricle of the heart, which forces blood into the **aorta** and major arteries. **Diastole** is the amount of pressure needed to keep the arteries open while the left ventricle of the heart refills with blood. Blood pressure is generally higher during activity, stress, or excitement, and decreases with rest or sleep. Blood pressure is affected by the person's age, gender, race, physical health, mental and emotional stress levels, and altitude. Blood pressure readings consist of obtaining two separate numbers: systolic, which has a normal range of 100 to 140, and diastolic, which has a normal range of 60 to 90. Blood pressure is written as a biphasic number, such as 120/90 (systolic/diastolic). (See Figure 22-1.)

STATISTICS

Hypertension affects an estimated 15 to 30% of the entire adult population in the United States. Of the 60 million people in the United States affected with hypertension, approximately 50% are unaware that they have high blood pressure.

Catecholamines – examples of catecholamines include epinephrine and norepinephrine; increase heart rate and act as vasoconstrictors

Sedentary – life style that includes very little physical labor, exertion, or exercise; inactive

Intima – lining of the blood vessels

Coarctation – narrowing of the lumen of a vessel; frequently refers to the aorta

Pheochromocytoma – tumor located in the adrenal medulla that secretes epinephrine and norepinephrine

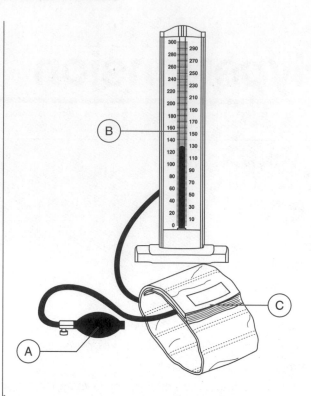

Figure 22-1 Blood pressure equipment: (a) bulb, (b) mercury manometer, (c) blood pressure cuff (From Hegner, *Assisting in Long-Term Care, 2nd edition Workbook,* copyright © 1992, Delmar Publishers)

RISK FACTORS FOR ESSENTIAL HYPERTENSION

Essential hypertension accounts for 90 to 95% of all people with diagnosed hypertension. Factors which predispose a person to essential hypertension are:

1. Obesity—Hypertension is most common in people who are overweight
2. Stress—An increase in the release of **catecholamines** elevates blood pressure
3. Smoking—nicotine acts as a vasoconstrictor, which elevates blood pressure
4. Heredity
5. **Sedentary** life style
6. Diabetes mellitus—People with diabetes mellitus have blood vessel scar formation in the **intima** of the vessel, which reduces elasticity of the vessel, elevating blood pressure
7. Race—Note that hypertension is most common in African-Americans
8. Age—Blood vessels lose their elasticity with age, which increases blood pressure
9. High dietary intake of sodium or fats and cholesterol
   - Sodium retains fluid in the body which increases the circulating fluid volume and elevates blood pressure
   - Cholesterol builds up in the lining of the blood vessels causing narrowed vessels and elevating blood pressure

RISK FACTORS FOR SECONDARY HYPERTENSION

Secondary hypertension accounts for 5 to 10% of all people diagnosed with hypertension. Factors that predispose a person to secondary hypertension are:

1. **Coarctation** of the aorta—Narrowing of the aorta due to malformation
2. **Pheochromocytoma**—A tumor of the adrenal gland that secretes large amounts of epinephrine and norepinephrine; generally these tumors are benign (See Figure 22-2)

Cushing's syndrome – overproduction and secretion of glucocorticoids from the adrenal glands

Glucocorticoids – hormones secreted by the adrenal gland that affect the metabolism of carbohydrates and proteins in the body

Hyperaldosteronism – condition during which an abnormally large amount of aldosterone is manufactured and secreted by the adrenal glands

Congenital – present from the time of birth

Pyelonephritis – inflammation of the kidney(s)

Glomerulonephritis – inflammation of the glomeruli of the kidney

Hyperthyroidism – condition during which an abnormally large amount of thyroid hormones is manufactured and secreted by the thyroid

Eclampsia – complication of pregnancy that develops during the last portion of the pregnancy; characterized by hypertension, weight gain, headaches, and edema; severe cases may lead to seizures, coma, and possible death

Neurological – refers to the nervous system

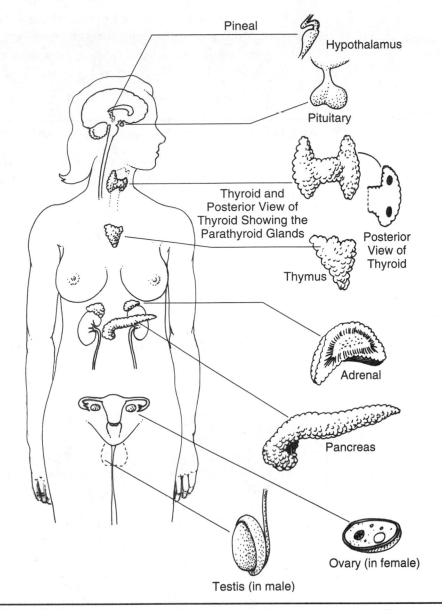

Figure 22-2 Endocrine glands in the body (From Burke, *Human Anatomy and Physiology in Health and Disease, 3rd edition,* copyright © 1992, Delmar Publishers)

3. **Cushing's syndrome**—Secretion of large amounts of **glucocorticoids** from the adrenal gland due to stimulation from the pituitary gland

4. **Hyperaldosteronism**—Production of large amounts of aldosterone by the adrenal gland

5. **Congenital** renal abnormalities—Kidney abnormalities that are present at birth and lead to fluid retention

6. **Pyelonephritis**—Inflammation of the kidney caused from bacterial infection

7. **Glomerulonephritis**—Inflammatory disease of the glomeruli of the kidneys that has the potential to lead to kidney failure

8. **Hyperthyroidism**—Increased production of hormones by the thyroid gland

9. Pregnancy—**Eclampsia**, a severe condition that can occur in the last half of pregnancy, causes fluid retention, hypertension, seizures, coma, and possible death

10. **Neurological** disorders—Brain tumors, increased intracranial pressure, head injury, cerebrovascular disease, strokes, and cerebral aneurysm are examples of neurological disorders that can cause hypertension

11. Diabetes mellitus—Diabetes mellitus can damage the intima (lining) of the blood vessels of the body, that can cause hypertension

12. Oral contraceptive use—Oral contraceptives contain estrogen and/or progestin and have the potential to elevate blood pressure

SIGNS, SYMPTOMS, AND ASSOCIATED CARE

Elevated blood pressure often has no symptoms and has been termed "the silent killer." When symptoms are present, they are generally indicative of organ or vascular involvement and include the following:

1. Headache
2. Vertigo
3. Palpitations
4. Nosebleeds
5. Impotence

The signs and symptoms of this disease are signals that hypertension should be considered as a diagnosis. Associated care for these signs and symptoms is aimed at patient comfort measures and staff protection measures.

DIAGNOSIS

Hypertension is diagnosed by obtaining an accurate blood pressure and monitoring the blood pressure on a routine basis. Hypertension is divided into several categories. (See Table 22-1.)

Diagnosis of secondary hypertension is also obtained with an accurate blood pressure reading and monitoring the blood pressure on a routine basis. Other tests that are performed help to diagnose the cause for secondary hypertension.

1. *EKG* will aid in the determination of heart-related causes
2. *CXR* is used to determine the presence of cardiac disease
3. *Urinalysis* is used to determine the presence of diabetes mellitus or renal disease
4. *Intravenous pyelography* is used to determine the presence of chronic renal disease
5. Thyroid function tests are used to determine the presence of thyroid disease, e.g. *Thyroxine, T3*, and *TSH*
6. *BUN* and *creatinine* to determine the presence of renal disease

Table 22-1 Systolic and Diastolic Blood Pressures			
Category	Systolic Range	Diastolic Range	Example
Normal	100–140	60–90	120/75
Mild hypertension	140–159	90–104	150/100
Moderate hypertension	160–199	105–114	180/110
Severe hypertension	200 or higher	115 or higher	200/115

Calcium channel blocker – medication that dilates vessels of the heart and reduces the oxygen requirements of the heart muscle; also used in the treatment of arrhythmias

Beta blockers – medications that decrease blood pressure and heart rate; may also be used for the treatment of angina

Peripheral – refers to a part of the body away from the midline

Angiotensin – vasoconstrictor in the bloodstream that is produced by the kidney

Encephalopathy – refers to any disease or disorder of the brain

Hypertrophy – enlarged size of a tissue or organ

Proteinuria – increased amounts of protein or albumin in the urine

TREATMENT

The goal of treatment is to maintain blood pressure at optimal level with a minimum of side effects and prevent complications.

1. Weight loss to desirable level
2. Stress reduction
3. Low-fat diet; calories from fat should make up less than 30% of total daily calories
4. Low-sodium diet of less than 2500 milligrams daily
5. Alternate form of birth control to replace oral contraceptives
6. Exercise program of 30 minutes of exercise 3 to 5 times per week
7. Relaxation techniques such as biofeedback, deep breathing, and meditation
8. Treatment of causes of secondary hypertension
9. Limit alcohol intake to no more than one ounce of alcohol daily
10. Smoking cessation
11. Medications

    - Diuretics to decrease total blood volume and blood pressure. It is necessary to monitor for sodium and potassium depletion, e.g. Hygroton, Hydrodiuril, Lasix, Aldactone
    - **Calcium channel blockers** to produce vasodilation, e.g. Verapamil, Nifedipine, Diltiazem
    - **Beta blockers** to lower blood pressure by decreasing cardiac output, e.g. Aldomet, Minipress, Inderal, Lopressor
    - Vasodilators to dilate vessels thereby decreasing **peripheral** vascular resistance, e.g. Apresoline, Corgard
    - Angiotensin converting enzyme (ACE) inhibitors reduce blood pressure by decreasing the production of **angiotensin**, e.g. Captopril, Enalapril, Lisinopril

COMPLICATIONS OF HYPERTENSION

Complications of hypertension result when the elevated blood pressure damages the intima of the blood vessels causing scar tissue formation, loss of elasticity of blood vessels, and decreased blood flow to the specific parts of the body. Following are complications that can result to specific organs of the body as a result of hypertension.

1. Brain—**encephalopathy**, stroke (cerebrovascular accident [CVA])
2. Heart—left ventricular **hypertrophy**, left ventricular failure, myocardial infarction (heart attack), congestive heart failure (CHF), coronary artery disease, and arrhythmias
3. Kidneys—decreased blood flow to kidneys, **proteinuria**, renal failure, and edema
4. Eyes—blindness

HYPERTENSIVE CRISIS

Hypertensive crisis is a life-threatening elevation in blood pressure and is considered a medical emergency. Precipitating factors include sudden cessation of medications, extreme salt intake, and stress.

CONSIDERATIONS FOR CARE

1. Educate patient and family regarding the disease process.

2. Educate patient and family regarding forms of treatment as well as side effects of medications.

3. Provide emotional support to patient.

4. Educate patient regarding importance of follow-up care and routine blood pressure monitoring.

5. Educate patient that hypertension generally is not associated with specific symptoms until complications arise.

6. Instruct patient regarding importance of following medication prescription as directed by physician.

7. Be aware that medications that can be taken on a daily basis will be easier for the patient to remember.

8. Instruct patient to report side effects to physician as there may be other options for medications to control blood pressure or methods to control side effects.

9. Assist patient and family in dietary education.

10. Consult dietitian as necessary.

11. Consult physical therapist as needed to recommend exercise program.

12. Educate patient and family regarding the need for life style changes as related to exercise, diet, and stress.

13. Monitor blood pressure using the following guidelines:

    - Obtain medication history from patient

    - Measure blood pressure under the same conditions each time

    - Use correct size of blood pressure cuff. Too large of cuff may give false low reading and too small of cuff may give false high reading.

    - Adjust position for patient comfort

    - Allow patient to rest if recent exertion or stress

    - Record blood pressure reading correctly

    - Record blood pressure for patient information and instruct regarding need for further monitoring

    - Report promptly to physician any person with a diastolic pressure of 120 or greater

14. Educate patient and family that blood pressure can be controlled but not cured.

15. Educate patient that medication control may result in orthostatic hypotension and he should get up slowly from lying position and sit or lay down promptly if experiencing vertigo.

16. Educate patient and family regarding need to carry a medical alert card and wear a medical alert bracelet or necklace.

17. Identify and modify patient risk factors for hypertension as well as monitoring for complications resulting from hypertension.

18. Educate patient and family regarding monitoring blood pressure at home on a routine basis.

FOR MORE INFORMATION

National High Blood Pressure Education Program
120/80 National Institutes of Health
Bethesda, MD 20892
(301) 496-1809

National Council on Patient Information and Education
Suite 1010
1625 I Street NW
Washington, DC 20006
(202) 466-6711

National Cholesterol Education Program
National Heart, Lung, and Blood Institute
C-200
Bethesda, MD 20892
(301) 230-1340

ASSIGNMENT SHEET: HYPTERTENSION

Short Answer

1. Write a brief definition for the terms listed throughout the chapter.

2. Describe normal blood pressure readings and what each of the readings indicates.
   a. Systolic
   b. Diastolic

3. Write a brief definition for hypertension.

4. Describe the incidence of hypertension.

5. List nine (9) risk factors associated with essential hypertension.

6. List twelve (12) risk factors associated with secondary hypertension.

7. Describe five (5) signs and symptoms associated with hypertension and describe the implications this could have.

8. Identify specific methods of diagnosis for hypertension.

9. Identify six (6) specific methods used to diagnose the cause of secondary hypertension.

10. Describe the goal of treatment for hypertension.

11. List eleven (11) specific methods of treatment used for hypertension.

12. Describe the cause of the complications associated with hypertension.

13. Describe complications associated with four (4) specific organs due to hypertension.
    a. Brain
    b. Heart
    c. Kidney
    d. Eye

14. Define hypertensive crisis.

15. List eighteen (18) specific considerations for caring for a patient with hypertension.

16. Describe each of the following procedures used in the diagnosis of the cause of secondary hypertension.

    a. Electrocardiogram (EKG)
    b. Chest x-ray (CXR)
    c. Intravenous pyelography (IVP)

17. Write the normal ranges for each of the following laboratory tests.

    a. Thyroid tests
       • Thyroxine
       • T3
       • TSH
    b. BUN
    c. Creatinine
    d. UA
       • Color
       • Specific gravity
       • pH

KNOWLEDGE INTO ACTION

1. Helen Franzen, a 58-year-old, comes into your clinic for a yearly physical examination. You are doing the initial assessment and obtain a blood pressure reading of 198/124. Mrs. Franzen's physician chooses to try nonmedication forms of treatment initially for her hypertension. List six methods of nonmedication forms of treatment, which could be used initially to treat Mrs. Franzen's hypertension.

2. Mrs. Franzen returns to your clinic in 3 months to recheck her blood pressure. At this time, her blood pressure is 172/104. At this point, her physician chooses to add a medication to her treatment. List the categories of medications that could be used to lower Mrs. Franzen's blood pressure and describe the rationale of why each of the medications would lower blood pressure.

3. Mrs. Franzen is ready to leave the clinic and comments to you, "What could happen to me if this blood pressure got out of hand?" What will your response be?

4. You are assisting a new staff member to take blood pressures. List four (4) guidelines you would want to stress to the new staff member in obtaining correct blood pressures.

23 Myocardial Infarction

OBJECTIVES

Upon completion of this chapter, the student should be able to:

- Define the key terms listed throughout the chapter
- Describe the physiology of the heart
- State a specific definition for myocardial infarction
- Describe the incidence of myocardial infarction
- List the cause of myocardial infarction
- List the risk factors for myocardial infarction and methods to reduce or eliminate these risk factors
- Describe the symptoms of myocardial infarction
- Identify specific methods for diagnosis of myocardial infarction
- Identify specific methods for treatment of myocardial infarction
- Describe complications that may result after a myocardial infarction and associated care for these complications
- Describe specific considerations for caring for a patient with myocardial infarction

KEY TERMS

Myocardial infarction (MI) – heart muscle death due to complete or partial obstruction of the coronary arteries that supply the specific regions of the heart muscle with blood; also known as heart attack

Ischemia – diminished blood supply to a portion of the body

Artery – blood vessel that carries blood away from the heart

Septum – division between two cavities or spaces within the body; frequently refers to the septum of the heart or the nasal septum

Atria (atrium) – upper chambers of the heart

Tricuspid valve – valve located between the right atrium and right ventricle of the heart

INTRODUCTION

Myocardial infarction (MI) is **ischemia** and necrosis of the heart muscle caused by insufficient coronary **artery** blood flow to keep the heart muscle alive. The site of the necrosis depends on which coronary arteries are involved. (See Figure 23-1.)

PHYSIOLOGY OF THE HEART

The heart is a hollow organ that is responsible for pumping oxygenated blood to the entire body. The heart is divided into right and left sides by a muscular wall called the **septum**. There are two upper chambers of the heart called the **atria (atrium)**, and the lower chambers of the heart are called the ventricles. Blood enters the right atrium of the heart after delivering oxygen and nutrients to the tissues of the body. It is squeezed into the right ventricle through the **tricuspid valve** where it then travels through the **pulmonary semilunar valve** through the **pulmonary artery** into the lungs, where it becomes oxygenated. Blood returns from the lung through the **pulmonary vein** into the left atrium. It travels through the **mitral valve (bicuspid)** into the left ventricle. Blood leaves the left ventricle through the **aortic semilunar valve**, through the aorta, and begins its journey back through the body to deliver its supply of oxygen and nutrients. The heart itself is supplied with oxygenated blood from arteries that branch off the aorta. (See Figure 23-2.)

STATISTICS

Heart disease is the leading cause of death in the United States. More than 50% of heart attack deaths occur within the first 60 minutes after the onset of symptoms; approximately 67% of deaths occur prior to the patient arriving at the hospital. Care is often

Pulmonary semilunar valve – valve located between the right ventricle of the heart and the pulmonary artery

Pulmonary artery – artery that carries blood to the lungs from the right ventricle of the heart

Pulmonary vein – vein that carries blood from the lungs to the left atrium of the heart

Mitral valve (bicuspid) – valve located in the heart between the left atrium and the left ventricle

Aortic semilunar valve – valve connecting the left ventricle of the heart and the aorta

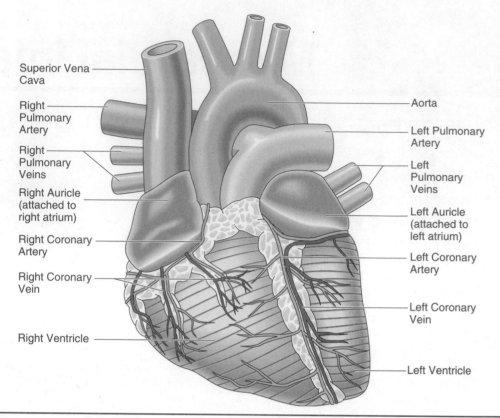

Superior Vena Cava

Right Pulmonary Artery

Right Pulmonary Veins

Right Auricle (attached to right atrium)

Right Coronary Artery

Right Coronary Vein

Right Ventricle

Aorta

Left Pulmonary Artery

Left Pulmonary Veins

Left Auricle (attached to left atrium)

Left Coronary Artery

Left Coronary Vein

Left Ventricle

Figure 23-1 External heart structures (From Layman, *The Medical Language,* copyright © 1995, Delmar Publishers)

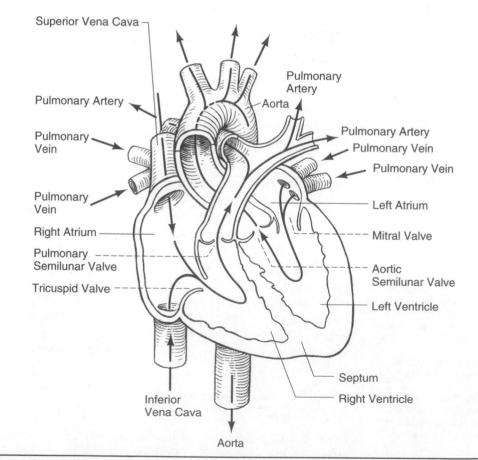

Superior Vena Cava

Pulmonary Artery

Pulmonary Vein

Pulmonary Vein

Right Atrium

Pulmonary Semilunar Valve

Tricuspid Valve

Inferior Vena Cava

Pulmonary Artery

Aorta

Pulmonary Artery

Pulmonary Vein

Pulmonary Vein

Left Atrium

Mitral Valve

Aortic Semilunar Valve

Left Ventricle

Septum

Right Ventricle

Aorta

Figure 23-2 Internal heart structures and blood flow (From Ehrlich, *Medical Terminology for Health Professions,* copyright © 1988, Delmar Publishers)

delayed due to denial on the part of the patient, thereby prolonging the length of time between onset of symptoms and seeking medical attention. About 8 hours is the average amount of time for a patient to be admitted to a coronary care unit (CCU) after the onset of symptoms. More than 1,500,000 people have heart attacks every year in the United States with approximately 650,000 dying from the myocardial infarction itself or associated complications.

CAUSE

Myocardial infarction is caused when any part of the heart does not get adequate blood, nutrient, and oxygen perfusion, therefore causing tissue death. (See Figure 23-3.) When the heart muscle dies (necrosis), it is less effective as a pump and blood flow is reduced to the heart as well as to the rest of the body. Myocardial infarction is caused by one of several factors.

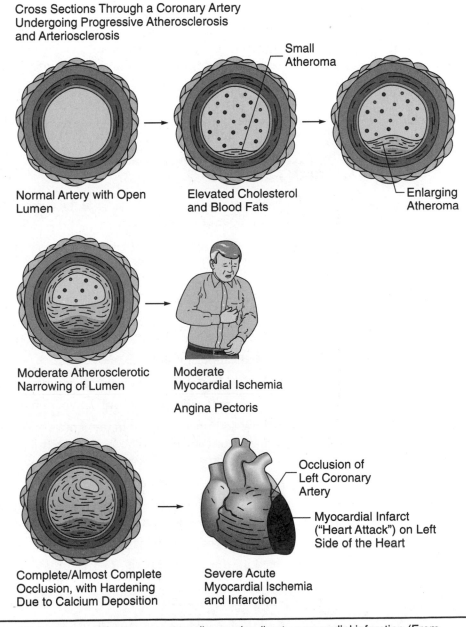

Cross Sections Through a Coronary Artery Undergoing Progressive Atherosclerosis and Arteriosclerosis

Small Atheroma

Normal Artery with Open Lumen

Elevated Cholesterol and Blood Fats

Enlarging Atheroma

Moderate Atherosclerotic Narrowing of Lumen

Moderate Myocardial Ischemia

Angina Pectoris

Complete/Almost Complete Occlusion, with Hardening Due to Calcium Deposition

Severe Acute Myocardial Ischemia and Infarction

Occlusion of Left Coronary Artery

Myocardial Infarct ("Heart Attack") on Left Side of the Heart

Figure 23-3   Phases of coronary artery disease leading to myocardial infarction (From Layman, *The Medical Language*, copyright © 1995, Delmar Publishers)

Spasm – uncontrolled movement caused by contraction of the muscles

Inferior – below another part

Vasoconstriction – constriction of the vessels of the body or a specific area of the body

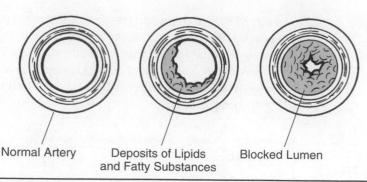

Normal Artery   Deposits of Lipids and Fatty Substances   Blocked Lumen

Figure 23-4 Atherosclerosis of an artery (From Keir et al., *Medical Assisting: Administrative and Clinical Competencies*, *3rd edition*, copyright © 1993, Delmar Publishers)

1. Coronary artery thrombosis precipitated by coronary artery disease, plaque build-up, or coronary artery **spasm** (See Figure 23-4)
2. Coronary artery inflammatory disease caused by infection

The area of the myocardial infarction depends on which coronary artery is damaged.

1. Inferior myocardial infarction results when the right coronary artery is occluded. An **inferior** MI damages the inferior wall of the left ventricle.
2. Anterior myocardial infarction results when the left anterior descending artery is occluded. An anterior MI damages the anterior wall of the left ventricle as well as the septum.

RISK FACTORS

1. Heredity—cannot be changed, but the person should have regular physicals and reduce other risk factors
2. Males are at greater risk than females—cannot be changed, but males should have regular physicals and reduce other risk factors
3. Age—cannot be changed, but since 55% of MIs occur in people over the age of 65, those people should also have regular physicals and reduce other risk factors
4. High blood pressure (hypertension)—methods of control include:
   - Medications to control blood pressure
   - Weight loss as needed to control hypertension
   - Exercise to aid in the control of hypertension
   - Low-sodium diet to aid in the control of hypertension. Foods that are high in sodium and should be avoided include processed foods, cured meats, salted chips and crackers, pickles, and table salt.
   - Minimize stress to aid in the control of hypertension
   - Stop smoking to aid in the control of hypertension. The nicotine in cigarettes is a vasoconstrictor and elevates blood pressure.
   - Have blood pressure checked regularly
5. Smoking—increases the risk of myocardial infarction by 2 to 4 times due to the **vasoconstrictive** properties of nicotine
   - Smoking cessation
   - If unable to cease smoking, switch to a low-nicotine brand of cigarette or decrease the number of cigarettes smoked

6. Blood cholesterol levels—although blood cholesterol has been shown to be predispositioned by heredity to a certain extent, there are methods to control certain factors as listed:
   - Low-saturated fat and low-cholesterol diet. Items that are high in saturated fats and cholesterol and should be avoided or eaten in moderate amounts include egg yolks, butter, cheese, and red meats.
   - Weight loss to aid in the control of elevated blood cholesterol levels
   - Exercise to aid in the control of elevated blood cholesterol levels
   - Medications as needed to aid in the control of moderate- to high-risk levels of blood cholesterol

7. Obesity
   - Weight loss under the direction of a physician
   - Exercise to aid in the reduction of weight
   - Lifelong eating habits that meet the nutritional requirements of the individual

8. Diabetes mellitus
   - Control blood sugar levels by diet, exercise, and medications as prescribed by the physician

9. Inactivity (sedentary life style)
   - Exercise to improve cardiovascular circulation
   - Develop lifelong exercise and fitness habits

10. Stress
    - Decrease stress levels as possible
    - Realize and set priorities
    - Psychological help as needed to manage stress
    - Change in life stressors as indicated, e.g. employment
    - Get adequate sleep and rest
    - Participate in regular exercise
    - Eat well-balanced meals

11. Oral contraceptives
    - Consider alternative form of birth control under advice of physician

SIGNS, SYMPTOMS, AND ASSOCIATED CARE

1. Persistent pain, pressure, or fullness in the chest
2. Pain that spreads to the neck, shoulders, or arms
3. Pain not relieved by rest
4. Nausea or vomiting
5. Diaphoresis
6. Light-headedness
7. Syncope
8. Hypotension or hypertension
9. Palpitations
10. Bradycardia or tachycardia
11. Dyspnea

The signs and symptoms of this disease are signals that myocardial infarction should be considered as a diagnosis. Associated care for these signs and symptoms is aimed at patient comfort measures and staff protection measures. The patient exhibiting these

Congestive heart failure (CHF) – disease caused by inadequate pumping action of the heart resulting in fluid accumulation within the body

Dressler's syndrome – syndrome occurring after a myocardial infarction (heart attack) characterized by fever, chest pain, pleuritis, and pericarditis

signs and symptoms should be treated as though he is having a myocardial infarction until the diagnosis has been ruled out. See the section entitled Treatment for further care information.

DIAGNOSIS

1. Symptoms
2. *Electrocardiogram (EKG)* (See Figure 23-5)
3. Serum enzyme (*LDH* and *CPK*) elevation
4. *Echocardiogram*
5. Elevated *white blood cell count (WBC)*
6. Elevated *ESR*

COMPLICATIONS OF MYOCARDIAL INFARCTION

1. **Congestive heart failure (CHF)** due to the weakened heart muscle
   - Monitor for symptoms of CHF, e.g. dyspnea, cough, edema, and weight gain
   - Monitor vital signs (See Appendix D)
   - Diuretics to eliminate fluid accumulation in body tissue
2. Dysrhythmia
   - Monitor heart rhythm with heart monitor system
   - Administer medications to control dysrhythmias
3. **Dressler's syndrome** may occur several days to several weeks after MI. It is characterized by pericarditis, fever, chest pain, pleurisy, and joint pain.
   - Monitor for and report any symptoms of Dressler's syndrome
   - Instruct patient to report any unusual symptoms upon discharge from the hospital

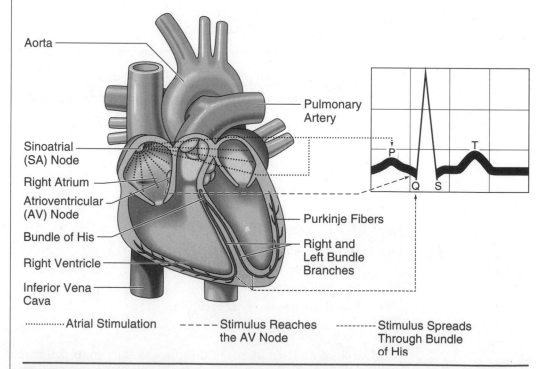

Aorta
Pulmonary Artery
Sinoatrial (SA) Node
Right Atrium
Atrioventricular (AV) Node
Bundle of His
Right Ventricle
Inferior Vena Cava
Purkinje Fibers
Right and Left Bundle Branches

P   Q S   T

·········· Atrial Stimulation   – – – – Stimulus Reaches the AV Node   ---------- Stimulus Spreads Through Bundle of His

Figure 23-5   Electrical pathway of the heart and tracing of the heart rhythm (From Layman, *The Medical Language*, copyright © 1995, Delmar Publishers)

Thromboembolism – blood clot that has moved from its site of origin

TED hose – elastic stockings used to aid in venous return of blood to the heart and decrease or prevent edema

Cardiogenic shock – shock that results due to severely compromised cardiac output

4. **Thromboembolism**
   - Administer blood thinners as directed by physician to prevent blood clot formation
   - Encourage range of motion (ROM) exercise and rehabilitative exercises as soon as able to prevent clot formation
   - Monitor for symptoms of clot formation in various body systems, e.g. symptoms of blood clots include ankle edema, chest pain, dyspnea, calf pain, and swelling
   - Encourage the use of antiembolism stockings (**TED hose**) as directed by physician

5. Depression
   - Monitor for symptoms of depression
   - Allow patient as much control as possible over various aspects of hospitalization care
   - Offer comfort and reassurance

6. **Cardiogenic shock**, due to decreased cardiac output due to the damaged heart muscle
   - Monitor for symptoms of cardiogenic shock. Symptoms of cardiogenic shock include chest pain, decreased urine output, dyspnea, diaphoresis, cyanosis, hypotension, and weak and irregular pulse (See Figure 23-6)
   - Treat with intravenous (IV) fluids and vasodilators

TREATMENT

1. Oxygen—needed by heart muscle and other organs of the body
2. Medications
   - Nitroglycerin to relieve pain caused by vasoconstriction
   - Morphine sulfate to relieve pain and improve cardiac output
   - Anticoagulant therapy to prevent thromboembolism formation
   - Lidocaine to decrease ventricular irritability

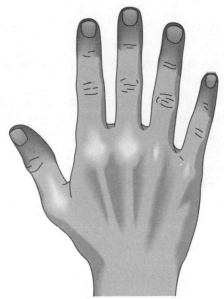

Acrocyanosis–Cyanosis
Blueness of the Extremities

Figure 23-6   Cyanosis of the hand (From Smith et al., *Medical Terminology: A Programmed Text, 7th edition*, copyright © 1995, Delmar Publishers)

Angina – chest pain caused by decrease in oxygen supply to the heart muscle without causing muscle necrosis; angina pain is similar to the pain experienced with a myocardial infarction

Atherosclerosis – hardening of the arteries due to accumulation of fat and plaque within the lining of the arterial walls

Table 23-1   Cholesterol and Fat Content of Foods

Food	Serving Size	Cholesterol (mg)	Fat (grams)
Whole milk	1 cup	34	8.3
1% milk	1 cup	18	4.8
Ice cream	1 cup	87	24.2
Frozen yogurt	1 cup	11	2.5
Chicken with skin	3 oz	73	9
Chicken without skin	3 oz	71	3
Turkey (dark)	3 oz	74	8.5
Turkey (white)	3 oz	60	2.6
Butter	1 tsp	12	4.2
Margarine	1 tsp	0	3.7

- Calcium channel blockers, which dilate arteries that supply blood to the heart and help prevent spasm of coronary arteries
- Beta blockers are used to control hypertension, **angina**, and dysrhythmias
- Digitalis slows and strengthens heart contractions making them more effective
- Thrombolytic therapy (Streptokinase or TPA) restores perfusion through an occluded artery by dissolving the clot that is blocking it. It is important to watch for signs of bleeding after administration of thrombolytic therapy, e.g. bleeding gums, nosebleeds, vaginal bleeding, blood in urine, blood in stool, bloody emesis, intraperitoneal bleeding, CNS bleeding, hemoptysis, or bruising. It is important to prevent injury to patient after administration of thrombolytic therapy.

3. Bedrest is usually recommended as exercise increases heart rate, which in turn increases cardiac workload and decreases cardiac output

4. A special diet should be included in the hospital care as well as education for the patient and family about lifelong dietary habits

   - Easy-to-chew-and-digest food initially to decrease circulatory needs for digestive tract
   - Low-cholesterol diet to prevent further **atherosclerosis** and decrease serum blood cholesterol levels (See Table 23-1)
   - Low-sodium diet as prescribed by physician due to increased fluid retention
   - Caffeine restricted initially due to the vasoconstriction effects of caffeine and CNS stimulant effects of caffeine

5. *Coronary artery bypass graft*

CONSIDERATIONS FOR CARE

1. Monitor medications and their effects on pain, vital signs, cardiac rhythm, and comfort level.
2. Instruct patient regarding the importance of reporting pain, dyspnea, or any other problems they may experience.
3. Schedule care and treatments around the patient's rest periods.
4. Monitor visitors due to the increased rest needs of the patient.
5. Obtain baseline vital signs and monitor on routine basis.

6. Alleviate anxiety by explaining care, equipment, and procedures.

7. Be alert for symptoms of fluid retention, e.g. weight gain, elevated blood pressure, decreased urine output, edema, dyspnea, crackles in lungs, cough, or cyanosis.

8. Offer emotional support to the patient and family.

9. Educate patient and family regarding the need to change life style, diet, exercise, and medications as well as the significance of quitting smoking.

10. Decrease incidence of constipation by increasing fiber in the diet, exercise, fluids, and stool softeners. Straining with a bowel movement increases vagal nerve stimulation which may cause severe bradycardia.

11. After a heart attack, the person should start exercising to rehabilitate and strengthen the heart muscle, increase lung capacity, increase circulation to the body, and increase longevity and chance of survival in the instance of a future heart attack. The rehabilitation should be continued upon discharge from the hospital and should be directed by the physician.

12. Monitor cardiac rhythm to detect change.

13. Educate client and family regarding medications, dosages, and possible side effects.

FOR MORE INFORMATION

American Heart Association
National Center
7320 Greenville Avenue
Dallas, TX 75231

ASSIGNMENT SHEET: MYOCARDIAL INFARCTION

Short Answer

1. Write a brief definition for the terms listed throughout the chapter.

2. Write a brief definition for myocardial infarction.

3. Describe the rationale behind seeking medical attention immediately if a person thinks she is having a heart attack.

4. List eleven (11) risk factors of a heart attack and methods to eliminate or reduce each of the risk factors.

5. List eleven (11) signs and symptoms of a possible heart attack.

6. Describe why bedrest would decrease cardiac workload.

7. List eight (8) possible symptoms of fluid retention.

8. Describe the rationale behind each of the following diets for a patient with a heart attack.

    a. Low cholesterol
    b. Low sodium
    c. Caffeine free

9. Describe three (3) life style changes a patient may need to make following a heart attack.

10. Describe ten (10) symptoms that might indicate bleeding after giving streptokinase.

11. Describe each of the following tests used to diagnose or treat a myocardial infarction.

    a. EKG (Electrocardiogram)
    b. Echocardiogram
    c. Coronary artery bypass graft

12. List the normal range for each of the following serum laboratory tests used in the diagnosis of myocardial infarction or that is associated as a risk factor.

    a. Cholesterol
    b. CPK
    c. Blood sugar (BS)
    d. WBC
    e. ESR

KNOWLEDGE INTO ACTION

1. Jonna Shriver, a 54-year-old housekeeper, is admitted to your hospital to rule out a myocardial infarction. List six symptoms Mrs. Shriver could have had that would have prompted her to seek medical attention.

2. Mrs. Shriver's physician orders laboratory tests to help determine whether Mrs. Shriver's symptoms were caused from a myocardial infarction. List three (3) laboratory tests that could be performed to aid in the diagnosis of myocardial infarction and their normal ranges.

3. You are aware that patients may encounter complications following a myocardial infarction. For each of the complications that follows, describe what symptoms to monitor for with each as well as associated care to eliminate or reduce the risk of the complication or methods to control the symptoms of the complication.

    a. Congestive heart failure
    b. Dysrhythmia
    c. Dressler's syndrome
    d. Thromboembolism
    e. Depression
    f. Cardiogenic shock

4. Mrs. Shriver's physician requests a dietary consult. Describe the type of diet that could possibly be ordered for Mrs. Shriver and the rationale for three (3) specific portions of the diet.

5. Mrs. Shriver's physician is concerned that she may retain fluid due to the location of her heart attack as well as her history. List six (6) symptoms of fluid retention that need to be monitored not only in the hospital but also by Mrs. Shriver once she returns home.

Congestive Heart Failure

OBJECTIVES

Upon completion of this chapter, the student should be able to:

- Define the key terms listed throughout the chapter
- Describe the physiology of the heart
- State a specific definition for congestive heart failure
- Describe the incidence of congestive heart failure
- List signs and symptoms associated with left-sided heart failure versus right-sided heart failure, the rationale for these symptoms, and associated care
- List risk factors associated with the development of congestive heart failure
- Identify specific methods for diagnosis of congestive heart failure
- List the specific goals for treatment of congestive heart failure
- Identify specific methods for treatment of congestive heart failure
- Describe specific considerations for caring for a patient with congestive heart failure

KEY TERMS

Contraction – any shortening of a muscle

Constriction – narrowing of a lumen or opening

INTRODUCTION

Congestive heart failure (CHF) results when the heart muscle is unable to pump oxygenated blood to the body. This is caused by damage to the heart muscle or weakening of the heart muscle. The body and heart attempt to compensate for this decreased pumping action by an increase in the heart rate (**contractions**), **constriction** of blood vessels, and enlargement of the heart. The heart is a muscle. With increased workload, as with any muscle, it will increase in size and strength. Congestive heart failure is further divided into left-sided heart failure and right-sided heart failure.

PHYSIOLOGY OF THE HEART

The heart is a hollow organ that is responsible for pumping oxygenated blood to the entire body. The heart is divided into right and left sides by a muscular wall called the septum. There are two upper chambers of the heart called the atria (atrium), and the lower chambers of the heart are called the ventricles. Blood enters the right atrium of the heart after delivering oxygen and nutrients to the tissues of the body. It is squeezed into the right ventricle through the tricuspid valve where it then travels through the pulmonary semilunar valve through the pulmonary artery into the lungs, where it becomes oxygenated. Blood returns from the lung through the pulmonary vein into the left atrium. It travels through the mitral valve (bicuspid) into the left ventricle. Blood leaves the left ventricle through the aortic semilunar valve, through the aorta, and begins its journey back through the body to deliver its supply of oxygen and nutrients. The heart itself is supplied with oxygenated blood from arteries, which branch off the aorta.

STATISTICS

Approximately 4 million people in the United States have a diagnosis of congestive heart failure (CHF).

Coronary – heart

COPD – chronic obstructive pulmonary disease

Emphysema – chronic lung disease; airways of the lungs become distended and lose their elasticity

Arteriosclerosis – hardening of the arteries

Lumen – diameter of the interior of a vessel or duct

Valvular – related to structures in the body that allow blood or other fluids in the body to flow in a single direction

Vascular – refers to the blood vessels of the body

Pulmonary – refers to the lung

Veins – blood vessels that return blood to the heart

Capillaries – smallest of the blood vessels forming the junction of arteries and veins; also refers to the smallest of the lymphatic system vessels

Respiration – process of breathing in (inspiration) and out (expiration) that brings oxygen into the body (inspiration) and releases the waste product of carbon dioxide (expiration)

RISK FACTORS

Heart failure occurs when a disease or illness causes the heart muscle to be damaged and, therefore, loses ability to contract efficiently; by increased pulmonary pressure, which impairs cardiac output; and also by increased systemic vascular pressure, which impairs cardiac output. Another cause of congestive heart failure is increased metabolic (oxygen) needs of a diseased body system. Examples of these include:

1. Myocardial infarction (MI)—heart attack
2. **Coronary** heart disease
3. Chronic lung disease (**COPD, emphysema**)
4. Pulmonary embolism
5. Hypertension—approximately 75% of patients with CHF have a history of hypertension
6. Age due to decreased contractility and efficiency of the heart muscle with advancing age
7. Smoking due to vasoconstrictive action of nicotine
8. **Arteriosclerosis** due to increased contraction force of the heart needed to overcome arteriosclerosis
9. High-cholesterol diet due to decreased **lumen** size of the vessels and a subsequent need for the heart to contract with more force to overcome vascular resistance
10. Diabetes mellitus due to vascular deterioration caused by diabetes mellitus
11. **Valvular** disease of the heart

SIGNS AND SYMPTOMS

Left-sided heart failure is the most common type of heart failure. Right-sided heart failure often occurs as a result of left-sided heart failure but will occasionally occur by itself. CHF is generally a chronic problem with symptoms developing insidiously. (See Figure 24-1.)

Left-Sided Heart Failure

Symptoms of left-sided heart failure occur as a result of the left ventricle being unable to contract with enough force to expel the blood into the **vascular** system of the body. As a result, the blood backs up into the **pulmonary** system (**veins** and **capillaries**). The increased pressure causes serum to leak out of the capillaries and accumulate in the alveoli.

1. Dyspnea due to the congestion in the lungs from the accumulation of fluid
   - Assist with position for patient comfort (See Figure 24-2)
   - Assist with activities of daily living (ADLs) as necessary
   - Monitor ease of **respirations** and respiratory rate
   - Observe frequent rest periods to conserve energy
   - Do as many activities as possible in a sitting position, e.g. dressing, bathing, cooking, and cleaning
   - Avoid constrictive garments or undergarments
   - Provide oxygen as needed and as directed by physician
   - Utilize fan in room to circulate air and assist in making breathing easier
   - Arrange schedule of activities around patient rest periods
   - Assess breath sounds on routine basis

- Observe for signs of hypoxia, e.g. cyanosis, decreased level of consciousness, confusion, and diaphoresis
- Humidify air as needed
- Provide reassurance to patient
- Treat cause of dyspnea

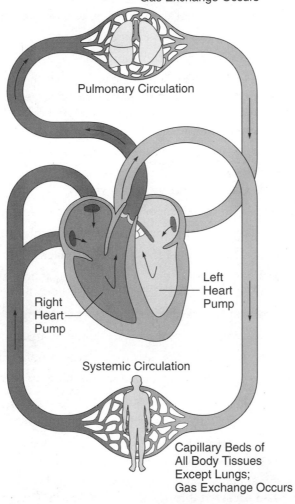

Capillary Beds of Lungs; Gas Exchange Occurs

Pulmonary Circulation

Left Heart Pump

Right Heart Pump

Systemic Circulation

Capillary Beds of All Body Tissues Except Lungs; Gas Exchange Occurs

■ Oxygen-poor Blood ▢ Oxygen-rich Blood

Figure 24-1 The circulatory system (From Layman, *The Medical Language,* copyright © 1995, Delmar Publishers)

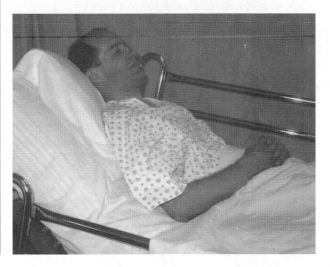

Figure 24-2 Fowler's position

Rales – abnormal respiratory sound that occurs as a result of air moving within lungs that have an increased amount of secretions present within them

Orthopnea – difficulty breathing unless in an upright position

Engorgement – process by which blood vessels become filled with blood

Mucous – fluid secreted by the mucous membranes of the body

Paroxysmal – sudden exacerbation of symptoms of a short duration

Nocturnal – refers to night time

2. **Rales** due to congestion in the lungs from the accumulation of fluid
   - Monitor breath sounds at frequent intervals
   - Assist with position for patient comfort
   - Assess for signs of hypoxia
   - Provide oxygen as needed and directed by physician
   - Assess for need for diuretics as ordered
   - Monitor for effectiveness of diuretics as evidenced by decreased rales

3. **Orthopnea** due to congestion in the lungs from the accumulation of fluid
   - Assist with position for patient comfort
   - Monitor patient for ease of respirations

4. Cough due to the congestion in the lungs from the accumulation of fluid. The cough is often productive and may be blood-tinged due to irritation in the alveoli from the fluid accumulation and irritation of the capillaries due to the **engorgement** with fluid.
   - Utilize *postural drainage technique* to facilitate drainage of **mucous** from lungs
   - Dispose of tissues and sputum correctly
   - Encourage patient to cover mouth when coughing
   - Observe sputum for signs of hemoptysis or infection
   - Educate regarding effective coughing to facilitate productiveness of cough
   - Offer fluids as tolerated to thin mucous secretions while monitoring intake and output (I and O). Fluids may accumulate within the tissues.
   - Humidify air to prevent respiratory tract drying
   - Splint chest to assist patient in coughing more effectively
   - Provide container for patient to cough secretions into
   - Administer expectorants to aid in coughing up secretions
   - Provide frequent mouth care
   - Utilize meticulous handwashing by patient, visitors, and staff members
   - Utilize universal precautions at all times when coming in contact with blood or body fluids (See Appendix C)

5. **Paroxysmal nocturnal** dyspnea due to the reabsorption of edematous fluid which had occurred throughout the day; this reabsorption is due to the increased cardiac output which occurs with rest
   - Monitor respiratory ease during night
   - Establish method for patient to call for assistance as needed during the night
   - Assist with position for patient comfort
   - Monitor intake and output (I and O)

6. Fatigue due to decreased oxygenation of body tissues due to decreased cardiac output
   - Assist patient with ADLs as necessary
   - Schedule care, activities, and treatment around patient's rest schedule
   - Monitor phone calls and visitors around patient's energy level and rest schedule
   - Encourage frequent rest periods
   - Provide assistance as needed to prevent injury due to weakness

Contractility – able to contract or shorten in length

Telemetry – transmission of heart rhythm to a distant screen through the use of electronics while the patient wears a small, portable monitor

Cardiomegaly – enlargement of the heart

- Provide method for patient to call for assistance
- Encourage patient to set realistic goals of activities
- Allow adequate time to do activities and procedures to avoid frustration or possible injury
- Encourage exercise to maintain muscle strength
- Provide cane or walker for ambulation and transfer
- Provide private room to promote rest periods

7. Tachycardia due to the compensatory method of the heart due to decreased **contractility** of the heart muscle
   - Utilize heart monitor (**telemetry**) to monitor heart rhythm and pulse rate
   - Instruct patient to report periods of palpitations
   - Educate patient and family regarding method to take patient pulse rate
   - Assess heart rate and rhythm changes with exertion and rest
   - Encourage relaxation techniques for patient use
   - Provide calm, quiet, relaxed atmosphere for patient

8. Insomnia due to dyspnea and nocturia
   - Encourage relaxation techniques, music, or other methods to relax patient at bedtime
   - Avoid caffeine and other stimulants prior to bedtime
   - Avoid distractions and noise once the patient is in bed
   - Avoid large meals close to bedtime
   - Schedule medications and treatments at times other than bedtime
   - Exercise at regular intervals throughout the day
   - Avoid sleeping throughout the day as able

9. Restlessness due to decreased oxygenation of body tissues due to decreased cardiac output
   - Administer oxygen as needed and directed by physician
   - Provide activities throughout the day that the patient enjoys
   - Offer regular exercise routines for the patient

10. **Cardiomegaly** due to the increased work load of the ventricles as they attempt to compensate for the inefficient contractility of the heart muscle
    - Monitor cardiomegaly with the use of CXR on routine basis
    - Monitor for chest pain

11. Cyanosis due to decreased oxygenation of body tissues due to decreased cardiac output; also due to blood that is directed toward the vital organs and away from the extremities
    - Monitor skin color
    - Monitor *arterial blood gases (ABGs)*
    - Administer oxygen as needed and as directed by physician

12. Chest pain due to decreased oxygenation of the cardiac muscle caused by decreased cardiac output
    - Administer oxygen as needed and as directed by physician
    - Rest periods as needed
    - Monitor for activities that cause an exacerbation of chest pain
    - Schedule activities around rest periods to avoid overworking the heart muscle

Sacral – the five vertebrae located at the distal end of the spinal column directly above the coccyx

Ascites – accumulation of fluid within the peritoneal cavity

Peritoneal – refers to peritoneum

Gastrointestinal – refers to the system of the body that includes the mouth, esophagus, stomach, small intestine, and large intestine; function is to digest foods and remove the nutrients and fluids from them for use in the tissues of the body

Right-Sided Heart Failure

Symptoms of right-sided heart failure occur as a result of the right ventricle being unable to contract with enough force to expel the blood into the pulmonary system. As a result, the blood backs up into the vascular system of the body (veins and capillaries).

1. **Sacral** and ankle edema due to accumulation of fluid in the tissues of the body caused by pressure within the blood vessels
   - Avoid constrictive clothing or undergarments
   - Restrict salt in diet as prescribed by physician. Foods that are high in sodium and should be avoided include processed foods, cured meats, salted chips and crackers, pickles, and table salt.
   - Provide elastic stockings (TED hose) or Jobst stockings may be necessary to reduce swelling
   - Monitor edema on routine basis
   - Encourage patient to elevate edematous extremity above the level of the heart to reduce swelling
   - Monitor for skin breakdown in edematous areas
   - Monitor for symptoms of decreased circulation in edematous areas, e.g. cool to touch, cyanotic, and decreased sensation
   - Obtain baseline weight and monitor on a routine basis
   - Monitor intake and output (I and O)

2. Weight gain due to fluid accumulation
   - Obtain baseline weight and monitor on routine basis
   - Monitor intake and output (I and O)
   - Provide low-salt diet
   - Limit fluid intake as directed by physician

3. Neck vein distention due to venous accumulation of fluid and the inability of the neck veins to empty completely into the superior vena cava due to fluid congestion within the right atrium of the heart
   - Monitor for neck vein distention

4. Hepatomegaly due to fluid accumulation within the liver
   - Monitor for hepatomegaly
   - Avoid abdominal injury in the presence of hepatomegaly
   - Monitor liver function with laboratory tests, e.g. *SGOT, SGPT, bilirubin, albumin, alkaline phosphatase, prothrombin time*
   - Educate to avoid use of alcohol and medications metabolized in the liver
   - Monitor for jaundice

5. **Ascites** due to fluid accumulation within the **peritoneal** cavity
   - Assist with position for patient comfort
   - Measure abdominal girth on routine basis, with area marked so same area is measured each time for accuracy
   - Provide nonconstrictive clothing and undergarments
   - Assist in draining fluid from abdominal cavity

6. Nausea and vomiting due to hepatomegaly and ascites pressure; also due to decreased blood flow to the **gastrointestinal** system
   - Administer antiemetics before meals as prescribed by physician
   - Offer food choices according to patient preference
   - Control odors and unpleasant sights in room

Hypoxemia – decreased amounts of oxygen in the bloodstream and, therefore, decreased amounts of oxygen available to the tissues of the body

- Offer fluids frequently to prevent dehydration. Symptoms of dehydration include decreased urine output, hypotension, concentrated urine, weight loss, constipation, dry skin, dry mouth, confusion, and tenting of skin.
- Monitor intake and output to avoid dehydration
- Monitor serum electrolytes (*sodium, potassium,* and *chloride*)
- Observe rest periods after meals
- Avoid foods that are spicy, rich, or previously disagreeable to patient
- Provide receptacle for patient to vomit into as needed; this should be cleaned whenever used and changed on a frequent basis
- Provide meticulous mouth care
- Prevent aspiration of vomit
- Utilize universal precautions at all times when coming in contact with blood or body fluids (See Appendix C)
- Avoid greasy foods as they tend to stay in the stomach for a long period of time
- Avoid cooking food if possible due to increased nausea with odors of foods
- Avoid hot foods as necessary due to the increased odors of hot foods
- Eat in well-ventilated area to decrease the accumulation of odors of foods while eating

7. Nocturia due to reabsorption of edematous fluid that had occurred throughout the day; this reabsorption is due to the increased cardiac output that occurs with rest
   - Assist patient to bathroom as needed
   - Monitor patient during night if going to bathroom
   - Provide night light, especially if in new surrounding or confusion
   - Provide a urinal or commode for patient use
   - Provide method for patient to contact staff if assistance is needed

8. Cardiomegaly due to the increased work load of the ventricles as they attempt to compensate for the inefficient contractility of the heart muscle
   - Monitor cardiomegaly through the use of CXR
   - Monitor for chest pain

DIAGNOSIS

Diagnosis of CHF includes the following methods.

1. Signs and symptoms
2. Physical examination
3. *EKG (electrocardiogram)*
4. *Chest x-ray (CXR)* shows pulmonary congestion
5. Neck vein distention
6. *Echocardiogram*
7. *Arterial blood gases* shows **hypoxemia**
8. *Electrolytes*, with sodium and potassium decreased

TREATMENT

Treatment of CHF has four main goals.

1. Decreased accumulation of fluid in the various parts of the body

Antihypertensive – medication used in the treatment of high blood pressure (hypertension)

Lassitude – extreme fatigue

2. Improved oxygenation to body tissues
3. Decreased cardiac workload
4. Treatment of the primary cause of CHF

Specific methods of treatment include the following.

1. Diuretics—eliminate the accumulation of fluid in the various parts of the body, primarily pulmonary congestion and edema occurring in the ankles, sacrum, peritoneal cavity, and body organs, e.g. Lasix
2. Low-sodium diet used to minimize retention of fluid
3. Oxygen therapy
4. Treatment of the underlying cause of the CHF
5. Weight reduction to normal or near-normal range to reduce the workload of the heart
6. Smoking cessation due to vasoconstriction caused by nicotine
7. Vasodilators are given to increase cardiac output by decreasing vascular resistance
8. Fluid restriction
9. Digoxin is used to strengthen the contractility of the heart muscle
10. Severe CHF may require heart transplantation
11. **Antihypertensives** used to promote vasodilation, e.g. Apresoline

CONSIDERATIONS FOR CARE

1. Educate patient and family regarding the disease process.
2. Educate patient and family regarding forms of treatment as well as side effects of medications.
3. Provide emotional support to patient and family.
4. Nonjudgmental acceptance of emotions and behavior of patient and family.
5. Educate patient and family regarding importance of taking medications at scheduled time.
6. Educate patient and family regarding the importance of follow-up care.
7. Obtain baseline vital signs and respiratory status and monitor on routine basis.
8. Encourage patient to perform activities and care around periods of peak energy and to rest according to fatigue or increase of dyspnea.
9. Educate patient and family regarding importance of monitoring weight on routine basis at home and reporting significant weight gain to physician.
10. Educate patient and family regarding importance of monitoring for and reporting symptoms of worsening CHF to physician, e.g. increased dyspnea, fatigue, cyanosis, weight gain, and mental confusion.
11. Facilitate obtaining oxygen for home use as necessary.
12. Facilitate obtaining home assistance, such as home health agency, public. health agency, meal delivery system, or help with home care.
13. Educate regarding low-salt diet to follow at home; facilitate dietary consult as needed and as available.
14. Educate regarding importance of checking pulse rate prior to administration of Digoxin.
15. Educate regarding symptoms of electrolyte imbalance due to diuretic use, e.g. **lassitude**, mental changes, change in level of consciousness, and arrhythmias.

16. Educate regarding methods to achieve or maintain weight within normal range to decrease cardiac workload.

17. Educate regarding methods or programs to assist in smoking cessation.

18. Facilitate obtaining antiembolism stockings or Jobst stockings for home use.

19. Educate patient regarding importance of routine blood pressure checks and facilitate obtaining home blood pressure equipment. Educate regarding use and make patient aware of alternative methods of getting blood pressure checked routinely.

20. Educate patient and family regarding monitoring for signs of decreased peripheral circulation, e.g. cyanosis to extremities, diminished sensation to extremities, numbness or tingling to extremities, extremities cool to touch, and presence or absence of peripheral pulses. (See Figure 24-3.)

21. Facilitate obtaining a hospital bed or similar with adjustable head elevation to aid in position of comfort for breathing.

22. Educate patient and family regarding importance of small meals to avoid placing additional pressure on the stomach due to ascites.

23. Facilitate admission into wellness program or cardiac rehabilitation program to have exercise program monitored by health care professionals.

24. For patients with decreased mobility, stress the importance of observing for and preventing skin breakdown. Signs of skin breakdown (decubitus ulcers) include redness, swelling, warm or hot to touch, open sores, cyanosis, pain, and blisters. Prevention measures include frequent reposition (minimum of every 1 to 2 hours); meticulous skin care; massage areas at bony prominences; encourage activity as able; alternating pressure mattresses; prevent pressure from appliances or tubing; prevent friction when repositioning by using a lift sheet and adequate assistance; and linens must be clean, dry, and wrinkle-free.

25. Educate client and family regarding low-sodium diet.

26. Oxygen as needed.

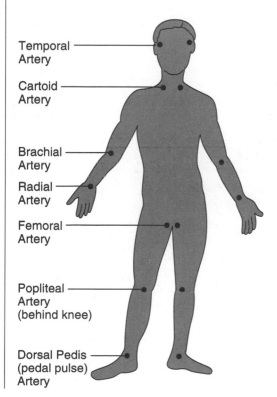

Temporal Artery

Cartoid Artery

Brachial Artery

Radial Artery

Femoral Artery

Popliteal Artery (behind knee)

Dorsal Pedis (pedal pulse) Artery

Figure 24-3   Pulse sites of the body (Adapted from Simmers, *Diversified Health Occupations, 3rd edition*, copyright © 1993, Delmar Publishers)

27. Monitor telemetry for heart rate and rhythm changes.

28. Monitor intake and output (I and O).

29. Monitor for neck vein distention.

FOR MORE INFORMATION

American Heart Association
National Center
7320 Greenville Avenue
Dallas, TX 75231

ASSIGNMENT SHEET: CONGESTIVE HEART FAILURE

Short Answer

1. Write a brief definition for the terms listed throughout the chapter.

2. Describe the physiology of the heart.

3. Write a brief definition for congestive heart failure (CHF).

4. Describe the incidence of congestive heart failure (CHF).

5. List twelve (12) signs and symptoms of left-sided heart failure, the rationale, and associated care for each of the symptoms.

6. List eight (8) signs and symptoms of right-sided heart failure, the rationale, and the associated care for each of the symptoms.

7. List eleven (11) risk factors associated with the development of congestive heart failure (CHF).

8. Identify eight (8) specific methods used to aid in the diagnosis of congestive heart failure (CHF).

9. List four (4) specific goals of treatment for congestive heart failure (CHF).

10. Identify eleven (11) specific methods of treatment used for congestive heart failure (CHF).

11. List twenty-nine (29) considerations for caring for a patient with congestive heart failure (CHF).

12. Describe what is meant by universal precautions. (See Appendix C.)

13. Write the normal range for each of the following vital signs. (See Appendix D.)

    a. Temperature
    b. Pulse
    c. Respirations
    d. Blood pressure

14. Describe each of the following procedures used in the diagnosis or treatment of congestive heart failure (CHF).

    a. Postural drainage
    b. Electrocardiogram (EKG)
    c. Chest x-ray (CXR)
    d. Echocardiogram
    e. Arterial blood gases (ABGs)

15. Write the normal range for each of the following laboratory tests.

    a. Arterial blood gases (ABGs)
       - pCO_2
       - pH
       - pO_2
       - HCO_3
    b. Sodium (Na)
    c. Potassium (K)
    d. Chloride (Cl)
    e. SGOT
    f. SGPT
    g. Bilirubin
    h. Albumin
    i. Alkaline phosphatase
    j. Prothrombin time

KNOWLEDGE INTO ACTION

1. Chiang Ling, a 68-year-old restaurant owner, is admitted to your facility with CHF. He is on Lasix 20 mg daily. (Lasix is a diuretic.) You are aware that you need to monitor for dehydration as well as electrolyte imbalance when a patient is taking diuretics. Describe the symptoms of dehydration and electrolyte imbalance, and what is included in electrolytes.

2. Mr. Ling becomes increasingly weak during his hospital stay. You are discussing methods of dealing with his nocturia as associated with his weakness with other staff members during a staff meeting. List three (3) methods of associated care to help Mr. Ling in dealing with his problem of nocturia associated with weakness.

3. There are numerous risk factors that could have increased Mr. Ling's chances of developing CHF. List five (5) of those risk factors.

4. Part of Mr. Ling's treatment includes the following: diuretics, oxygen, smoking cessation, vasodilators, and Digoxin. Describe the rationale for each of the listed methods of treatment prescribed for Mr. Ling.

   a.   Diuretics
   b.   Oxygen
   c.   Smoking cessation
   d.   Vasodilators
   e.   Digoxin

5. Mr. Ling is a slender man and due to his weakness has limited ability to be out of bed. You are concerned that Mr. Ling may develop a decubitus ulcer. List symptoms of decubitus ulcers as well as methods to prevent the formation of decubitus ulcers.

6. Mr. Ling has vital signs ordered to be checked every 8 hours. List the vital signs, what each of the vital signs is measuring, and the normal range for each of the vital signs.

	Vital Sign	Meaning of Measurement	Normal Range
1.			
2.			
3.			
4.			

UNIT 6

RESPIRATORY DISEASES

CHAPTER
25
Asthma

OBJECTIVES

Upon completion of this chapter, the student should be able to:

■ Define the key terms listed throughout the chapter

■ Describe the physiology of the respiratory system

■ State a specific definition for asthma

■ Describe the incidence of asthma

■ List the precipitating factors for asthma and describe how to reduce or eliminate these factors

■ Describe the symptoms of asthma and associated care for these symptoms

■ Identify specific methods for diagnosis of asthma

■ Identify specific methods for treatment of asthma

■ Describe specific considerations for caring for a person with asthma

■ State a definition for status asthmaticus, symptoms for status asthmaticus, and associated care

KEY TERMS

Bronchospasm – spasm or constriction of the bronchus causing a narrowing of the lumen of the bronchus; often occurs in asthma and decreases the exchange of oxygen and carbon dioxide

Extrinsic – outside

Dander – small particles released from the hair or feathers of animals

Intrinsic – within the body

Nasal – nose

Sinus – hollow space or cavity

INTRODUCTION

Asthma is a chronic disease that is characterized by episodes of reversible airway obstruction. The manifestations of the disease include **bronchospasm**, increased mucous production, mucosal inflammation, and edema. The patient's airways, for reasons that are not entirely known, have an increased sensitivity to allergies, infection, weather, irritants, and exercise. **Extrinsic** asthma refers to asthma attacks that are precipitated by specific external allergens, such as animal **dander**, molds, pollens, and feathers. **Intrinsic** asthma refers to asthma attacks that are precipitated from internal or nonallergenic factors, such as respiratory infections, stress, exhaustion, hormonal, or endocrine changes as well as changes in temperature and humidity.

PHYSIOLOGY OF THE RESPIRATORY SYSTEM

The respiratory system is made up of the nose and **nasal** cavity, **sinuses**, pharynx, larynx, trachea, bronchi, bronchioles, and alveoli. (See Figure 25-1.) The purpose of the respiratory system is to draw oxygen-rich air into the lungs (inspiration) to be transported to the body system through the blood vessels. The waste product, carbon dioxide (CO_2), is then released through the lungs (expiration). The respiratory system is lined with mucous membrane, which moistens the respiratory tract as well as assists in trapping and removing foreign particles from entering the lungs. Also located along the respiratory system are cilia, tiny hairlike structures, that also function to trap and remove foreign particles from the airway. Up to one quart of mucous is normally secreted daily by the mucous membranes of the respiratory tract.

STATISTICS

Asthma affects an estimated 12 to 15 million people in the United States to varying degrees, with an estimated $4.5 billion spent annually on medical care for patients with

Allergen – substance an individual is allergic to that causes allergic symptoms (sneeze, cough, watery eyes, and hives)

External – exterior or outside

Immunotherapy – therapy that builds up the body's natural immune system by injecting small amounts of antibodies, which have been produced by a donor, into the person's system

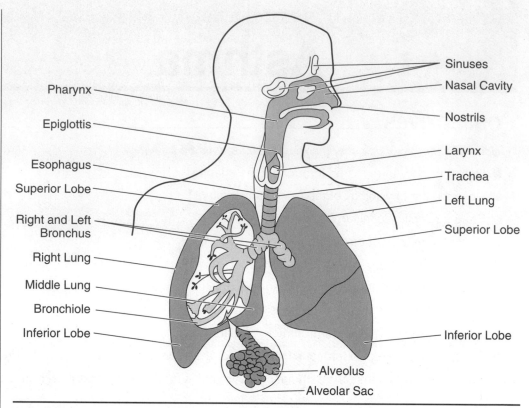

Figure 25-1   The respiratory system

asthma. A total of 4 to 7% of the population in the United States is affected by asthma. Asthma can begin at any age, though 3.9 million people with asthma are under the age of 18, and 50% are under the age of 10. Asthma is the major cause of absenteeism from school.

Peaks of the disease occur during the fall and winter with these peaks thought to be due to the temperature changes, humidity changes, amount of allergens in the environment, and the increase of respiratory infections during these seasons. More than 9 million days of work are lost annually due to the symptoms associated with asthma. Approximately 4,000 to 5,000 people die from asthma annually in the United States, and 150,000 people are hospitalized annually in the United States for a total of 1 million hospital days.

PRECIPITATING FACTORS FOR ASTHMA ATTACKS

1. **Allergens**, e.g. dust, molds, animal dander, pollen, feathers, and foods. Approximately 50 to 70% of patients with asthma have allergies.

    * Avoid **external** allergens, which trigger attacks
    * Administer allergy injections as indicated (**immunotherapy**)
    * Practice environmental control
    * Stay indoors when air pollution or allergen index level is high
    * Educate that if an animal continues in the home, the pet should have weekly baths and should not sleep in the bedroom of the person with allergies or asthma
    * Wash bedding at least weekly
    * Avoid upholstered furniture
    * Avoid vacuuming if possible

Bronchodilator – medication that dilates the bronchus

- Avoid knick-knacks that collect dust
- Use pillows and bedding filled with synthetic fibers rather than feathers or down

2. Viral infections, e.g. common cold, viral infections, and influenza
   - Avoid infected people as much as possible
   - Administer influenza and pneumonia vaccinations as directed by physician
   - Maintain optimal physical health to prevent infection
   - Administer **bronchodilators** and corticosteroids as directed by physician
   - Encourage fluids to thin secretions
   - Encourage adequate rest

3. Exercise
   - Avoid outdoor exercise in cold weather
   - Maintain exercise program as prescribed by physician to maintain optimal health benefits
   - Administer bronchodilator after exercise to prevent post-exercise bronchospasm
   - Experiment with different types of exercise to find which type is most easily tolerated

4. Environmental factors, e.g. air pollution, cigarette smoke, paint, and cleaners
   - Practice environmental control
   - Stay indoors when air pollution level is high
   - Avoid smoking by the patient and the family
   - Avoid fireplaces and wood stoves

5. Weather
   - Wear a mask or loose-fitting scarf around the mouth and nose on cold days
   - Avoid being outdoors in windy weather due to increased allergens in the air
   - Educate that heavy rain may clean the air of allergens
   - Educate that air-conditioning helps by reducing the amount of pollens and mold spores that come inside; air-conditioning also lowers the humidity, which helps to control the amount of mold and dust mites
   - Provide careful cleaning of bathrooms and basements to decrease the amount of mold formation
   - Clean dehumidifiers often to prevent mildew from forming

6. Emotions—emotional factors do *not* cause asthma but can trigger an asthma attack
   - Teach relaxation techniques
   - Educate those around the person to remain calm during an asthma attack
   - Avoid situations that may increase stress and, therefore, trigger an attack
   - Facilitate psychological treatment if needed to deal with stress and the disease itself

7. Drugs, e.g. aspirin
   - Avoid aspirin and medications containing aspirin
   - Wear a medical alert identification at all times
   - Instruct health care personnel of allergies to specific medications
   - Educate that Tartrazine (yellow dye #5) may trigger an asthma attack in aspirin-sensitive patients

Histamine – protein substance that is normally present in the body and is released in response to injury or inflammation

Mast cells – cells present in the connective tissues that are responsible for manufacturing and storing histamine; stimulated as part of the inflammatory response of the body

SIGNS, SYMPTOMS, AND ASSOCIATED CARE

During an allergic reaction, **histamines** are released from **mast cells**. This release of histamines causes swelling of the mucous membranes, increased mucous production, edema of the airway, and bronchospasms.

1. Wheezing due to constriction of the airway can often be heard without a stethoscope
   - Administer bronchodilators to reduce spasm
   - Administer oxygen (O_2) as directed by physician
   - Provide reassurance to patient
   - Assist with position for patient comfort
   - Humidify air as needed
   - Monitor breathing, skin color, and level of consciousness
   - Avoid constrictive clothing or linens

2. Coughing due to constriction of the airway, inflammation, and increased mucous production. Coughing is common for asthmatic children after exercising or crying (occurs in 80% of children with asthma). Bronchodilators prior to exercise can reduce or prevent these coughing episodes. Coughing at night is common due to symptoms worsening at night.
   - Humidify air as needed
   - Encourage fluids to thin mucous secretions to expel more easily
   - Administer expectorants as needed to aid in coughing up secretions
   - Splint chest to assist patient to cough more effectively
   - Provide container for patient to cough secretions into
   - Dispose of tissues and sputum properly
   - Provide frequent mouth care
   - Utilize meticulous handwashing by patient, visitors, and staff members
   - Provide postural drainage technique to facilitate drainage of mucous from lungs
   - Encourage patient to cover mouth when coughing
   - Observe sputum for signs of hemoptysis or infection
   - Educate regarding effective coughing techniques to facilitate productiveness of cough
   - Utilize universal precautions when handling any blood or body fluids (See Appendix C)

3. Frequent respiratory infections due to increased mucous production and trapped stale air in the airways
   - Avoid people with respiratory infections
   - Maintain optimal health to fight off infections
   - Administer influenza and pneumonia vaccinations as directed by physician
   - Educate patient and family regarding symptoms of respiratory infection such as cough, phlegm production, chest pain, fever, chills, dyspnea, and diaphoresis
   - Educate patient and family to report symptoms of respiratory infection to physician
   - Educate patient regarding importance of completing medication prescribed for respiratory infection
   - Encourage fluids to thin secretions and make them easier to expel

Semi-Fowler's position – position of sitting up in bed with the back supported

Chest physiotherapy (chest percussion) – technique used to drain mucous from the lungs using manual vibration while the patient is in specific positions to enhance the effect of gravity on the mucous and secretions

Hyperventilation – rapid rate of respirations that increases the amount of air in the lungs; often seen in stress or with lung diseases

- Prevent transmission of infection by handwashing and correctly disposing of tissues and phlegm
- Avoid crowded areas, which increase the likelihood of contracting a respiratory infection

4. Dyspnea due to constriction of airways, inflammation, and increased mucous production
   - Administer O_2 as needed
   - Assist with position for patient comfort, e.g. **semi-Fowler's position**
   - Humidify air as needed
   - Provide reassurance to patient
   - Treat cause of dyspnea
   - Avoid constrictive garments and undergarments
   - Provide fan in room to circulate air and assist in making breathing easier
   - Encourage frequent rest periods to conserve energy
   - Arrange schedule of activities around patient rest periods
   - Assist with activities of daily living (ADLs) as necessary
   - Assess breath sounds on routine basis
   - Observe for signs of hypoxia, e.g. cyanosis, diaphoresis, decreased level of consciousness, and confusion
   - Monitor ease of respirations and respiratory rate
   - Do as many activities as possible in a sitting position, e.g. dressing, bathing, cooking, and cleaning

5. Spitting up mucous due to increased mucous production
   - Encourage fluids to loosen respiratory secretions
   - Provide tissues and dispose of properly
   - Provide frequent oral care
   - Provide **chest physiotherapy** and postural drainage

6. Diaphoresis due to increased respiratory effort
   - Apply cool cloth to face or forehead as desired by patient
   - Change clothing and linens as indicated
   - Bathe frequently with partial baths as needed
   - Provide deodorant or antiperspirant to minimize odors and perspiration

7. Pallor due to decreased air exchange in the lungs
   - Provide reassurance to patient
   - Encourage clothing and makeup to enhance coloring

8. Chest tightness due to bronchial constriction and decreased air exchange in the lungs
   - Provide reassurance
   - Administer medications to relieve chest tightness
   - Monitor for adequate oxygenation
   - Monitor for increased respiratory distress

9. **Hyperventilation** due to decreased air exchange in the lungs
   - Provide encouragement to patient
   - Monitor rate, depth, and character of respirations

10. Anxiety due to dyspnea and hypoxia
    - Provide reassurance to patient
    - Employ relaxation techniques

Flaring – spread outward

Sternal retraction – retraction of the sternum during periods of extreme respiratory difficulty in children

Cytology – study of the cell

- Provide calm, quiet atmosphere
- Inform patient what will be done to increase compliance
- Refrain from leaving patient alone during an acute asthma attack

11. Restlessness due to dyspnea and hypoxia
    - Provide reassurance to patient
    - Provide methods of quiet diversion
    - Administer medications to make breathing easier

12. Nostril **flaring** due to increased respiratory effort
    - Provide reassurance to patient
    - Administer medications to make breathing easier
    - Monitor rate, depth, and character of respirations
    - Monitor for symptoms of respiratory failure

13. **Sternal retraction** (in children) due to increased respiratory effort
    - Provide reassurance to patient
    - Administer medications to make breathing easier
    - Monitor, rate, depth, and character of respirations
    - Monitor for symptoms of respiratory failure

14. Tachycardia due to increased respiratory effort and decreased air exchange in the lungs
    - Monitor pulse rate
    - Provide reassurance to patient
    - Educate regarding relaxation techniques

15. Use of accessory respiratory muscles due to increased respiratory effort
    - Provide reassurance to patient
    - Assist with position for patient comfort
    - Humidify oxygen as indicated

DIAGNOSIS

1. Symptoms
2. History of family member(s) with allergies or asthma (30 to 40%)
3. Physical examination
4. *Pulmonary function studies* to determine the reversibility and severity of the obstruction. Note that pulmonary function studies are often normal between attacks.
5. Skin testing for identification of allergens
6. *Chest x-ray (CXR)* used to indicate areas of hyperinflation as well as possible infection
7. Sputum and nasal **cytology** will show increased number of eosinophils
8. *CBC* will show increased *eosinophil* count
9. *Serum IgE levels* elevated due to allergic response
10. *Arterial blood gases (ABGs)* indicate hypoxemia

TREATMENT

1. Avoid factors that trigger an asthma attack
2. Medications to treat the symptoms of asthma

Respiratory arrest – respirations cease

Mechanical ventilation – providing oxygenation of the lungs through artificial methods with the use of an endotracheal tube (intubation) and the use of an ambu bag or mechanical ventilator (respirator)

- Bronchodilators are used to open the airways that are constricted by asthma. Bronchodilators can be either inhaled or taken systemically, e.g. Metaproterenol, Albuterol, Terbutaline, Theophylline
- Inhaled anti-inflammatory medications are used to decrease inflammation and airway hyper-reactivity (prevents release of histamines) associated with asthma, e.g. Cromolyn, Beclomethasone
- Corticosteroids are used to decrease airway inflammation, irritability, and mucous production, e.g. Prednisone, Methylprednisolone, Dexamethasone

3. Allergy injections (immunotherapy)—small amounts of the allergen are given in gradually increasing doses to decrease the allergy antibody level, increase the blocking antibody level, and make the patient better able to tolerate the allergies

4. Chest physiotherapy and postural drainage

5. Maintain weight at normal range due to increased pressure obese abdomen puts on diaphragm

6. Encourage fluids to keep respiratory secretions thin

Some children "outgrow" asthma due to the increased size of the airways as they grow older. Estimates show that approximately 50% of children become symptom-free before adulthood and only 5 to 10% remain asthmatic throughout their entire adult life.

CONSIDERATIONS FOR CARE

1. Educate patient and family regarding the disease and treatment.
2. Provide emotional support for patient and family.
3. Observe patient's respiratory depth, rate, and character for symptoms of problems.
4. Auscultate chest for lung sounds and wheezing.
5. Monitor vital signs (see Appendix D).
6. Observe skin color and character.
7. Encourage fluids.
8. Educate regarding avoidance of asthma triggers .
9. Teach avoidance of sleeping pills as they decrease the respiratory rate.
10. Educate patient and family regarding need to carry a medical alert card and wear a medical alert bracelet or necklace.
11. Patients with inhalers should be educated regarding having them on hand at all times.

STATUS ASTHMATICUS

Status asthmaticus is a severe form of asthma that does not respond to conventional treatment. Symptoms continue for more than 24 hours. This is caused by infections, overuse of medications, dehydration, or medication noncompliance. The symptoms are similar to asthma, though more severe, and can lead to **respiratory arrest** and death. Treatment of status asthmaticus includes intravenous (IV) aminophylline, oxygen administration, chest physiotherapy, increased fluid intake, and possibly **mechanical ventilation**. Arterial blood gases are drawn on a frequent basis to monitor the levels of oxygen (O_2) and carbon dioxide (CO_2) in the blood.

FOR MORE INFORMATION

Asthma and Allergy Foundation of America
Suite 502
1125 15th Street NW
Washington, DC 20005
(202) 466-7643 or 1-800-7ASTHMA

American Lung Association
1740 Broadway, 14th Floor
New York, NY 10019-4374

ASSIGNMENT SHEET: ASTHMA

Short Answer

1. Write a brief definition for the terms listed throughout the chapter.

2. Describe the physiology of the respiratory system.

3. Write a brief definition for asthma.

4. Describe the incidence of asthma.

5. Describe the seven (7) precipitating factors for asthma and associated care.

6. List fifteen (15) symptoms that are often associated with asthma and associated care for these symptoms.

7. Describe ten (10) specific methods used to diagnose asthma.

8. Describe six (6) specific methods of treatment used for asthma.

9. Describe eleven (11) considerations for caring for a patient with asthma.

10. Describe the following associated with status asthmaticus:
    a. Definition
    b. Symptoms
    c. Treatment

11. List seven (7) symptoms of a respiratory infection.

12. Describe the following procedures used in the diagnosis or treatment of asthma.
    a. Arterial blood gases (ABGs)
    b. Pulmonary function studies
    c. Chest physiotherapy (percussion)
    d. Postural drainage
    e. Chest x-ray (CXR)

13. Write the normal ranges for each of the following serum laboratory tests.
    a. CBC
       - Hematocrit
       - Hemoglobin
       - Platelet count
       - Red blood cell count (RBC)
       - White blood cell count (WBC)
    b. Serum IgE
    c. ABGs
       - pCO_2
       - pH
       - pO_2
       - HCO_3
    d. Eosinophil

KNOWLEDGE INTO ACTION

1. Sandy Graham, a 12-year-old, comes in to the emergency room (ER) with a severe asthma attack. She has previously not had an asthma attack. The physician, in trying to distinguish the precipitating cause for her attack, asks her to write an approximate accounting of how her day was spent. It is a cold, windy day. The Grahams live in a city of 90,000 people with much industry.

   8:20 Get out of bed and shower
   8:45 Eat breakfast
   9:00 Help mother vacuum and dust the house
   11:30 Play outside with the dog
   12:00 Lunch
   12:45 Go to friend's house and play with her cat
   2:30 Return home. Headache and sneezing. Felt like a cold coming on. Took aspirin.
   4:00 Trouble breathing
   4:10 Came to ER

   Evaluate the scene, including the paragraph as well as Sandy's schedule, and list as many possible precipitating factors as you can find. (List at least five [5] possible factors.)

2. For each of the precipitating factors listed in the previous question, list two (2) methods of associated care to decrease the risk of precipitating an asthma attack.

3. Describe four (4) procedures or methods that could be used to aid in the diagnosis of Sandy's asthma.

4. Sandy is admitted to the pediatric ward of your hospital. The physician is worried about complications due to the sudden onset of her symptoms

and writes the order to "Monitor for symptoms of respiratory infection, hypoxia, and status asthmaticus." List the symptoms you would need to monitor for with each of the complications listed.

5. Sandy's physician orders the following treatment initially for the treatment of her asthma: (a) Theophylline (bronchodilator), (b) postural drainage, (c) Prednisone (corticosteroid), and (d) encourage fluids. Describe the rationale for each of the methods of treatment ordered.

6. You have been instructed to educate Sandy and her family prior to discharge about possible symptoms of an asthma attack for which they should monitor. List seven (7) symptoms to educate Sandy and her family about, as well as methods of associated care that correspond with each of the symptoms.

7. Upon discharge, the school nurse is notified so she can assist Sandy in educating her teachers and classmates. List seven (7) pieces of information that would be important to tell Sandy's teachers and classmates.

8. After the educational presentation has been given to Sandy's teachers and classmates, one of the teachers pulls you aside and says, "Sandy is such a hyperactive child, always looking for attention. Don't you think she could be doing this all just for attention?" What will your response be?

Chronic Obstructive Pulmonary Disease (COPD)

OBJECTIVES

Upon completion of this chapter, the student should be able to:

- Define the key terms listed throughout the chapter
- Describe the physiology of the respiratory system
- State a specific definition for COPD
- List and describe the diseases that are the main causes of COPD
- Describe the incidence of COPD
- List the risk factors for COPD
- List signs and symptoms associated with COPD and associated care for each of these symptoms
- Describe specific causes for exacerbations of the symptoms of COPD
- Identify specific methods for diagnosis of COPD
- Identify specific methods for treatment of COPD
- Describe the goals of treatment for COPD
- List complications associated with COPD
- Describe specific considerations for caring for a patient with COPD

KEY TERMS

Chronic obstructive pulmonary disease (COPD) – chronic lung disease that is the result of asthma, chronic bronchitis, and/or emphysema

Bronchitis – inflammation of the bronchial tubes

Asthma – disease characterized by reversible bronchospasm in the airway characterized by cough, dyspnea, wheezing, and increased mucous production

Tenacity – sticky or adhering

Alveolar sacs (alveoli) – small air sacks of the lungs in which carbon dioxide and oxygen exchange takes place during the process of respiration

Fibrosis – fibrous tissue formation

INTRODUCTION

Chronic obstructive pulmonary disease (COPD) is a chronic disease resulting in airway obstruction and decreased oxygenation. COPD is a result of the following three diseases: emphysema, chronic **bronchitis**, and **asthma**. The changes that occur in the airway due to COPD include decreased number and effectiveness of cilia, increased mucous production, **tenacity** of mucous, destruction, and scar formation of the **alveolar sacs** and **fibrosis** of the bronchial tubes.

Emphysema is when the alveoli of the lungs are overinflated and lose their elasticity due to the formation of scar tissue. Due to the overinflation, the lungs are less effective in the exchange of oxygen and carbon dioxide (CO_2). (See Figure 26-1.) Chronic bronchitis is defined as a chronic infection of the respiratory tract. Asthma is a chronic respiratory disease characterized by bronchospasms, dyspnea, and wheezing.

PHYSIOLOGY OF THE RESPIRATORY SYSTEM

The respiratory system is made up of the nose and nasal cavity, sinuses, pharynx, larynx, trachea, bronchi, bronchioles, and alveoli. (See Figure 25-1.) The purpose of the respiratory system is to draw **oxygen (O_2)**-rich air into the lungs (inspiration) to be transported to the body system through the blood vessels. The waste product, carbon dioxide (CO_2), is then released through the lungs (expiration). The respiratory system is lined with mucous membrane, which moistens the respiratory tract as well as assists in trapping and removing foreign particles from entering the lungs. Also located along the respiratory system are cilia, tiny hairlike structures, that also function to trap and

Oxygen (O₂) – gas present in the atmosphere that is necessary for the respiratory process of humans and other animals

Alpha 1-antitrypsin – protein that is often deficient in patients with emphysema

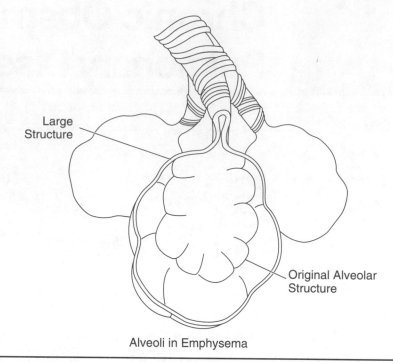

Alveoli in Emphysema

Figure 26-1 Overinflation of alveoli seen with emphysema (From Badasch, *Essentials for the Nursing Assistant in Long-Term Care, 2nd edition,* copyright © 1994, Delmar Publishers)

remove foreign particles from the airway. Up to one quart of mucous is normally secreted daily by the mucous membranes of the respiratory tract. (See Figure 26-2.)

STATISTICS

COPD affects approximately 15 million people in the United States, most of whom are males. It is the second leading cause of disability in the United States and the fourth leading cause of death. More than 84,000 die annually of complications associated with COPD. Approximately 434,000 people in the United States die annually due to diseases associated with cigarettes at a cost of greater than $55 billion. The cost associated with COPD alone is greater than $7.7 billion annually.

RISK FACTORS

The most common cause of COPD is cigarette smoking. Smoking is the cause of 82% of the chronic lung diseases. The other predisposing factors to COPD are:

1. Chronic respiratory infections
2. Allergies
3. Industrial pollutants
4. Heredity
5. **Alpha 1-antitrypsin** protein deficiency, which is known to be a cause of emphysema
6. Autoimmunity

SIGNS, SYMPTOMS, AND ASSOCIATED CARE

The following are symptoms that are commonly seen with COPD.

1. Dyspnea with mild to moderate exertion
   - Assist with position for patient comfort

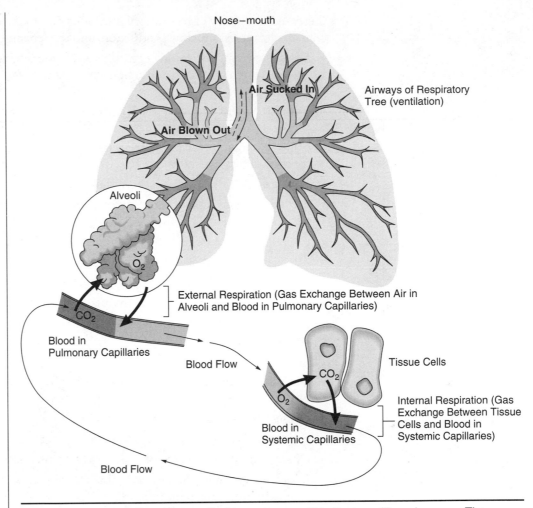

Figure 26-2   Oxygen and carbon dioxide exchange within the lung (From Layman, *The Medical Language*, copyright © 1995, Delmar Publishers)

- Monitor ease of respirations and respiratory rate
- Encourage frequent rest periods to conserve energy
- Encourage to do as many activities as possible in a sitting position, e.g. dressing, bathing, cooking, and cleaning
- Avoid constrictive garments and undergarments
- Administer oxygen as needed and directed by physician
- Provide fan in room to circulate air and assist in making breathing easier
- Arrange schedule of activities around patient rest periods
- Assist with activities of daily living (ADLs) as necessary
- Assess breath sounds on routine basis
- Observe for signs of hypoxia, e.g. cyanosis, decreased mental status, and confusion
- Humidify air as needed
- Provide reassurance to patient
- Treat cause of dyspnea

2. Cyanosis
- Monitor skin color
- Monitor *arterial blood gases (ABGs)*
- Assist patient to increase oxygenation
- Administer oxygen as needed and directed by physician

3. Increased frequency of respiratory infections due to the decreased number of cilia, the increased mucous production, and the tenacity of the mucous
   - Educate patient and family regarding symptoms of respiratory infection, such as cough, phlegm production, chest pain, fever, chills, dyspnea, and diaphoresis
   - Educate patient and family to report symptoms of respiratory infection to physician
   - Educate patient regarding importance of completing medication prescribed for respiratory infection
   - Encourage fluids to thin secretions and make them easier to cough up
   - Prevent transmission of infection by handwashing, correctly disposing of tissues and phlegm
   - Provide proper care and disposal of tissues and container to spit into
   - Avoid people with respiratory infections
   - Maintain optimal health to fight off infections
   - Administer influenza and pneumonia vaccinations as directed by physician
   - Avoid crowded areas, which increase the likelihood of contracting a respiratory infection

4. Productive cough
   - Facilitate *postural drainage* technique to facilitate drainage of mucous from lungs
   - Dispose of tissues and sputum correctly
   - Encourage patient to cover mouth when coughing
   - Observe sputum for signs of hemoptysis or infection
   - Educate regarding effective coughing techniques to facilitate productiveness of cough
   - Encourage fluids to thin mucous and facilitate drainage from lungs
   - Humidify air to prevent drying out of respiratory tract
   - Provide container for patient to cough secretions into
   - Administer expectorants as needed to aid in coughing up secretions
   - Provide frequent mouth care
   - Employ meticulous handwashing by patient, visitors, and staff members
   - Utilize universal precautions when handling any blood or body fluids (See Appendix C)

5. Structural changes of the chest, often referred to as "barrel chest"
   - Avoid constrictive garments and undergarments
   - Avoid clothing that accents the structural changes

6. Weight loss due to anorexia, difficulty eating due to dyspnea, as well as the increased energy needs due to difficulty breathing
   - Obtain baseline weight and monitor weight on routine basis
   - Encourage patient to participate in dietary choices
   - Offer nutritional supplements and vitamins
   - Encourage family and friends to bring in food that is appealing to patient as dietary restrictions allow
   - Administer parenteral fluids
   - Monitor intake and output (I and O)
   - Encourage rest periods before and after meals
   - Avoid unpleasant sights and odors in room to make meals more appealing

- Provide meticulous mouth care
- Monitor for skin breakdown due to loss of body tissue
- Encourage clothing styles that do not draw attention to weight loss
- Monitor for symptoms of dehydration, e.g. decreased urine output, constipation, dry skin, tenting of skin, dry mouth, dry eyes, concentrated urine, hypotension, and confusion
- Restrict sodium if patient is retaining fluid. Foods that are high in sodium and should be avoided include processed foods, cured meats, salted chips and crackers, pickles, and table salt.

7. Use of accessory breathing muscles
   - Avoid constrictive garments and undergarments
   - Assist with position for patient comfort
   - Be aware that touch may not be comfortable for patient as touch may feel constrictive

8. Wheezing or rales
   - Monitor breath sounds at frequent intervals
   - Assist with position for patient comfort
   - Assess patient skin color for signs of hypoxia (cyanosis)
   - Administer oxygen as needed and directed by physician

EXACERBATIONS

Exacerbations of COPD are caused by several physical as well as emotional factors.

1. Extremely hot or cold temperatures
2. Strong winds
3. Aerosol sprays, including perfumes, hairspray, cooking spray, and paint
4. Environmental chemicals
5. Perfumed lotions, deodorants, or cosmetics
6. Dust from outdoors or from cleaning
7. Stress
8. Exercise
9. Humidity

DIAGNOSIS

Diagnosis is often delayed due to denial on the part of the patient as well as a tendency for patients to minimize their symptoms as they learn to adjust to them. Diagnosis of COPD includes the following methods.

1. Symptoms
2. *Chest x-ray (CXR)*
3. *Pulmonary function test* to measure air exchange and lung capacity
4. *Arterial blood gases (ABGs)* show decreased O_2 (oxygen) levels and increased CO_2 (carbon dioxide) levels
5. *Spirometer*
6. *Peak-flow meter*

Respiratory failure – increase in carbon dioxide levels in the blood and decreased levels of oxygen in the blood due to poor air exchange within the lungs

TREATMENT

Treatment is based on the following goals.

1. Prevention of exacerbations
2. Improving air exchange
3. Removing secretions from respiratory tract
4. Prevention of complications

Methods of treatment include the following.

1. Quit smoking
2. Oxygen therapy for patients with decreased levels of oxygen
3. Medications

   - Bronchodilators used to treat bronchospasm and open bronchial tubes, e.g. Theodur, Brethine, Alupent, Theophylline, Aminophylline
   - Corticosteroids to reduce inflammation and open bronchial tubes, e.g. Prednisone, Beclomethasone, Vanceril
   - Antibiotics to treat respiratory infections, e.g. Vibramycin, Erythromycin, Bactrim
   - Vaccinations, such as influenza and pneumococcal vaccines
   - Expectorants to loosen and help remove mucous secretions

4. Regular exercise program
5. Lung transplant

COMPLICATIONS

1. Frequent respiratory infections leading to pneumonia
2. **Respiratory failure**

CONSIDERATIONS FOR CARE

1. Universal precautions should be used at all times (see Appendix C).
2. Educate patient and family regarding the disease process.
3. Educate patient and family regarding forms of treatment as well as side effects of treatment.
4. Provide emotional support to patient and family.
5. Encourage proper nutrition and fluid intake.
6. Educate patient and family regarding the importance of taking medications at the scheduled time and to complete the entire regimen of prescribed medications.
7. Educate patient and family regarding the importance of follow-up care.
8. Monitor for symptoms of complications.
9. Monitor for symptoms of dehydration, e.g. decreased urine output, dry mucous membranes, dry skin, concentrated urine, constipation, decreased level of consciousness, hypotension, confusion, and tenting of skin.
10. Educate patient regarding method of coughing effectively.
11. Monitor patient level of comfort and offer comfort measures such as relaxation techniques, imaging, massage, and warm packs.
12. Monitor intake and output (I and O).
13. Provide calm, relaxed atmosphere for patient to rest.

14. Assist in position for patient comfort.

15. Dispose of sputum and tissues correctly.

16. Encourage patient to cover mouth while coughing.

17. Encourage patient and family members to quit smoking.

18. Educate patient to avoid irritants that may cause an exacerbation of the symptoms.

19. Educate patient regarding breathing exercises which are designed to prolong expiration.

20. Provide assistance, encouragement and community resources for necessary life style changes due to the disease.

21. Facilitate support group contacts for patient and family.

22. Contact community resources as necessary for financial assistance for patient and family.

23. Obtain baseline vital signs and monitor at frequent intervals.

24. Assist patient in obtaining self-help devices, such as long-handled shoehorns, reaching devices, elastic shoelaces, and velcro fasteners for clothing.

25. Educate patient to avoid doing activities that raise dust, such as dusting, sweeping, and vacuuming.

26. Assist patient in securing a handicapped parking permit if necessary.

27. Assist patient in setting up a method of notifying someone in case of emergency, e.g. signal to neighbors, have someone call at set time each day, or emergency alert system.

28. Educate patient and family regarding need to carry a medical alert card and wear a medical alert bracelet or necklace.

29. Suction equipment should be available at bedside.

30. Increase fluid intake to liquefy secretions.

31. Humidify air to liquefy secretions.

32. Obtain baseline lung sounds on admission to hospital and monitor on routine basis.

33. Monitor ABGs.

34. Educate client and family regarding diet high in carbohydrates and protein. Foods high in carbohydrates include fruits, vegetables, and whole grains. Foods high in protein include meats, eggs, poultry, cheese, and milk.

35. Avoid crowded places and people with respiratory infections or other forms of infection.

FOR MORE INFORMATION

Asthma and Allergy Foundation of America
Suite 305
1717 Massachusetts Avenue, NW
Washington, DC 20036
1-800-7ASTHMA (727-8462)

National Jewish Center for Immunology and Respiratory Medicine
1400 Jackson Street
Denver, CO 80206
LUNGLINE 1-800-222-LUNG (5864)

ASSIGNMENT SHEET: COPD

Short Answer

1. Write a brief definition for the terms listed throughout the chapter.

2. Describe the physiology of the respiratory system.

3. Write a brief definition for COPD.

4. List and describe the three (3) diseases that are the main causes of COPD.

5. Describe the incidence of COPD.

6. List the six (6) risk factors for COPD.

7. List eight (8) signs and symptoms of COPD and associated care for these symptoms.

8. List nine (9) common causes associated with exacerbations of the symptoms of COPD.

9. List six (6) specific methods used to aid in the diagnosis of COPD.

10. Describe the four (4) specific goals of treatment for COPD.

11. List five (5) specific methods used in the treatment of COPD.

12. List two (2) complications associated with COPD.

13. List thirty-five (35) considerations for caring for a patient with COPD.

14. Describe what is meant by universal precautions. (See Appendix C.)

15. Describe each of the following procedures used in the diagnosis or treatment of COPD.

    a. Arterial blood gases (ABGs)
    b. Chest x-ray (CXR)
    c. Spirometer
    d. Postural drainage
    e. Peak-flow meter
    f. Pulmonary function test

KNOWLEDGE INTO ACTION

1. Harold Deibert, a 72-year-old retired grain storage elevator operator, is admitted to the hospital to rule out COPD. He has smoked since he was in the service, more than 50 years ago. Helen Deibert, Harold's wife, is present in the room. They are aware that the doctor is ruling out COPD and that Harold's lungs are involved. Mrs. Deibert asks you, "What exactly is COPD, and how are my husband's lungs affected by this disease?" What will your response be?

2. Mr. Deibert was admitted to the hospital with the following symptoms: dyspnea, increased frequency of respiratory infection, productive cough, and weight loss. List three (3) methods of associated care for each of the symptoms that could be incorporated into Mr. Deibert's hospital care and three (3) methods of associated care that could be incorporated into a plan of care once Mr. Deibert is discharged to home.

3. When Mr. Deibert was admitted to the hospital, the physician wrote many orders. For each of the orders written by the physician, describe the rationale behind the order.

    a. Assess breath sounds every 8 hours.
    b. Arterial blood gases on admission. Repeat in 24 hours.
    c. Temperature every 4 hours.
    d. Respiratory therapy to facilitate postural drainage as needed.
    e. Influenza and pneumonia vaccinations on admission.
    f. Monitor intake and output.
    g. Low-sodium diet.
    h. Chest x-ray on admission.
    i. Oxygen as needed.
    j. Aminophylline (bronchodilator) twice daily.

4. Mr. Deibert was discharged from the hospital two weeks ago. You have been assigned to see if he has any questions. He comments to you, "The doctor sent me home on these antibiotics. I felt so much better, I quit taking them." Upon further questioning, you find out that Mr. Deibert has taken 6 days of a 10-day prescription of antibi-

otics. What will your response be and why would you respond this way?

5. Approximately 6 weeks after discharge, Mrs. Deibert calls the doctor's office and is quite concerned. She says her husband is cyanotic, confused, sleeps most of the time, and hasn't urinated since early this morning, at which time his urine was very dark. Based on Mr. Deibert's history of COPD, what two (2) complications are you concerned about? (Choose the best answer.)

   a. Pneumonia and bladder infection
   b. Dehydration and hypoxia
   c. Meningitis and hypoxia
   d. Kidney failure and a heart attack

6. Once again, Mr. Deibert is admitted to the hospital. Prior to discharge, you have been asked to tell Mrs. Deibert some considerations for care for taking care of her husband. List two (2) considerations for care Mrs. Deibert should keep in mind for each of the following areas of care.

   a. Fluids and nutrition
   b. Emergency care
   c. Personal care
   d. Prevention of complications

Pneumonia

Upon completion of this chapter, the student should be able to:

- Define the key terms listed throughout the chapter
- Describe the physiology of the respiratory system
- State a specific definition for pneumonia
- Describe the incidence of pneumonia
- List the causative organisms for pneumonia
- List signs and symptoms associated with pneumonia and associated care for these symptoms
- List the specific types of pneumonia associated with the modes of transmission
- Describe the risk factors for pneumonia and the rationale and associated care for each of the factors
- Describe the risk factors for aspiration pneumonia, the rationale, and associated care for each of the factors
- Identify specific methods for diagnosis of pneumonia
- Identify specific methods for treatment of pneumonia
- Describe available vaccinations that can decrease the risk of pneumonia
- Describe complications associated with pneumonia and list the symptoms for each of the complications
- Describe specific considerations for caring for a patient with pneumonia

INTRODUCTION

Pneumonia is defined as an acute infection of the lung tissue causing inflammation. It can involve the bronchi and bronchioles (bronchial pneumonia) or the lobes of the lung itself (lobar pneumonia). The inflammation of the bronchial or lung tissue impairs the exchange of carbon dioxide (CO_2) and oxygen (O_2).

PHYSIOLOGY OF THE RESPIRATORY SYSTEM

The respiratory system is made up of the nose and nasal cavity, sinuses, pharynx, larynx, trachea, bronchi, bronchioles, and alveoli. (See Figure 25-1.) The purpose of the respiratory system is to draw oxygen-rich air into the lungs (inspiration) to be transported to the body system through the blood vessels. The waste product, carbon dioxide (CO_2), is then released through the lungs (expiration). The respiratory system is lined with mucous membrane, which moistens the respiratory tract and assists in trapping and removing foreign particles before entering the lungs. Also located along the respiratory system are cilia, tiny hairlike structures, that also function to trap and remove foreign particles from the airway. Up to one quart of mucous is normally secreted daily by the mucous membranes of the respiratory tract. (See Figure 27-1.)

STATISTICS AND RISK FACTORS

Pneumonia is the sixth leading cause of death in the United States, with more than 76,500 deaths annually due to pneumonia. The illness is more common in males than in

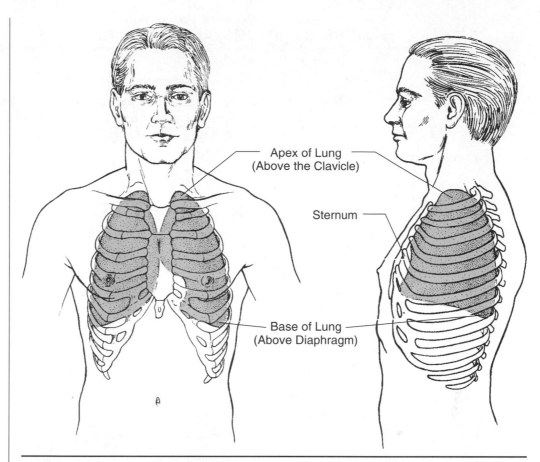

Figure 27-1   Location of the lungs within the chest (From Kinn, *Medical Terminology: Building Blocks for Health Careers*, copyright © 1990, Delmar Publishers)

females and occurs frequently in the very young, the elderly, and those with an impaired immune system, due to chemotherapy, corticosteroids, radiation therapy, or organ transplant. More than 3.9 million people develop pneumonia annually in the United States. The total cost associated with pneumonia exceeds $6 billion annually.

CAUSATIVE ORGANISMS

The causative organisms for pneumonia are many. The most common organisms are as follows, with approximately 90% of all pneumonia caused by bacterial organisms.

1. *Streptococcus pneumoniae* (See Figure 27-2a)
2. *Haemophilus influenzae*
3. *Staphylococcus aureus* (See Figure 27-2b)
4. *Legionella pneumophilia*
5. *Mycoplasma pneumoniae*
6. *Pnuemocystis carinii pneumonia*
7. *Klebsiella*
8. *Pseudomonas*

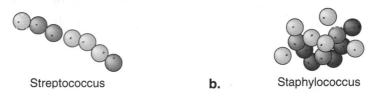

a.   Streptococcus   **b.**   Staphylococcus

Figure 27-2   (a) Streptococcus and (b) Staphylococcus (From Smith et al., *Medical Terminology: A Programmed Text, 7th edition*, copyright © 1995, Delmar Publishers)

SIGNS, SYMPTOMS, AND ASSOCIATED CARE

1. Fever
   - Monitor temperature at routine intervals
   - Provide comfort measures for patient with elevated temperature such as cool cloth to forehead, partial or complete bath as needed, clothing and bedding changed frequently due to diaphoresis, and encourage fluids to prevent dehydration
   - Avoid exposing patient to a draft
   - Cover with blankets as necessary
   - Monitor intake and output (I and O)
   - Maintain comfortable room temperature for patient
   - Avoid plastic mattresses and plastic bed protectors as they increase perspiration
   - Use antiperspirant or deodorant to minimize sweating and odor

2. Cough
   - Encourage fluids to thin mucous secretions to cough up more easily
   - Administer expectorants as needed to aid in coughing up secretions
   - Educate regarding effective coughing techniques to facilitate productiveness of cough
   - Provide container for patient to cough secretions into
   - Dispose of tissues and sputum properly
   - Provide frequent mouth care
   - Employ meticulous handwashing by patient, visitors, and staff
   - Utilize universal precautions when handling any blood or body fluids (See Appendix C)
   - Provide postural drainage technique to facilitate drainage of mucous from lungs
   - Encourage patient to cover mouth when coughing
   - Observe sputum for signs of hemoptysis or infection
   - Humidify air as needed

3. Chest pain
   - Assist with position for patient comfort
   - Provide warm packs to chest
   - Offer pain control methods such as relaxation techniques, imaging, or pain medications as prescribed by physician

4. Sputum production that may be yellow-green or occasionally blood tinged
   - Dispose of tissues and sputum correctly
   - Utilize universal precautions when handling any blood or body fluids (See Appendix C)
   - Employ meticulous handwashing by patient and staff
   - Encourage fluids to thin secretions and cough up more easily
   - Obtain sputum samples as needed for culture, sensitivity, and gram stain

5. Tachypnea
   - Monitor respiratory rate routinely
   - Monitor skin color for cyanosis
   - Assist with position for patient comfort

- Monitor for complications of hypoxemia
- Monitor for nasal flaring and sternal retraction, especially in infants and children

6. Dyspnea
   - Administer oxygen as needed and as directed by physician
   - Avoid constrictive garments and undergarments
   - Provide fan in room to circulate air and assist in making breathing easier
   - Encourage frequent rest periods to conserve energy
   - Arrange schedule of activities around patient rest periods
   - Assist with activities of daily living (ADLs) as necessary
   - Assess breath sounds on routine basis
   - Observe for signs of hypoxia, e.g. cyanosis, diaphoresis, decreased level of consciousness, and confusion
   - Monitor ease of respirations and respiratory rate
   - Do as many activities as possible in a sitting position, e.g. dressing, bathing, cooking, and cleaning
   - Humidify air as needed
   - Provide reassurance to patient
   - Treat cause of dyspnea

TYPES OF PNEUMONIA

1. Primary pneumonia is caused by inhalation of the causative pathogen.
2. Secondary pneumonia is pneumonia caused by the spread of the pathogen from a distant site.
3. Aspiration pneumonia results when a foreign substance is drawn into the lungs causing inflammation and allowing a pathogen to reproduce and cause the pneumonia.

PREDISPOSING FACTORS FOR PNEUMONIA

1. Long-term illness and debilitating illness
   a. Due to immobilization the secretions pool in the lungs, which provides a perfect medium for pathogens to reproduce; during immobilization the patient frequently does not breathe deeply and effectively
   b. During long-term illness, a person often has decreased nutritional status, which predisposes them to pneumonia and other illness
   c. Due to the long-term illness, a person may have a compromised immune system, which makes them a perfect candidate for pneumonia, since the body is less able to fight off infections
   - Encourage ambulation and activities as possible
   - Reposition patient at least every 2 hours
   - Encourage coughing and deep-breathing exercises
   - Encourage proper nutrition and adequate fluid intake
   - Monitor for symptoms of pneumonia and other illness
   - Encourage pneumococcal and influenza vaccinations for patients who have chronic illness
   - Provide humidified air for patient to breathe

2. Surgery to the abdomen or **thoracic** region

   a. Anesthesia decreases the person's respiratory ability, allowing secretions to pool in the lungs and providing a medium for pathogens to grow

   b. Patient may not cough and deep breathe effectively due to pain or due to sedation

   c. Due to immobilization post-operatively, patient may have buildup of secretions in the lungs

- Encourage coughing and deep-breathing exercises
- Administer pain medications as needed to encourage coughing and deep breathing
- Splint chest and/or abdomen to promote coughing and deep breathing
- Encourage patient to be up as soon as possible post-operatively
- Reposition patient at least every 2 hours
- Monitor for symptoms of pneumonia
- Provide humidified air for patient to breathe

3. Lung cancer or other neoplastic diseases

   a. Lung cancer has deteriorated the lung tissue, which allows pathogens to multiply

   b. With cancer and cancer treatment, the immune system often is compromised, which decreases the body's ability to fight infections

   c. With cancer and cancer treatment, the person often has a decreased nutritional status, which predisposes them to pneumonia and other illness

   d. With cancer and cancer treatment, the patient often becomes dehydrated, which causes the mucous in the lungs to thicken and "trap" organisms, allowing them to reproduce freely; thick mucous is also more difficult to expectorate from the lungs

- Monitor patient for symptoms of pneumonia or other illness
- Encourage proper nutrition and adequate fluid intake
- Encourage pneumococcal and influenza **vaccine** for patients with lung cancer or other neoplastic diseases
- Encourage coughing and deep-breathing exercises
- Encourage patient to be as active as possible
- Reposition patient at least every 2 hours while in bed
- Provide humidified air for patient to breathe

4. **Malnutrition**

   a. With decreased nutritional status, the patient is predisposed to pneumonia and other illness

   b. In the presence of dehydration, mucous in the lungs becomes thicker, which "traps" the pathogens and allows them to grow freely; thick mucous is also more difficult to expectorate from the lungs

- Educate and encourage proper nutrition and adequate fluid intake
- Monitor intake and output (I and O)
- Monitor for symptoms of dehydration, e.g. decreased urine output, constipation, dry skin, tenting of skin, dry mouth, dry eyes, concentrated urine, hypotension, and confusion
- Monitor weight on a routine basis to assess adequacy of nutrition
- Provide humidified air for patient to breathe
- Monitor for symptoms of pneumonia or other illness

Cystic fibrosis – disease affecting the respiratory tract and exocrine glands of the body; characterized by increased mucous production in the lungs and increased perspiration

5. Asthma and chronic respiratory disease, e.g. COPD, chronic bronchitis, and emphysema

   a. Diminished airway associated with asthma decreases air exchange in the lungs

   b. Decreased number of cilia or impaired function of cilia in asthma impairs the filtering function of the cilia allowing pathogens to enter more freely

   c. Increased mucous production and thicker mucous "trap" the pathogens in the lungs and allow them to grow freely

   • Encourage coughing and deep-breathing exercises

   • Encourage patient to be as active as tolerated

   • Encourage adequate fluid intake

   • Encourage to avoid people with respiratory infections or other infections

   • Encourage pneumococcal and influenza vaccinations

   • Employ meticulous hand care on the part of patient, staff, and visitors to avoid transmission of illness

   • Administer breathing treatments and medications as prescribed by physician

6. **Cystic fibrosis**

   a. The increased mucous production associated with cystic fibrosis "traps" the pathogens in the lungs and allows them to grow freely

   b. Mucous in the lungs is thicker in consistency and difficult to expectorate from the lungs

   • Encourage adequate fluid intake

   • Provide humidified air for the patient to breathe

   • Administer breathing treatments and medications as prescribed by physician

7. Drug abuse and alcoholism

   a. Often accompanied by a decreased nutritional status, which predisposes the patient to pneumonia as well as other illness

   b. With decreased mental alertness accompanied by vomiting, patient is at risk for aspiration and progression into pneumonia

   • Educate regarding options and availability for alcohol and drug counseling and treatment

   • Encourage proper nutrition and adequate fluid intake

   • Provide nutritional supplements and vitamins to patient with decreased nutritional intake

   • Monitor patient with history of drug or alcohol ingestion for possibility of vomiting with aspiration

   • Monitor for symptoms of pneumonia or other illness

   • If decreased mental alertness, position patient on side to diminish possibility of aspiration

   • Utilize suction equipment as needed

8. Medical treatments that cause immunosuppression, e.g. chemotherapy, radiation therapy, and corticosteroids. With an impaired immune system, the patient is unable to fight off infections

   • Monitor for symptoms of pneumonia or other illness

   • Encourage pneumococcal and influenza vaccines as advised by physician

   • Encourage proper nutrition and adequate fluid intake

   • Avoid people with infections

Noxious – poisonous or harmful

Intubation – insertion of a hollow tube through the nose or mouth into the trachea for the purpose of delivering oxygen to a patient in an emergency

- Employ meticulous handwashing on the part of the patient, staff, and visitors
- Provide private room or isolation for the patient

9. Industrial pollution and exposure to **noxious** chemicals causes inflammation to the respiratory tract, leading to a decrease in the number of cilia to filter pathogens; an increase in the amount of mucous, which traps pathogens; thicker mucous, which is more difficult to expectorate and results in a tendency to trap pathogens
   - Educate regarding importance of avoiding industrial pollutants and noxious chemicals
   - Educate regarding proper ventilation and the use of masks when possible in the presence of industrial pollutants and noxious chemicals

10. Prolonged **intubation** or presence of tracheostomy (See Figure 27-3)
   a. Irritation of the respiratory tract causes impairment of the cleansing function of the cilia as well as increased mucous production
   b. With a tracheostomy, the patient has loss of the cleansing function in the nose and upper airway
   - Employ sterile technique for suctioning and other treatments
   - Utilize meticulous skin care around the tracheostomy
   - Monitor for symptoms of pneumonia or other illness
   - Provide humidified air for patient to breathe
   - Educate to avoid people with infections
   - Employ meticulous handwashing on the part of the staff and visitors
   - Dispose of suctioned secretions properly
   - Utilize universal precautions when in contact with any blood or body fluids (See Appendix C)
   - Educate patient and family regarding proper care of the tracheostomy for the patient requiring long-term care at home

PREDISPOSING FACTORS FOR ASPIRATION PNEUMONIA

1. Diminished level of consciousness due to disease, trauma, or anesthesia
   a. Loss of control of oral secretions
   b. Possibility of vomiting and inability for patient to remove from mouth
   - Utilize suction equipment as needed
   - Position patient on side or sitting up to avoid aspiration

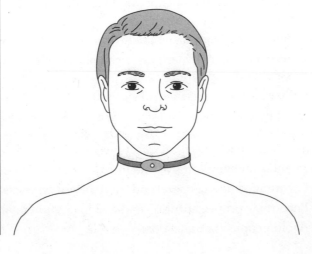

Figure 27-3 Position of a tracheostomy

Debilitating – causing extreme weakness

Myasthenia gravis – disease of the muscular system caused by a lack of acetylcholine

Hemiparesis – paralysis of one half of the body

Culture – growth of organisms obtained from a specimen in the body as a method of diagnosis of the causative pathogen of a disease; examples include sputum and wound drainage

Sensitivity – determining which treatment would be most effective in treating the microorganism that has been cultured

Gram stain – procedure of staining a smear on a slide to determine the type of bacteria; gram-positive bacteria organisms stain dark purple in reaction to the crystal violet iodine solution and safranin O, gram-negative bacteria organisms stain pink or red

Oximeter – noninvasive machine used to determine the amount of oxygen in the blood

Antimicrobial – substance used in the treatment of microbes

- Provide adequate hydration
- Provide frequent oral care

2. **Debilitating** illness, e.g. Alzheimer's disease, **myasthenia gravis**, multiple sclerosis, Parkinson's disease, and stroke
   a. Loss of control of oral secretions
   b. Impaired ability to chew and swallow food
   c. Inability to maintain correct posture with eating and drinking
   d. Lack of awareness of surroundings
   e. Diminished cough reflex in the presence of choking
   - Utilize suction equipment as needed
   - Position patient on side or in an upright position to diminish possibility of aspiration
   - Provide upright position for patient for eating or drinking
   - Encourage patient to chew food thoroughly
   - Diminish outside distractions for patient when eating
   - Educate that foods may need to be ground, chopped, or pureed
   - Place food on the unaffected side of the mouth in the presence of **hemiparesis**
   - Educate that liquids may need to be thickened

3. Nutrition via nasogastric tube (NG)
   a. Impaired gag reflex due to placement in back of throat
   b. Possibility of vomiting and inability for patient to remove from mouth
   - Monitor correct tube placement frequently in the presence of continuous nasogastric feeding
   - Place patient in an upright position for tube feeding if possible
   - Monitor for vomiting

DIAGNOSIS

1. Symptoms
2. Physical examination to include auscultation of breath sounds
3. *Chest x-ray (CXR)*
4. *Sputum specimen for **culture**, **sensitivity**, and **gram stain***
5. *CBC will show elevated WBC*
6. *Arterial blood gases (ABGs) will indicate presence of hypoxemia*
7. **Oximeter** will indicate presence of diminished levels of oxygen in the blood

TREATMENT

1. Treatment with **antimicrobial** medications depending on causative organism
2. Encourage fluids
   - Thins mucous in respiratory tract to ease expectoration
   - Possibility of dehydration due to decreased appetite and diaphoresis
3. Oxygen therapy dependent upon arterial blood gas (ABG) levels obtained and condition of the patient
4. Bedrest in initial stages of disease; gradually increasing activity until patient has reached former state of activity
5. *Postural drainage* and *chest percussion* to loosen secretions

Atelectasis – collapsed lung

Mucous plug – hardened mucous secretions that block a portion of the airway within the lung

Pleural effusion – fluid accumulation in the cavity surrounding the lung

Empyema – pus-filled cavity, generally located in the lung

Meningitis – inflammation of the meninges of the brain and spinal cord

6. Medications for pain may be required

7. Cough suppressants may be prescribed in the presence of a severe nonproductive cough; important not to suppress a productive cough

8. Medications to reduce fever, e.g. Aspirin, Acetaminophen

9. Ventilatory assistance may be necessary in severe cases

10. Cough expectorant medications to aid in expelling secretions from the lungs

AVAILABLE VACCINATIONS

1. Polyvalent pneumococcal polysaccharide vaccine is used in the prevention of pneumococcal pneumonia
   - High-risk groups include persons with chronic illness, persons over the age of 65, health care workers, children with chronic illness, and persons with impaired immune systems due to medications or disease
   - Has shown to be up to 90% effective with the vaccine protecting the person for 5 to 10 years

2. Influenza vaccine
   - High-risk groups include persons with chronic illness, persons over the age of 65, health care workers, children with chronic illness, and persons with impaired immune systems due to medications or disease
   - Has been shown to be 80% effective

COMPLICATIONS

1. Hypoxemia

   Symptoms: confusion, dyspnea, cyanosis, diaphoresis, and decreased level of consciousness

2. **Atelectasis** caused from **mucous plug** in the airway

   Symptoms: diminished or absent breath sounds over a portion of the lung, cyanosis, dyspnea, cyanosis, tachycardia, and tachypnea

3. **Pleural effusion**

   Symptoms: dyspnea, increased cough, chest pain, and diminished or absent breath sounds over a portion of the lung

4. **Empyema**

   Symptoms: increased fever, malaise, and chest pain

5. Pericarditis

   Symptoms: chest pain radiating to shoulders, and neck and back, which often intensifies with inspiration and diminishes with upright position

6. Bacteremia

   Symptoms: fever, cyanosis, reduced level of consciousness, and joint pain

7. **Meningitis**

   Symptoms: nuchal rigidity, headache, irritability, delirium, seizures, and fever

8. Death

CONSIDERATIONS FOR CARE

1. Educate patient and family regarding the disease process.

2. Educate patient and family regarding forms of treatment as well as side effects of treatment.

3. Provide emotional support to patient and family.
4. Encourage proper nutrition and increased fluid intake.
5. Educate patient and family regarding the importance of taking medications at the scheduled time and to complete the entire regimen of prescribed medications.
6. Educate patient and family regarding the importance of follow-up care.
7. Monitor for symptoms of complications.
8. Monitor for symptoms of dehydration as follows: decreased urine output, dry mucous membranes, dry skin, concentrated urine, constipation, decreased level of consciousness, hypotension, tenting of skin, and confusion.
9. Educate patient regarding method of coughing effectively.
10. Monitor patient level of comfort and offer comfort measures such as relaxation techniques, imaging, massage, warm packs, and medications as prescribed by physician.
11. Monitor intake and output (I and O).
12. Provide calm, relaxed atmosphere for patient to rest.
13. Encourage meticulous handwashing on the part of the patient, staff, and visitors.
14. Assist in position for patient comfort.
15. Dispose of sputum and tissues correctly.
16. Encourage patient to cover mouth when coughing.
17. Masks and a private room may be necessary for the patient while in the hospital.
18. Educate patient and family regarding the availability of influenza vaccine and pneumovax vaccine.
19. Monitor ABG and oximeter levels.
20. Monitor lung sounds on routine basis.

FOR MORE INFORMATION

Department of Public Health and Human Services
Centers for Disease Control
Atlanta, GA 30333

CHAPTER 27 REVIEW

ASSIGNMENT SHEET: PNEUMONIA

Short Answer

1. Write a brief definition for the terms listed throughout the chapter.

2. Describe the physiology of the respiratory system.

3. Write a brief definition for pneumonia.

4. Describe the incidence of pneumonia.

5. List eight (8) causative organisms for pneumonia.

6. List six (6) signs and symptoms associated with pneumonia and associated care for these symptoms.

7. List the three (3) types of pneumonia according to their mode of transmission.

8. List ten (10) predisposing factors for pneumonia, the rationale, and associated care for each of these factors.

9. List three (3) predisposing factors for aspiration pneumonia, the rationale, and associated care for each of these factors.

10. List seven (7) specific methods used to aid in the diagnosis of pneumonia.

11. List ten (10) specific methods used to treat pneumonia.

12. Describe two (2) available vaccinations that could decrease the incidence of pneumonia.

13. List eight (8) complications associated with pneumonia and the symptoms associated with each of the complications.

14. List twenty (20) considerations for caring for a patient with pneumonia.

15. Describe each of the following procedures used in the diagnosis or treatment of pneumonia.

    a. Sputum culture, sensitivity, and gram stain
    b. Chest x-ray (CXR)
    c. Postural drainage
    d. Chest percussion

16. Write the normal ranges for each of the following laboratory tests.

    a. CBC
       - Hematocrit
       - Hemoglobin
       - Platelet count
       - Red blood cell count (RBC)
       - White blood cell count (WBC)
    b. Arterial blood gases (ABGs)
       - pCO_2
       - pH
       - pO_2
       - HCO_3

KNOWLEDGE INTO ACTION

1. Erika Mercado, a 78-year-old from your neighborhood, is admitted to the hospital with pneumonia. Her symptoms include the following: fever, cough, tachypnea, chest pain, and dyspnea. Describe how you would assist Mrs. Mercado with each of these symptoms and how you would monitor to see if there was improvement in these symptoms.

2. You have just finished making Mrs. Mercado's bed and are washing your hands. Mrs. Mercado says to you, "Everybody is always washing their hands. Is there something wrong with me that you're not telling me?" What will your response be?

3. You are helping a friend study for a test on pneumonia. You ask your friend to tell you the rationale behind each of the predisposing factors as well as associated care to reduce or eliminate these predisposing factors. What should the response be?

    a. Long-term illness and debilitating illness
    b. Surgery to abdomen or thoracic region
    c. Lung cancer or other neoplastic diseases
    d. Malnutrition
    e. Asthma and chronic respiratory disease
    f. Cystic fibrosis
    g. Drug abuse and alcoholism
    h. Medical treatments that cause immunosuppression

    i.   Industrial pollution and exposure to noxious chemicals

    j.   Prolonged intubation or presence of tracheostomy

4. Your friend has completed all of the rationales and associated care items for predisposing factors for pneumonia. Now you ask your friend to do the same for predisposing factors for aspiration pneumonia.

    a.   Diminished level of consciousness

    b.   Debilitating illness

    c.   Nutrition via nasogastric tube

5. Mrs. Mercado's physician asks for a stethoscope to auscultate her lungs. Describe the importance of this procedure.

6. On Mrs. Mercado's chart, the physician writes an order to obtain a sputum specimen for culture, sensitivity, and gram stain. When you go into the room to obtain the sputum specimen, Mrs. Mercado asks what the purpose of "having me cough up into a cup" is. What will your response be?

7. Mrs. Mercado is on a "force fluid" diet. She says to you, "I feel like I'm getting waterlogged. What docs he want me to drink all this fluid for anyway?" What will your response be?

8. Prior to discharge, Mrs. Mercado's physician writes the order to give Mrs. Mercado a polyvalent pneumococcal polysaccharide vaccine. What would the purpose of this vaccine be?

9. Mrs. Mercado has been taking very limited fluids during her hospitalization. Her physician is concerned that she may become dehydrated once she returns home and asks you to teach Mrs. Mercado specific symptoms of dehydration to watch for. What symptoms would you teach her about? (List 6.)

UNIT 7

GENETIC AND CONGENITAL DISORDERS

Cerebral Palsy

OBJECTIVES

Upon completion of this chapter, the student should be able to:

- Define the key terms listed throughout the chapter
- State a specific definition for cerebral palsy
- Describe the incidence of cerebral palsy
- List the categories of cerebral palsy
- Describe the causes of cerebral palsy
- List signs and symptoms associated with cerebral palsy
- Identify specific methods used in the diagnosis of cerebral palsy
- Identify specific methods for treatment of cerebral palsy
- Describe specific considerations for caring for a patient with cerebral palsy

KEY TERMS

Neuromuscular – refers to a combination of the muscles and the nerves

Prenatal – refers to the period before birth

Perinatal – refers to the time directly before, during, and after birth

Postnatal – refers to the period after birth

Anoxia – deficiency or absence of oxygen leading to tissue death

Athetoid – specific category of cerebral palsy in which the motor cortex of the brain is damaged resulting in difficulty with smooth coordination and involuntary movement

Ataxia – lack of muscle coordination with voluntary or involuntary movement

INTRODUCTION

Cerebral palsy is a nonprogressive **neuromuscular** disorder resulting from damage to the brain before (**prenatal**), during (**perinatal**), or after (**postnatal**) birth. The damage may also occur later in life due to head trauma. This damage results from **anoxia**. The disability caused by the anoxia may be slight or completely disabling.

STATISTICS

Cerebral palsy occurs in two to six children out of 1,000 live births per year in the United States. More than 90% of the time, the damage occurs during the prenatal or perinatal period.

TYPES OF CEREBRAL PALSY

There are three main types of cerebral palsy. (See Figure 28-1.)

They are classified according to their main characteristics as follows.

1. Spastic includes 70% of patients with diagnosis of cerebral palsy; the part of the brain that controls voluntary movement is damaged

2. **Athetoid** includes 20% of patients with diagnosis of cerebral palsy; the motor cortex of the brain is damaged resulting in difficulty with smooth coordination and involuntary movement

3. **Ataxia** includes 10% of patients with cerebral palsy; the portions of the brain that control voluntary and involuntary movement are both involved

Maternal – refers to the mother

Toxoplasmosis – infection caused from the *Toxoplasma gondii* organism that can cause infections of the lungs, liver, immune system, and central nervous system

Rubella – infectious disease of short duration caused by a virus characterized by rash and fever; also known as German measles

Umbilical cord – network of blood vessels that connects the placenta to the fetus

Toxin – poisonous substance

Toxemia – toxic substances present in the blood that cause generalized symptoms due to their disbursement throughout the body

Placenta previa – placental attachment near the opening of the uterus (cervix) rather than the normal position higher on the uterine wall

Abruptio placenta – premature separation of the placenta

Breech – refers to presentation or delivery of a fetus buttocks first

Forceps – instrument used to grasp or hold an object

Anomalies – contrasts from what is normally expected; congenital anomalies are generally due to faulty fetal development in the uterus

Bilirubinemia – accumulation of bilirubin in the blood

Kernicterus – buildup of bilirubin in the brain and spinal cord of an infant

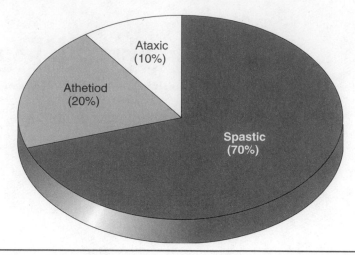

Figure 28-1   Types of cerebral palsy

RISK FACTORS

1. Prenatal causes include the following
   - **Maternal** infection, e.g. **toxoplasmosis** and **rubella**
   - Compression of the **umbilical cord**
   - Maternal exposure to drugs, alcohol, or **toxins**
   - **Toxemia**
   - Maternal malnutrition
2. Perinatal causes include the following.
   - **Placenta previa**
   - **Abruptio placenta**
   - **Breech** delivery
   - **Forceps** delivery
   - Multiple births
   - Anesthesia or medications used during delivery
3. Postnatal causes include the following.
   - Infant infections, e.g. encephalitis or meningitis
   - Vascular **anomalies**
   - Cerebral hemorrhage or thrombosis
   - Anoxia
   - **Bilirubinemia (kernicterus)**
4. Trauma due to head injury, e.g. falls, motor vehicle accidents, head wounds, or abuse

SIGNS AND SYMPTOMS

Signs and symptoms are variable with each person affected by cerebral palsy. They may have the symptoms in varying degrees or complete lack of certain symptoms. A generalized list of signs and symptoms associated with cerebral palsy is as follows.

1. Irritability
2. Shrill or abnormal cry
3. Absent or poor sucking reflex
4. Poorly developed gross motor and fine motor movements

Dyskinesia – impairment of voluntary movement

Paralysis – loss of feeling or movement to a certain portion of the body

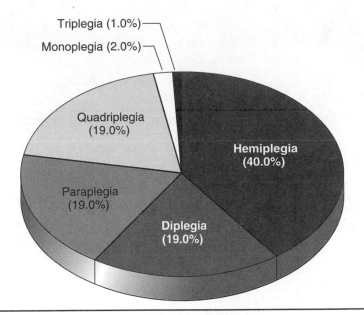

Figure 28-2   Types of paralysis

5. Weakness
6. Extreme preference for one side of the body
7. Dysphagia
8. Mental retardation present in 50 to 75% of patients with cerebral palsy
9. Seizures present in 20 to 25% of patients with cerebral palsy
10. Spasticity present in 50 to 70% of patients with cerebral palsy
11. **Dyskinesia** present in 20 to 25% of patients with cerebral palsy
12. Ataxia present in 5 to 10% of patients with cerebral palsy
13. Speech disorders present in 70 to 80% of patients with cerebral palsy
14. Difficulty spreading legs for diaper change
15. Abnormal reflexes
16. **Paralysis** (See Figure 28-2)

DIAGNOSIS

Diagnosis is made on the evaluation of the presence of symptoms and history. There is no specific diagnostic test to determine a diagnosis of cerebral palsy. The following methods aid in the diagnosis of cerebral palsy.

1. Signs and symptoms
2. History of prenatal, perinatal, and postnatal period
3. History of trauma and brain injury
4. *Neurological examination*—a baseline neurological examination should be completed on admission to the hospital and monitored on a routine basis. Basic areas of the neurological examination include the following.
   - Check patient level of consciousness (LOC)
   - Cranial nerve check
   - Check patient orientation to time, place, and person with questions to determine the presence of short-term and long-term memory
   - Check muscle strength, movement, and coordination as well as tendon reflexes
   - Check sensations to heat, cold, touch, and pain

Habilitation – process of improving the functional ability of a person with a disability

Orthotics – appliances used in the treatment or rehabilitation of neuromuscular illness or disorders

Mobility – the capability of movement or of being mobile

Gastrostomy – opening from the abdomen to the stomach for the purpose of feeding

5. Physical examination
6. Diagnostic procedures to rule out other causes of symptoms, e.g. *CT scan*; presence of infections; or neoplasm
7. Testing to determine physical, mental, and social functioning
8. Auditory and visual testing to determine hearing and vision loss
9. Social testing to determine coping strategies and abilities on the part of the patient and family

TREATMENT

Treatment is aimed at **habilitation**, helping the patient do as much as he can and as well as he can.

1. *Physical therapy*
2. *Occupational therapy*
3. *Speech therapy*
4. Vocational training
5. Adaptive equipment
6. **Orthotic** devices
7. Methods to aid in **mobility**

CONSIDERATIONS FOR CARE

1. Educate family regarding the disability.
2. Realize that there is a tremendous impact on a couple and family to learn that their child has cerebral palsy.
3. Encourage families to contact other families that also have children with cerebral palsy for support.
4. Encourage family to voice feelings and concerns.
5. Facilitate continuity of staff so family can get to know staff members better and feel more comfortable expressing feelings to them.
6. Encourage and assist parents in setting realistic goals for their child.
7. Encourage parents to include their other children in the care of the child and to make an effort to spend quality time with the other children specifically.
8. Make family aware of community resources for emotional support, educational support, or financial assistance as needed.
9. Help family realize that the child with cerebral palsy needs love and nurturing just as much as any other individual.
10. Make family aware of the importance of patience and understanding.
11. Help family to contact day-care providers and educational facilities.
12. Facilitate physical therapy, speech therapy, and occupational consults as needed.
13. Educate family regarding physical exercise program to do at home.
14. Educate family regarding care of the child during seizures as appropriate.
15. Educate family regarding need for appropriate nutrition and alternate ways of providing nutrition due to dysphagia, e.g. special methods of feeding, nasogastric tube (NG), or **gastrostomy** feeding.
16. Encourage the child to be as independent as possible in activities of daily living (ADLs).
17. Educate family regarding immunization schedule for their child. (See Table 28-1.)

Table 28-1   Child's Immunization Schedule

Child's Age	Immunization Needed
2 months	• **DTP** Immunization —**Diphtheria** —**Tetanus Toxoids** —**Pertussis Vaccine** • Oral Polio Vaccination
4 months	• **DTP** Immunization • Oral Polio Vaccination
6 months	• **DTP** Immunization
15 months	• **MMR** Immunization —**Measles** —**Mumps** —**Rubella Virus** • **DTP** Immunization • Oral Polio Vaccination
18 months	• **HbCV** Vaccination —**Haemophilus Influenza B** —**Polysaccharide Antigen**
4 to 6 years	• **DTP** Immunization • Oral Polio Vaccination

Source: The U.S. Public Health Service Centers for Disease Control
Note: The immunization schedule above is a recommended guide and should be applied based on medical and legal requirements for individual health needs.

FOR MORE INFORMATION

United Cerebral Palsy Association
#1112
1522 K Street
Washington, DC 20005
(800) 872-1827

National Easter Seal Society
70 East Lake Street
Chicago, IL 60601

American Academy of Cerebral Palsy and Developmental Medicine
Suite 118
1910 Byrd Avenue
Richmond, VA 23230

ASSIGNMENT SHEET: CEREBRAL PALSY

Short Answer

1. Write a brief definition for the terms listed throughout the chapter.

2. Write a brief definition for cerebral palsy.

3. Describe the incidence of cerebral palsy.

4. List the three (3) classifications of cerebral palsy.

5. Describe the four (4) causes (categories of causes) of cerebral palsy.

6. List sixteen (16) signs and symptoms of cerebral palsy.

7. List nine (9) methods used to aid in the diagnosis of cerebral palsy.

8. List seven (7) categories of treatment used for cerebral palsy.

9. Describe seventeen (17) considerations for caring for a patient with cerebral palsy.

10. Describe the specific methods of caring for a person during a seizure.

11. Describe the following procedures associated with the diagnosis of cerebral palsy.
    a. CT scan
    b. Neurological examination

KNOWLEDGE INTO ACTION

With a neurological examination, the presence of symptoms, as well as the history of the difficult labor and delivery the mother and infant have had, the physician determines a diagnosis of cerebral palsy. You have been asked to assist a social worker in working with the family regarding long-term care for the child and to help answer any questions the family may have. What will your response be for each of the following questions raised by the family? (The family has named their little girl Lauren.)

1. What are the chances that Lauren will be mentally retarded?
2. How can we determine if Lauren has any problems with her hearing?
3. Will Lauren have to have therapy?
4. Did we do something wrong during the pregnancy to have caused this to happen to Lauren?
5. What about our son? How do we explain this to him?
6. Won't our son be jealous of all the attention Lauren gets? How would it be best to handle that with him?
7. Lauren seems to have such a hard time sucking from her bottle. Is there any way we can make sure she is getting enough to eat?
8. Do we need to have Lauren get her shots when it's time?
9. The doctor talked about doing a CT scan on Lauren. What is that anyway?

Down Syndrome

OBJECTIVES

Upon completion of this chapter, the student should be able to:

■ Define the key terms listed throughout the chapter

■ State a specific definition for Down syndrome

■ Describe the incidence of Down syndrome and relate the incidence of Down syndrome to maternal age

■ Describe basic information regarding the chromosomal structure of cells

■ Describe the cause of Down syndrome as related to chromosomal abnormality

■ List risk factors associated with Down syndrome

■ List signs and symptoms associated with Down syndrome

■ List specific complications associated with Down syndrome

■ List specific methods used to aid in the diagnosis of Down syndrome

■ Identify specific methods for treatment of Down syndrome

■ Describe specific considerations for caring for a patient with Down syndrome

■ List specific areas of medical and physical problems associated with Down syndrome and associated care for these problems

KEY TERMS

Gene – hereditary unit that makes up DNA

INTRODUCTION

Down syndrome is a birth defect caused by a chromosomal abnormality that results in mental retardation and a variety of physical characteristics.

STATISTICS

One out of every fourteen births results in a child with a birth defect and is the leading cause of infant death in the United States. Down syndrome is the most common genetic birth defect, with 1 in 800 to 1,000 live births affected by the defect. Approximately 3,000 to 5,000 children are born annually in the United States with Down syndrome. As a woman gets older, her chances of having a child with Down syndrome increases dramatically. Approximately 80 to 85% of the children with Down syndrome are born to women under the age of 35. The probability of a child having Down syndrome versus age of the mother is described in Figure 29-1.

CHROMOSOME INFORMATION

Chromosomes are made up of **genes**, which determine the inherited characteristics we acquire. The cells of the body are normally made up of 46 chromosomes or 23 pairs. One of each of these pairs comes from each the mother and father. The chromosomes are numbered pairs from largest (pair #1) to smallest (#22). Pair #23 are the sex chromosomes. (See Figure 29-2.)

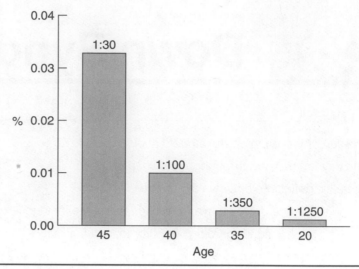

Figure 29-1 Down syndrome probability versus age of mother

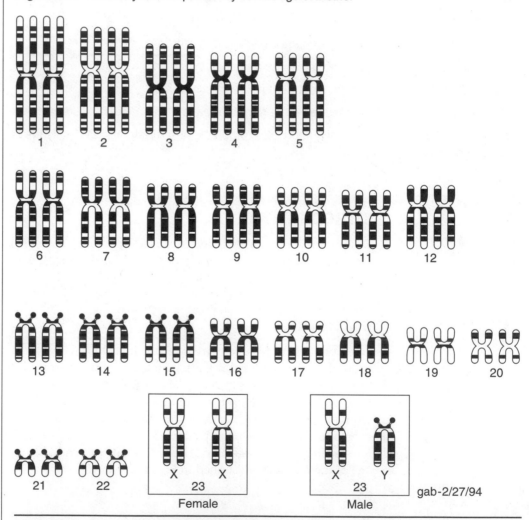

Figure 29-2 Karyotype of human chromosomes

There are several chromosomal possibilities that can cause Down syndrome. They are as follows. (See Figure 29-3.)

1. Trisomy 21, which results when there are three rather than two copies of chromosome #21; this results in 47 chromosomes rather than the normal 46; this type of Down syndrome is not inherited from the parents. Trisomy 21 accounts for approximately 95% of persons with Down syndrome.

Ovum – female reproductive cell or egg

Viruses – organisms that rely on other cells (hosts) for the nutrients necessary to sustain themselves

Paternal – refers to the father

Stature – height when in an upright position

Hypotonia – abnormal reduction in tone or strength of muscles

Brushfield spots – spots present on the iris of the eye, generally white, light gray, or yellow in color; often present in individuals with Down syndrome

Simian crease – crease present on the palm of the hand; a common symptom of Down syndrome

Umbilical hernia – herniation in the area of the umbilicus (navel or "belly button")

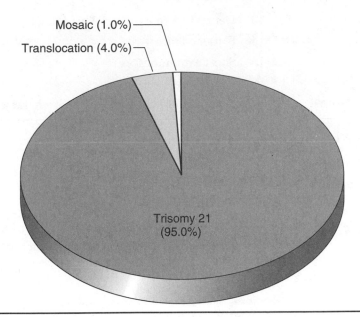

Figure 29-3   Down syndrome incidence by type

2. Translocation Down syndrome during which chromosome #21 attaches to another chromosome (usually #14, 21, or 22). This child will have the normal 46 chromosomes. This type of Down syndrome is inherited and accounts for approximately 4% of persons with Down syndrome.

3. Mosaic Down syndrome results when the child has both normal and abnormal chromosomes in cells and accounts for approximately 1% of persons with Down syndrome.

RISK FACTORS

1. Maternal age, due to the deterioration of the **ovum** due to age, although approximately 80 to 85% of children with Down syndrome are born to mothers under the age of 35

2. Effects of radiation, **viruses**, alcohol, or drugs

3. Increased **paternal** age, predominantly age 50 and older, increases the risk of Down syndrome

SIGNS AND SYMPTOMS

1. Mental retardation, mild to severe, with the mental developmental delay becoming more apparent as the child grows older

2. Oval-shaped eyes

3. Short **stature**

4. Small mouth

5. Large, protruding tongue

6. Small ears

7. Flattened nose with a wide bridge

8. **Hypotonia**

9. **Brushfield spots**

10. **Simian crease**, which is a single transverse crease on the palm of the hand

11. Short neck

12. **Umbilical hernia**

Clinodactyl – abnormal outward deviation of one or more fingers

Secondary sex characteristics – physical characteristics that develop at the time of puberty and were not present at birth; examples include development of breasts and pubic hair in females and development of facial hair and increased body hair in males

Brachycephalic – condition of a short head

Blepharitis – inflammation of the eyelid

Hyperextensible – more than normal extension of a joint, often causing injury

Hypotonic – decreased muscle tone

Leukemia – malignant disease characterized by uncontrolled growth of immature white blood cells

Hypothyroidism – decreased secretion of hormones by the thyroid gland

Karyotype – arrangement of the chromosomes according to order of size

Miscarriage – spontaneous expulsion of the fetus from the uterus prior to viability of the fetus

13. Dental problems, e.g. delayed development of teeth and malalignment
14. Flattened face
15. Short extremities
16. **Clinodactyl**
17. Underdeveloped **secondary sex characteristics**, e.g. genitalia, facial hair, and breasts
18. **Brachycephalic**
19. Thin hair
20. **Blepharitis**
21. Protruding abdomen
22. **Hyperextensible** joints
23. Tendency for skin to be dry and cracked
24. Broad, stubby hands and feet

COMPLICATIONS

Several complications that are frequently associated with Down syndrome are:

1. Congenital heart abnormalities occurring in approximately 40 to 45% of persons with Down syndrome with septal defects being the most common
2. Increased incidence of respiratory infections due to **hypotonic** chest and abdominal muscles
3. Decreased life expectancy with an average of approximately 50 years of age
4. Males with Down syndrome have been shown to be infertile
5. Females with Down syndrome have a 50% chance of having a child also with Down syndrome
6. Increased incidence of **leukemia** with a rate 15 to 20 times more common in persons with Down syndrome
7. Thyroid disorders occurring in 15 to 20% of all children with Down syndrome, e.g. **hypothyroidism**
8. Approximately 20 to 40% of children with Down syndrome do not survive the first few years of life
9. An average of 8 to 12% of children with Down syndrome have a congenital abnormality of the gastrointestinal tract
10. Approximately 60 to 80% of all people with Down syndrome have hearing deficits
11. An average of 3% of all people with Down syndrome have cataracts

DIAGNOSIS

1. Presence of physical characteristics
2. Genetic studies (**Karyotype**) at birth
3. *Amniocentesis* can detect presence of Down syndrome during the twelfth to sixteenth week of pregnancy. It takes approximately 2 to 4 weeks to obtain the results of this test.
4. *Chorionic villus sampling* can detect Down syndrome and other chromosomal disorders during the eighth to eleventh week of pregnancy. It takes an average of 1 to 3 weeks to obtain the results of this test. *This test can increase the risk of **miscarriage**.*

Cardiovascular – refers to the blood vessels of the heart

TREATMENT

Although there is no cure for Down syndrome, there are many things that can be done to promote the highest achievements for the person with Down syndrome.

1. **Cardiovascular** surgery to correct congenital heart defects
2. Plastic surgery to correct physical characteristics, e.g. protruding tongue often will be corrected due to impact on speech, eating, appearance, and dental problems

CONSIDERATIONS FOR CARE

1. Educate family regarding the defect.
2. Realize that there is a tremendous impact on a couple and family to learn that their new baby has Down syndrome.
3. Encourage families to contact other families that also have children with Down syndrome for support.
4. Encourage family to voice feelings and concerns.
5. Facilitate continuity of staff so family can get to know staff members better and feel more comfortable expressing feelings to them.
6. Encourage and assist parents in setting realistic goals for their child.
7. Encourage parents to include their other children in the care of the child and to make an effort to spend quality time with the other children specifically.
8. Make family aware of community resources for emotional support, educational support, or financial assistance as needed.
9. Make family aware of genetic counseling due to the increased risk of having another child with Down syndrome.
10. Help family realize that the child with Down syndrome needs love and nurturing just as much as any other individual.
11. Make family aware that the child with Down syndrome often learns best by imitation and will need frequent repetition and reinforcement.
12. Make family aware of the need to develop patience and understanding.
13. Most children with Down syndrome are very loving and affectionate.
14. Children with Down syndrome generally have a higher level of social development than that of their mental development.
15. Stress importance of providing a safe environment for the child as they are often very trusting, even of situations and persons that are not safe.
16. Due to decreased muscle tone, the child may have difficulty swallowing and will need to sit up to eat.
17. Medical staff need to examine their own feelings towards the child and treat them with dignity and respect.

METHODS OF ASSISTANCE DUE TO MENTAL AND PHYSICAL PROBLEMS ASSOCIATED WITH DOWN SYNDROME

1. Respiratory problems associated with (a) hypotonic chest and abdominal muscles and (b) mouth breathing due to flattened bridge of nose
    - Sit child up to feed to avoid aspiration
    - Provide small, frequent feeding as the child tires quickly due to mouth breathing

- Educate family regarding symptoms of a respiratory infection, e.g. cough, sputum, fever, chest pain, dyspnea, and diaphoresis
- Educate parents regarding postural drainage and chest percussion
- Provide humidified air for the child to breathe
- Suction the child as needed
- Change child's position frequently
- Provide meticulous mouth care

2. Difficulty obtaining adequate nutrition due to (a) protruding tongue, (b) mouth breathing due to flattened bridge of nose, (c) hypotonicity of muscles of mouth and gastrointestinal tract, and (d) difficulty controlling mucous

- Suction the nose and mouth prior to feeding
- Sit the child in an upright position to eat
- Offer small frequent feeding to reduce the fatigue from eating at one time
- Weigh child on routine basis to ensure appropriate growth and nutrition
- Use small spoon with a long, straight handle
- Utilize suction equipment as needed
- Instruct family members regarding Heimlich maneuver in the event of choking
- Allow ample time for the child to eat

3. Skin dryness and cracking due to the fact that people with Down syndrome tend to age more rapidly

- Encourage oral fluids
- Avoid harsh soaps for bathing
- Avoid bleach and irritating detergents in laundering
- Apply creams and moisturizing lotions to skin
- Apply lip balm for the treatment and prevention of cracked, dry lips
- Administer sunscreen to prevent sunburn
- Educate parents to monitor for skin irritation and infection, e.g. redness, rash, drainage, warm or hot to touch, red streaks going up the extremity, fever, pain, and decreased function

4. Slow or decreased mental and physical ability due to (a) mental retardation, (b) hypotonicity of muscles and joints, and (c) decreased nutritional status

- Educate parents/caregiver regarding methods to stimulate the child mentally and physically
- Facilitate physical therapy consult to assist the parents/caregiver with an exercise program appropriate for the child
- Facilitate occupational therapy consult to assist the parents/caregiver in setting up methods of assisting the child in self-care skills and activities of daily living (ADLs)
- Provide awareness of self-help items available for the child
- Provide awareness of community resources available for the child/family
- Facilitate social worker consult to make family/caregiver aware of community resources, financial resources, and support groups
- Assist the parents/caregiver in locating day-care if needed
- Assist parents/caregiver in exploring options in the public school system and make them aware of laws that govern education for children with handicaps. These laws state that every child is entitled to an education appropriate for him or her in the least restrictive environment.

- Encourage the parents/caregiver to set realistic goals for the child
- Encourage the family to locate a responsible person to stay with the child on occasion for the family to take a break from the responsibility of child-rearing
- Encourage frequent positive reinforcement for the child

FOR MORE INFORMATION

March of Dimes Birth Defects Foundation
1275 Mamaroneck Avenue
White Plains, NY 10605

National Down Syndrome Congress
Suite 250
1605 Chantilly Drive
Atlanta, GA 30324

National Down Syndrome Society
146 East 57th Street
New York, NY 10022

ASSIGNMENT SHEET: DOWN SYNDROME

Short Answer

1. Write a brief definition for the terms listed throughout the chapter.

2. Write a brief definition for Down syndrome.

3. Describe the incidence of Down syndrome and relate the incidence with maternal age.

4. Describe the normal relationship of genes, chromosomes, and cells of the human body.

5. Describe the three (3) causes of Down syndrome as related to chromosomal abnormalities.

6. Describe the three (3) groups of risk factors for Down syndrome.

7. List twenty-four (24) physical characteristics associated with Down syndrome.

8. Describe why mental developmental delays would become more apparent as the child grows older.

9. List four (4) specific methods used in the diagnosis of Down syndrome.

10. List two (2) specific methods used in the treatment of Down syndrome.

11. List seventeen (17) specific considerations for caring for a patient with Down syndrome.

12. Describe four (4) specific groups of medical and physical problems associated with Down syndrome, the rationale, and associated care for each of the groups.

13. Describe eleven (11) complications often associated with Down syndrome.

14. Describe each of the following procedures used in the diagnosis or treatment of Down syndrome.

    a. Amniocentesis
    b. Chorionic villus sampling
    c. Chest percussion
    d. Postural drainage

KNOWLEDGE INTO ACTION

1. One of the parents in a group you are giving a presentation on Down syndrome to has asked you if it would have been possible to know that their child had Down syndrome prior to being born. What will your response be? (Write a brief description for two [2] tests that could be done to detect Down syndrome in a child prior to birth.)

2. After you have described the above two tests, the same member of the group says she wishes she would have known that her child had Down syndrome prior to its birth as she would have had an abortion to end the pregnancy. She asks for your opinion on having an abortion to end a pregnancy if the child has Down syndrome. What will your response be?

3. To wrap up your session with these parents, you want to give them some helpful hints or considerations for care regarding methods of assistance due to the mental and physical problems often associated with Down syndrome. For each of the problems, list the rationale for the problem as well as five (5) methods of associated care.

    a. Respiratory problems
    b. Difficulty obtaining adequate nutrition
    c. Skin dryness and cracking
    d. Slow or decreased mental and physical ability

UNIT 8

GASTROINTESTINAL AND DIGESTIVE DISORDERS

Cirrhosis

OBJECTIVES

Upon completion of this chapter, the student should be able to:

■ Define the key terms listed throughout the chapter

■ State a specific definition for cirrhosis

■ Describe the physiology of the liver

■ Describe the incidence of cirrhosis

■ List the classifications of cirrhosis and the cause of each

■ List the signs and symptoms associated with cirrhosis and associated care for these symptoms

■ Identify specific methods for diagnosis of cirrhosis

■ Identify specific methods for treatment of cirrhosis

■ Identify complications associated with cirrhosis and symptoms of each

■ Describe specific considerations for caring for a patient with cirrhosis

KEY TERMS

Portal – refers to the vessel that carries blood to and through the liver

Spleen – organ located in the upper left quadrant of the abdomen that is necessary for the filtering, storage, and formation of blood and blood cells

Exocrine – gland that secretes directly to the surface of the skin or through ducts to the outside of the gland

Hepatic – refers to the liver

Bile – substance manufactured and secreted by the liver and stored in the gallbladder; the function of bile is to aid the body in digestion of fats

Gallbladder – organ located directly below the liver; function is to store and concentrate bile, which is manufactured by the liver

INTRODUCTION

Cirrhosis of the liver is a chronic disease with an insidious onset where the liver cells are destroyed and replaced with scar tissue. When the liver cells are destroyed, **portal** circulation is impaired, which causes blood to accumulate in the **spleen** and gastrointestinal tract.

PHYSIOLOGY OF THE LIVER

The liver is an **exocrine** gland located in the upper right quadrant of the abdomen. (See Figure 30-1.) The **hepatic** ducts drain **bile** out of the liver. The common hepatic duct leaving the liver and the cystic duct leaving the **gallbladder** join together to form the common bile duct. The common bile duct drains bile into the portion of the small intestine known as the **duodenum**. The three divisions of the small intestine are the duodenum, **jejunum**, and ileum. When a person eats foods that contain fat, they trigger the body to secrete a hormone called **cholecystokinin (CCK)** from the mucous membrane of the duodenum. The CCK stimulates the gallbladder to contract, which releases bile into the duodenum to begin the breakdown of the fat. (See Figure 30-2.)

The function of the gallbladder is to store and concentrate the bile that is produced by the liver. The function of the bile is to emulsify fats.

Other functions of the liver include:

1. Maintain normal *blood glucose* levels by storing sugar in the form of **glycogen** and releasing as necessary.

2. Production of *prothrombin* and *fibrinogen*, both plasma **proteins**, which are necessary for blood clotting.

3. Production of *albumin* (plasma protein), which is necessary for the maintenance of blood volume.

Duodenum – the first portion of the small intestine; approximately 10 to 12 inches in length

Jejunum – the middle portion of the small intestine; the small intestine is divided into three parts: the duodenum, jejunum, and ileum; the jejunum is approximately 8 feet in length

Cholecystokinin (CCK) – hormone secreted by the small intestine that stimulates contraction of the gallbladder, then releases enzymes secreted by the pancreas

Glucose – sugar manufactured in the body by the metabolism of carbohydrates; primary energy source for the body's cells

Glycogen – stored in the body and can be converted into glucose within the body during periods of hypoglycemia; glycogen is formed initially from carbohydrates

Prothrombin – part of the clotting factor that is converted to thrombin through interaction with thrombokinase

Fibrinogen – protein in the blood that is necessary for clotting

Protein – substance found in meats, vegetables, and dairy products; necessary for growth, energy, and muscle strength

Urea – presence of by-products of protein metabolism (carbonic acid) in the urine, blood, or lymph; carbonic acid is one of the main substances that make up urine

Bilirubin – product of hemoglobin breakdown; excreted by the liver; approximately 260 milligrams of bilirubin is produced daily, with the majority excreted through fecal material and the remainder (1%) excreted in urine

Detoxification – destruction, removal, or reduction of toxic substances

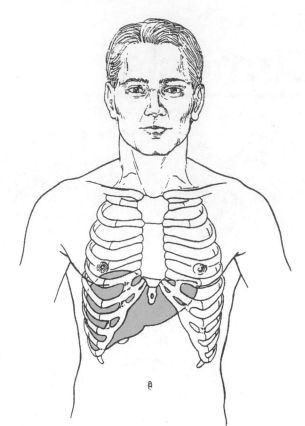

Figure 30-1   Location of the liver (From Kinn, *Medical Terminology: Building Blocks for Health Careers,* copyright © 1990, Delmar Publishers)

4. Storage of iron, Vitamin A, Vitamin B_{12}, and Vitamin D.

5. Breakdown of **urea**, which is transported to the kidneys for elimination from the body. Urea is a by-product of protein metabolism.

6. Breakdown of red blood cells releasing a substance called *bilirubin,* which gives stools their dark color.

7. **Detoxification** of alcohol and other toxic substances (e.g. drugs) in the blood.

STATISTICS

Cirrhosis is more common in men than women. The most common cause of cirrhosis is due to alcoholism. Approximately 80 to 90% of alcoholics will have a degree of cirrhosis. There is a mortality rate associated with cirrhosis, with cirrhosis being the ninth leading cause of death in the United States. (See Table 30-1.)

Table 30-1 Classifications of Cirrhosis		
Classification	**Percent**	**Cause**
Laennec's	30–50	Alcoholism and malnutrition
Postnecrotic	10–30	*Hepatitis*
Biliary	15–20	Bile duct disease
Pigment	5–10	*Hemochromatosis*
Idiopathic	5–10	Unknown
Cardiac	Rare	Right heart failure

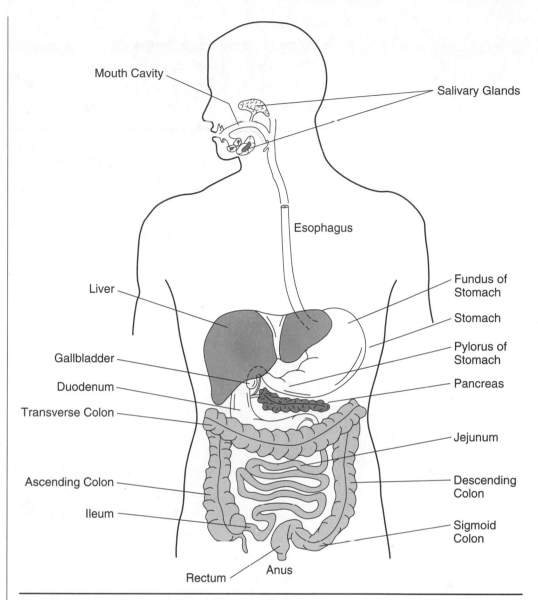

Mouth Cavity

Salivary Glands

Esophagus

Liver

Fundus of
Stomach

Stomach

Pylorus of
Stomach

Gallbladder

Duodenum

Pancreas

Transverse Colon

Jejunum

Ascending Colon

Descending
Colon

Ileum

Sigmoid
Colon

Rectum   Anus

Figure 30-2   Location of the abdominal organs (From Townsend, *Nutrition and Diet Therapy,
6th edition,* copyright © 1994, Delmar Publishers)

SIGNS, SYMPTOMS, AND ASSOCIATED CARE

1. Fatigue
    *   Assist patient with activities of daily living (ADLs) as necessary
    *   Schedule care, activities, and treatment around patient's rest schedule
    *   Monitor phone calls and visitors around patient's energy level and rest schedule
    *   Encourage frequent rest periods
    *   Provide assistance as needed to prevent injury due to weakness
    *   Provide method for patient to call for assistance
    *   Encourage patient to set realistic goals of activities
    *   Allow adequate time to do activities and procedures to avoid frustration or possible injury
    *   Encourage exercise to maintain muscle strength
    *   Provide cane or walker for ambulation and transfer
    *   Provide private room to promote rest periods

2. Anorexia
   - Obtain baseline weight and monitor on routine basis
   - Offer small, frequent meals as tolerated
   - Encourage patient to participate in dietary choices
   - Serve nutritional supplements and vitamins
   - Monitor for signs of dehydration, such as decreased urine output, concentrated urine, dry skin, tenting of skin, dry mucous membranes, dry mouth, dry eyes, confusion, hypotension, and constipation
   - Encourage family and friends to bring in food that is appealing to patient as dietary restrictions allow
   - Administer parenteral fluids as necessary
   - Monitor intake and output (I and O)
   - Encourage fluids to prevent dehydration
   - Avoid unpleasant sights and odors in room to make meals more appealing
   - Provide meticulous mouth care
   - Maintain social atmosphere for mealtimes to encourage the patient to eat
   - Encourage clothing that enhances patient appearance
   - Encourage exercise program as tolerated to increase appetite

3. Nausea and vomiting
   - Administer antiemetics before meals as prescribed by physician
   - Offer food choices according to patient preference
   - Control odors and unpleasant sights in room
   - Offer fluids frequently to prevent dehydration
   - Monitor intake and output to avoid dehydration
   - Monitor serum electrolytes (*sodium*, *potassium*, and *chloride*)
   - Encourage rest periods after meals
   - Avoid foods that are spicy, rich, or previously disagreeable to patient
   - Provide receptacle for patient to vomit into as needed; this should be cleaned whenever used and changed on a frequent basis
   - Provide meticulous mouth care
   - Prevent aspiration of emesis
   - Utilize universal precautions at all times when coming in contact with blood or body fluids (See Appendix C)
   - Avoid greasy foods as they tend to stay in the stomach a long period of time
   - Avoid cooking food if possible due to increased nausea with odors of foods
   - Avoid hot foods as necessary due to the increased odors of hot foods
   - Eat in well-ventilated area to decrease the accumulation of odors of foods while eating

4. Constipation
   - Encourage fluids
   - Encourage high-fiber diet. Foods that are high in fiber include fruits, vegetables, whole grains, prunes, and beans.
   - Increase exercise as tolerated
   - Administer enemas, suppositories, stool softeners, and laxatives as prescribed by physician
   - Monitor frequency, number, and consistency of stools

Rectal – refers to the rectum (distal 5 inches of the large intestine)

- Monitor for possible bowel obstruction. Avoid use of laxatives, enemas, or suppositories if bowel obstruction is suspected.
- Establish regular bowel routine
- Provide privacy for bowel routine

5. Diarrhea
   - Monitor number, amount, and consistency of stools
   - Monitor intake and output to avoid dehydration
   - Monitor serum electrolytes
   - Provide meticulous skin care, especially if incontinent
   - Monitor for presence of hemorrhoids
   - Monitor for rectal discomfort and offer Sitz baths, warm soaks, and topical ointments or suppositories
   - Administer antidiarrheal medications as prescribed by physician
   - Provide frequent skin care, especially to anal area to prevent skin breakdown
   - Monitor for presence of blood (*Hemoccult*®)
   - Offer reassurance to patient
   - Avoid foods that are too hot or too cold as they increase peristalsis

6. Bleeding tendencies
   - Observe for signs of abnormal bleeding and educate patient/family to observe and report any signs promptly to physician, e.g. hemoptysis, bloody emesis, bloody or tarry stools, nose bleeds, vaginal bleeding between menstrual cycles or postmenopausal, bleeding gums, or hematuria
   - Observe for signs of central nervous system (CNS) bleeding and educate patient/family to observe and report symptoms promptly to physician, e.g. altered level of consciousness, headache, vision changes, and vertigo
   - Prevent injury to patient who has thrombocytopenia, e.g. soft toothbrush, electric razor rather than straight-edge razor, wear seat belts in the car, elevated siderails, avoid straining with bowel movements, avoid vigorous nose-blowing, avoid intramuscular injections, avoid **rectal** temperatures, avoid use of tampons, and seek physician advice prior to vaginal or anal intercourse
   - Avoid products that contain aspirin, which alter normal platelet function
   - Monitor *platelet* count
   - Monitor *hemoglobin* and *hematocrit*
   - Apply pressure at sites of injection or blood drawing sites for minimum of 5 minutes or until bleeding stops

7. Weight loss
   - Obtain baseline weight and monitor weight on routine basis
   - Encourage patient to participate in dietary choices
   - Provide nutritional supplements and vitamins
   - Encourage family and friends to bring in food that is appealing to patient as dietary restrictions allow
   - Administer parenteral fluids as necessary
   - Monitor intake and output (I and O)
   - Encourage rest periods before and after meals
   - Avoid unpleasant sights and odors in room to make meals more appealing
   - Provide meticulous mouth care

- Monitor for skin breakdown due to loss of body tissue
- Encourage clothing styles that do not draw attention to weight loss
- Monitor for symptoms of dehydration, e.g. decreased urine output, constipation, dry skin, tenting of skin, dry mouth, dry eyes, concentrated urine, hypotension, and confusion

8. Hepatomegaly

- Monitor for hepatomegaly
- Avoid abdominal injury in the presence of hepatomegaly
- Monitor for signs of internal bleeding in the presence of hepatomegaly, such as abdominal pain, tachycardia, hypotension, and abdominal distention
- Monitor liver function with serum laboratory tests, e.g. *SGOT*, *SGPT*, *bilirubin*, *albumin*, *alkaline phosphatase*, and *prothrombin time*
- Monitor for bleeding tendencies in the presence of hepatomegaly
- Educate to avoid the use of alcohol and medications metabolized in the liver
- Monitor for jaundice

9. Pleural effusion

- Administer oxygen as needed
- Assist with position for patient comfort
- Employ sodium restriction. Foods high in sodium that should be avoided include processed foods, cured meats, salted chips and crackers, pickles, and table salt.
- Monitor for symptoms of hypoxia, e.g. cyanosis, decreased level of consciousness, confusion, and diaphoresis
- Run fan in room to circulate air to assist with dyspnea
- Drain fluid from abdomen to assist with breathing (paracentesis)

10. Mental changes

- Monitor for changes in mental status
- Protect patient from injury in the presence of decreased mental status
- Assist patient with ADLs as needed in the presence of decreased mental status
- Monitor for level of orientation
- Offer emotional support to patient and family in the event of confusion
- Provide calm, quiet environment for patient
- Avoid startling patient
- Allow family members or friends to stay with patient as much as needed if this is reassuring to patient

11. Anemia

- Administer blood transfusion and iron supplements as necessary for the treatment of anemia
- Monitor *hemoglobin* and *hematocrit*
- Monitor for weakness associated with anemia, assist with ADLs as necessary due to weakness, and protect from possible injury due to weakness
- Monitor physical symptoms of anemia, such as pallor, weakness, and vertigo

Esophageal varices –
dilation of the vessels of
the esophagus; may result
in inflammation and
bleeding; condition often
associated with cirrhosis
of the liver

Paracentesis – removal
of fluid from a cavity
through a surgically made
puncture site

Gynecomastia –
enlarged breasts in the
male

Spider angiomata – burst
capillaries located on the
skin; frequently seen in
patients with cirrhosis and
other forms of liver disease

12. **Esophageal varices**
    - Provide meticulous mouth care at frequent intervals through day
    - Offer food and beverages that are nonabrasive. Avoid spicy foods, acidic fruits and juices, carbonated beverages, highly salted foods, and foods that are extremely hot or cold.
    - Offer ice chips and fluids according to patient preference
    - Provide humidifier at bedside to humidify air
    - Monitor intake and output (I and O)
    - Administer nasogastric (NG) or parenteral fluids as necessary
    - Administer medications as prescribed by physician to treat any accompanying infection
    - Offer foods that are easy to chew and swallow
    - Monitor any emesis or bowel movements for the presence of blood
    - Monitor hemoglobin and hematocrit for the presence of anemia

13. Ascites—due to decreased albumin, lymph system involvement, and portal hypertension
    - Assist with position for patient comfort
    - Measure abdominal girth on routine basis, with area marked so same area measured each time for accuracy
    - Avoid constrictive clothing and undergarments
    - Assist with *paracentesis* as needed
    - Monitor abdominal distention

14. **Gynecomastia**
    - Encourage clothing to conceal enlargement of breasts
    - Offer emotional support to patient

15. Edema
    - Avoid constrictive clothing or undergarments
    - Restrict salt in diet as prescribed by physician
    - Apply elastic stockings (TED hose) or Jobst stockings to reduce swelling
    - Monitor edema on routine basis
    - Encourage patient to elevate edematous extremity above the level of the heart to reduce swelling
    - Monitor for symptoms of decreased circulation and skin breakdown in edematous areas, e.g. skin cool to touch, cyanosis, and decreased sensation
    - Obtain baseline weight and monitor on routine basis
    - Monitor intake and output (I and O)

16. **Spider angiomata**
    - Encourage clothing to assist in concealing vessels
    - Offer emotional support to patient

17. Jaundice
    - Monitor skin color
    - Monitor serum liver function tests
    - Provide low-fat diet. Items that are high in saturated fats and cholesterol and should be avoided or eaten in moderate amounts include egg yolks, butter, cheese, and red meats.

18. Right upper quadrant abdominal pain
    - Assist with position for patient comfort

- Monitor for pain and offer comfort measures as necessary
- Avoid constrictive garments and undergarments
- Offer methods to promote comfort, such as relaxation techniques, imaging, massage, and warm baths
- Administer medications as necessary and as prescribed by physician for the control of pain
- Encourage patient to request pain relief methods before pain becomes too severe

19. Amenorrhea
   - Monitor for amenorrhea
   - Monitor for frequency and duration of menstruation and monitor amount of vaginal flow

20. Testicular atrophy
   - Monitor for testicular atrophy
   - Offer emotional support
   - Facilitate counseling as necessary for patient and spouse or significant other due to changes in sexual function
   - Facilitate counseling as necessary for patients of child-bearing age due to the possibility of placing sperm in a sperm bank for future use

21. Impotence
   - Offer emotional support to patient
   - Facilitate sexual counselor or family counselor consult as needed

22. Pruritus
   - Provide meticulous skin care with mild, unscented soap
   - Avoid use of tapes and other adhesives on skin as able
   - Administer medications or creams to prevent itching
   - Utilize protective mittens for confused patient to prevent scratching and damage to skin
   - Encourage fluid intake
   - Pat skin gently dry
   - Avoid harsh soaps or bleach in clothing and linens
   - Avoid clothing and bedding that is irritating
   - Assess skin redness and irritation on routine basis
   - Observe for open areas and signs of infection
   - Avoid use of scented lotions and cosmetics
   - Administer antihistamines as necessary to relieve itching

DIAGNOSIS

1. Signs and symptoms
2. History
3. Physical examination
4. *Liver biopsy* used to detect liver tissue destruction and scar tissue formation
5. *CT scan* used to determine the extent of hepatomegaly
6. *Cholecystography* to determine gallbladder function
7. *Esophagoscopy* to determine presence of esophageal varices

Hyponatremia –
decreased amounts of
sodium in the blood

8. Laboratory tests to include:
   - *SGOT* (elevated)
   - *Alkaline phosphatase*
   - Bilirubin (elevated)
   - *SGPT* (elevated)
   - Serum vitamin levels (decreased levels of *Vitamins A, C,* and *K*)
   - *Albumin* (decreased)
   - *Prothrombin time* (prolonged)
   - *Hemoglobin* and *hematocrit*
   - Electrolytes (*sodium, potassium,* and *chloride*)
9. *Paracentesis* may also be used to reduce ascites
10. Presence of serum *hepatitis B surface antigen*

TREATMENT

1. Removal of causative factor, especially in cases of alcoholism and drug usage
2. Restricted sodium diet to 500 mg daily
3. Rest
4. Diuretics
5. Restricted fluid intake
6. Paracentesis
7. Antiemetics

COMPLICATIONS

1. Esophageal varices may cause hematemesis, bloody bowel movements, chest pain, pain with swallowing, and anemia
2. Bleeding tendencies, e.g. hemoptysis, bloody emesis, bloody or black tarry stools, nose bleeds, vaginal bleeding between menstrual cycles or post-menopausal, bleeding gums, bruising, or hematuria
3. **Hyponatremia** may cause convulsions, muscle spasms and twitching, increased tendon reflexes, or absence of urination

CONSIDERATIONS FOR CARE

1. Educate patient and family regarding the disease process.
2. Educate patient and family regarding forms of treatment as well as side effects of medications.
3. Provide emotional support for the patient and family.
4. Monitor for symptoms of complications.
5. Monitor intake and output (I and O).
6. Obtain baseline weight and monitor weight on a routine basis.
7. Measure abdominal girth routinely, with the area marked in such a way that the same area is measured.
8. Monitor level of comfort and offer comfort measures: relaxation techniques, positioning, massage, imaging, and medications as prescribed by physician.
9. Use universal precautions at all times (See Appendix C).

10. Obtain baseline vital signs (See Appendix D) and monitor on a routine basis during hospital stay.

11. Educate patient regarding the need to avoid all alcohol intake.

12. Educate patient to avoid medications that are metabolized by the liver.

13. Educate patient to avoid aspirin products, which alter normal platelet function.

14. Show nonjudgmental acceptance of emotions and behavior of patient and family.

15. Educate regarding proper nutrition.

16. Observe for signs of abnormal bleeding and educate patient/family to observe and report and signs promptly to physician, e.g. hemoptysis, bloody emesis, bloody or black tarry stools, nose bleeds, vaginal bleeding between menstrual cycles or postmenopausal, bleeding gums, bruising, and hematuria.

17. Observe for signs of CNS bleeding and educate patient/family to observe and report symptoms promptly to physician, e.g. altered level of consciousness, headache, vision changes, and vertigo.

18. Prevent injury to patient with cirrhosis due to increased incidence of bleeding, e.g. soft toothbrush, electric razor rather than straight-edge razor, wear seat belts in car, elevated siderails, avoid straining with bowel movements, avoid vigorous nose-blowing, avoid intra-muscular injections, and avoid rectal temperatures.

19. Encourage frequent rest periods as needed by patient.

20. Encourage patient to be as active as possible.

21. Assist with ADLs as needed.

22. Make patient and family aware of community resources and financial resources.

23. Assess the need for referral to Alcoholic's Anonymous or similar agency.

24. Monitor laboratory results for abnormal levels and report abnormalities to the physician.

25. Meticulous mouth care on routine basis.

FOR MORE INFORMATION

American Liver Foundation
998 Pompton Avenue
Cedar Grove, NJ 07009

ASSIGNMENT SHEET: CIRRHOSIS

Short Answer

1. Write a brief definition for the terms listed throughout the chapter.

2. Describe the physiology of the liver.

3. Describe the seven (7) main functions of the liver.

4. Write a brief definition for cirrhosis.

5. Describe the incidence of cirrhosis.

6. List the six (6) classifications of cirrhosis, and describe the cause of each classification.

7. List twenty-two (22) signs and symptoms associated with cirrhosis and associated care for these symptoms.

8. List and describe ten (10) methods used to aid in the diagnosis of cirrhosis.

9. List seven (7) specific methods used to treat cirrhosis.

10. List three (3) specific complications associated with cirrhosis and the symptoms of each.

11. List twenty-five (25) considerations for caring for a patient with cirrhosis.

12. Describe the importance of each of the following, and describe foods that are an important source of each.

    a. Iron
    b. Vitamin A
    c. Vitamin B_{12}
    d. Vitamin D
    e. Fiber

13. Describe each of the following procedures used in the diagnosis or treatment of cirrhosis.

    a. Paracentesis
    b. Liver biopsy
    c. CT scan
    d. Cholecystography
    e. Esophagoscopy

14. Describe what is meant by universal precautions, and describe the importance of it as associated with cirrhosis. (See Appendix C.)

15. List the normal ranges for each of the serum laboratory values.

    a. Sodium
    b. Potassium
    c. Chloride
    d. SGOT
    e. Alkaline phosphatase
    f. Bilirubin
    g. SGPT
    h. Vitamin levels
       • Vitamin A
       • Vitamin C
       • Vitamin K
    i. Hemoglobin
    j. Hematocrit
    k. Albumin
    l. Prothrombin time

KNOWLEDGE INTO ACTION

1. Raymond Larson, a 66-year-old, has been admitted to your facility with a diagnosis of cirrhosis of the liver. One of the admitting symptoms is thrombocytopenia. Describe what laboratory test could be done to diagnose and monitor thrombocytopenia, possible symptoms of thrombocytopenia, and methods to prevent injury to your patient who has thrombocytopenia.

2. Mr. Larson's physician has ordered the following items. Describe what each of the items means in relation to Mr. Larson's care and how each of the items would be carried out.

    a. Assist with ADLs
    b. Monitor I and O
    c. Utilize universal precautions
    d. Measure abdominal girth daily
    e. Low-sodium diet
    f. High-fiber diet
    g. Monitor for changes in mental status
    h. Low-fat diet

3. Mr. Larson's physician has ordered the following diagnostic tests to be done. Write a brief summary regarding your explanation to Mr. Larson for each of the ordered tests.

   a. Liver biopsy
   b. CT scan
   c. Cholecystography
   d. Esophagoscopy
   e. Paracentesis

4. Prior to Mr. Larson's discharge, he says to you, "My doctor told me not to have any alcoholic beverages. Why would he tell me to do that? I only drink at social occasions." What will your response be?

5. Mr. Larson's physician is concerned that Mr. Larson may develop the following complications associated with cirrhosis. Describe what symptoms he would want Mr. Larson to monitor for at home that could indicate the presence of esophageal varices and hyponatremia.

6. During Mr. Larson's hospital stay, you have been monitoring his vital signs. Circle the vital signs in each of the following lists that are in the normal range.

Blood pressures:
- 110/72
- 168/98
- 98/52
- 142/86

Temperatures:
- 98.6 orally
- 99.8 orally
- 99.0 rectally
- 99.6 axillary

Pulses:
- 72 per minute
- 98 per minute
- 66 per minute
- 54 per minute

Respirations:
- 16 per minute
- 22 per minute
- 12 per minute
- 34 per minute

OBJECTIVES

Upon completion of this chapter, the student should be able to:

- Define the key terms listed throughout the chapter
- Describe the physiology and function of the liver
- State a specific definition for hepatitis
- List additional names for the specific types of hepatitis
- Describe the route of transmission for the specific types of hepatitis
- Describe the vaccines available to aid in the prevention of hepatitis
- Describe the treatment for the specific types of hepatitis
- Describe the nonmedication forms of treatment for hepatitis
- Describe the incubation period for the specific types of hepatitis
- Identify methods to diagnose the specific types of hepatitis
- Identify additional tests performed during the diagnostic period for hepatitis
- Describe the prognosis associated with the specific types of hepatitis
- Describe the incidence of the specific types of hepatitis
- List the signs and symptoms associated with hepatitis and associated care for each of these symptoms
- Identify complications associated with hepatitis
- Describe methods of prevention for the specific types of hepatitis
- Describe specific considerations for caring for a patient with hepatitis

KEY TERMS

Cystic duct – gallbladder duct

Emulsify – breakdown of fats in the digestive system

INTRODUCTION

Hepatitis is an acute or chronic inflammation of the liver caused by either a virus or a nonviral cause, such as chemicals, drugs, or alcohol. There are five types of viral hepatitis categorized into the classifications of A, B, C, D, and E.

PHYSIOLOGY OF THE LIVER

The liver is an exocrine gland located in the upper right quadrant of the abdomen. (See Figure 30-1.) The hepatic ducts drain bile out of the liver. The common hepatic duct leaving the liver and the **cystic duct** leaving the gallbladder join together to form the common bile duct. The common bile duct drains bile into the portion of the small intestine known as the duodenum. The three divisions of the small intestine are the duodenum, jejunum, and ileum. When a person eats foods that contain fat, they trigger the body to secrete a hormone called cholecystokinin (CCK) from the mucous membrane of the duodenum. The CCK stimulates the gallbladder to contract, which releases bile into the duodenum to begin the breakdown of the fat. (See Figure 30-2.)

The function of the gallbladder is to store and concentrate the bile, which is produced by the liver. The function of bile is to **emulsify** fats.

Iron – mineral found in meats, legumes, and fortified grains that is necessary for the production of hemoglobin; hemoglobin is the protein portion of the red blood cell that transports oxygen

Vitamin A – vitamin present in green leafy vegetables, carrots, dairy products, and fish that is necessary for healthy gums, hair, nails, teeth, and function of the eyes

Vitamin B$_{12}$ – vitamin present in meats, eggs, and shellfish that is necessary for the function of the nervous system

Vitamin D – vitamin present in fortified dairy products, fish, and egg yolks that is necessary for the body's absorption of calcium

Infectious – ability to transmit a disease

Incubation – the length of time it takes from exposure to a disease to develop the symptoms of the disease

Symptomatic – presence of symptoms

Fulminant hepatitis – sudden onset of symptoms with hepatitis that usually results in death

Inanimate – refers to an object that is not alive

Immunity – the body's resistance to a disease or injury from a pathogen; most frequently refers to contagious diseases

Other functions of the liver include:

1. Maintain normal blood glucose levels by storing sugar in the form of glycogen and releasing as necessary.

2. Production of *prothrombin* and fibrinogen (both plasma proteins), which are necessary for blood clotting.

3. Production of *albumin* (plasma protein), which is necessary for the maintenance of blood volume.

4. Storage of *iron, Vitamin A, Vitamin B$_{12}$,* and *Vitamin D.*

5. Breakdown of urea that is transported to the kidneys for elimination from the body. Urea is a by-product of protein metabolism.

6. Breakdown of red blood cells, releasing a substance called *bilirubin,* which gives stools their dark color.

7. Detoxification of alcohol and other toxic substances (e.g. drugs) in the blood.

TYPE A HEPATITIS

- Additional names: **Infectious** hepatitis and short **incubation** hepatitis

- Route of transmission: Contaminated food or water (fecal-oral route); Hepatitis A has also been reported to have been transmitted through sexual contact and blood transfusion

- Vaccinations available: None

- Treatment: **Symptomatic**

- Incubation period: 3 to 7 weeks

- Diagnosis: Anti-HAV IgM determines presence of antibody during acute phase of the disease

- Prognosis: Immunity after infection; non-carrier; **fulminant hepatitis** may develop in 1% of patients; generally patients have a full recovery

- Incidence: Approximately 50% of Americans develop the disease in their lifetime

- Prevention: Immune globulin given within one week after exposure affords prevention in 80 to 90% who receive the immune globulin

TYPE B HEPATITIS

- Additional names: Serum Hepatitis and long incubation hepatitis

- Route of transmission: Contact with infected blood or body fluids; Hepatitis B virus can survive on **inanimate** objects for several days and has the possibility of being transmitted in that manner; the infection may also be passed on to an infant during birth. There are an estimated 1 million carriers of Hepatitis B in the United States.

- Vaccinations available: The only form of hepatitis for which a vaccine is available is Hepatitis B. The vaccine provides **immunity** from the disease for up to 5 years or longer. The series of three injections is administered over a 6-month period. The cost for the three injections ranges approximately from $150 to $200.

  1. Heptavax B
  2. Recombivax HB
  3. Engerix B
  4. Hepatitis Immune Globulin (HBIG)—after exposure

- Treatment: Symptomatic; Alphainterferon to reduce inflammation

- Incubation period: 4 weeks to 5 months

- Diagnosis: *HBsAg* determines presence of antibody during acute phase of the disease; *HBeAg* indicates a highly infectious state as well as the chance of developing chronic hepatitis; *anti-HBs* indicates immunity to Hepatitis B; *anti-HBc* indicates history of infection with Hepatitis B

- Prognosis: Possible immunity or may become carrier; 5 to 10% develop chronic hepatitis; high chance of mortality

- Incidence: There are an average of 300,000 new cases of Hepatitis B infections diagnosed annually in the United States. Of these, approximately 12,000 to 20,000 occur in health care workers. More than 500 health care workers are hospitalized annually due to Hepatitis B virus, and 200 to 300 die from the disease. Hepatitis B is the ninth leading cause of death in the world.

- Prevention: Routine screening of donated blood and blood products; vaccinations; caution with at-risk behaviors, e.g. multiple sexual partners and IV drug use

TYPE C HEPATITIS

- Additional names: Non-A, non-B hepatitis

- Route of transmission: Approximately 50% of cases by contact with infected blood or blood products; remaining 50% of spread unknown. Approximately 1% of the population in the United States are carriers of the Hepatitis C virus. Sexual contact and contaminated intravenous (IV) needles have also been shown to transmit Hepatitis C.

- Vaccinations available: None

- Treatment: Alphainterferon to reduce inflammation; symptomatic

- Incubation period: 2 weeks to 6 months

- Diagnosis: *Anti-HCV* indicates history of infection with Hepatitis C though may not appear until 2 to 6 months after initial exposure

- Prognosis: May become carrier; 50% develop chronic hepatitis of which 20% will develop cirrhosis

- Incidence: Approximately 150,000 to 170,000 cases diagnosed annually in the United States

- Prevention: Routine screening of donated blood and blood products

TYPE D HEPATITIS

- Additional names: Delta virus

- Route of transmission: Must have Hepatitis B to get Hepatitis D; contact with infected blood or body fluids

- Vaccinations available: None

- Treatment: Symptomatic

- Incubation period: 2 weeks to 2 months

- Diagnosis: *Anti-HDV* indicates acute phase of the disease or history of the infection

- Prognosis: Possible chronic carrier; if develop immunity to Hepatitis B will also be immune to Hepatitis D; high risk of chronic hepatitis with high chance of mortality

- Incidence: Rare

- Prevention: Routine screening of donated blood and blood products; vaccinations for Hepatitis B; caution with at-risk behaviors, e.g. multiple sexual partners and IV drug use

Enteric – refers to the intestine

Fatigue – feeling of tiredness or exhaustion

TYPE E HEPATITIS

- Additional names: **Enteric** non-A, non-B hepatitis
- Route of transmission: Contaminated food or water (fecal-oral route)
- Vaccinations available: None
- Treatment: Symptomatic
- Incubation period: 2 to 7 weeks
- Diagnosis: Symptoms
- Prognosis: 10% mortality during pregnancy
- Incidence: Hepatitis E is rare in the United States, generally occurring only with travelers to parts of the world where Hepatitis E is more common.
- Prevention: Caution to be aware of sanitary conditions, especially when traveling to countries that have a high rate of Hepatitis E, e.g. India, Asia, Mexico, and Africa

SIGNS, SYMPTOMS, AND ASSOCIATED CARE

The following symptoms pertain to all types of hepatitis unless specified. In certain types of hepatitis, such as A and C, the patient may have vague symptoms and not realize they have hepatitis, or they exhibit no symptoms at all.

1. **Fatigue**
   - Assist patient with activities of daily living (ADLs) as necessary
   - Schedule care, activities, and treatment around patient's rest schedule
   - Monitor phone calls and visitors around patient's energy level and rest schedule
   - Encourage frequent rest periods
   - Provide assistance as needed to prevent injury due to weakness
   - Provide method for patient to call for assistance
   - Encourage patient to set realistic goals of activities
   - Allow adequate time to do activities and procedures to avoid frustration or possible injury
   - Encourage exercise to maintain muscle strength
   - Provide cane or walker for ambulation and transfer
   - Provide private room to promote rest periods
2. Anorexia
   - Obtain baseline weight and monitor on routine basis
   - Encourage patient to participate in dietary choices
   - Administer nutritional supplements and vitamins
   - Monitor for signs of dehydration, such as decreased urine output, concentrated urine, dry skin, tenting of skin, dry mucous membranes, dry mouth, dry eyes, confusion, hypotension, and constipation
   - Encourage family and friends to bring in food that is appealing to patient as dietary restrictions allow
   - Encourage frequent, small meals as tolerated
   - Administer parenteral fluids as necessary
   - Monitor intake and output (I and O)
   - Encourage fluids to prevent dehydration
   - Avoid unpleasant sights and odors in room to make meals more appealing

Myalgia – muscle pain

- Provide meticulous mouth care
- Maintain social atmosphere for mealtimes to encourage the patient to eat
- Encourage clothing that enhances patient appearance
- Encourage exercise program as tolerated to increase appetite

3. Nausea and vomiting
   - Administer antiemetics before meals as prescribed by physician
   - Offer food choices according to patient preference
   - Control odors and unpleasant sights in room
   - Offer fluids frequently to prevent dehydration
   - Monitor intake and output to avoid dehydration
   - Monitor serum electrolytes (*sodium*, *potassium*, and *chloride*)
   - Frequent, small meals as tolerated
   - Encourage rest periods after meals
   - Avoid foods that are spicy, rich, or previously disagreeable to patient
   - Provide receptacle for patient to vomit into as needed; this should be cleaned whenever used and changed on a frequent basis
   - Provide meticulous mouth care
   - Prevent aspiration of vomit
   - Utilize universal precautions at all times when coming in contact with blood or body fluids (See Appendix C)
   - Avoid greasy foods as they tend to stay in the stomach a long period of time
   - Avoid cooking food if possible due to increased nausea with odors of foods
   - Avoid hot foods as necessary due to the increased odors of hot foods
   - Eat in well-ventilated area to decrease the accumulation of odors of foods while eating

4. **Myalgia**
   - Assist with position for patient comfort
   - Administer pain control methods, such as massage, relaxation techniques, imaging, and medications as prescribed by physician
   - Use pillows to offer support
   - Encourage patient to remain as active as possible
   - Assist with ADLs as necessary

5. Arthralgia
   - Administer heat or other methods of pain control, such as massage, relaxation, and imaging
   - Administer medications as prescribed by physician for pain control
   - Monitor level of comfort
   - Protect joints, immobilize joints, and decrease weight-bearing as able
   - Assist with ADLs as necessary due to pain
   - Assist with position for patient comfort
   - Encourage patient to keep as active as possible
   - Encourage frequent rest periods to provide joint rest and pain relief
   - Allow adequate time to do as much as possible for themselves, even though it may take longer
   - Use pillows to support extremities

6. Abdominal pain
   - Assist with position for patient comfort
   - Avoid constrictive garments and undergarments
   - Provide methods to promote comfort, such as relaxation techniques, imaging, massage, and warm baths
   - Monitor for level of pain and offer comfort measures as necessary
   - Administer medications as necessary and as prescribed by physician for the control of pain
   - Encourage patient to request pain relief methods before pain becomes too severe

7. Jaundice; note that with Hepatitis A, only 10% of patients will have jaundice
   - Monitor skin color
   - Monitor serum liver function tests

8. Dark-colored urine
   - Monitor color of urine
   - Monitor intake and output (I and O)
   - Save three consecutive voidings consistently to watch for change in color of urine

9. Clay-colored stools
   - Monitor color, frequency, and amount of stools
   - Monitor stools for bleeding (*Hemoccult®*)

10. Pruritus
    - Provide meticulous skin care with mild, unscented soap
    - Avoid use of tapes and other adhesives on skin as able
    - Apply medications or creams to prevent itching
    - Provide protective mittens to prevent scratching and damage to skin for confused patient
    - Encourage fluid intake
    - Pat skin gently dry
    - Avoid harsh soaps or bleach in clothing and linens
    - Avoid clothing and bedding that is irritating
    - Assess skin redness and irritation on routine basis
    - Observe for open areas and signs of infection
    - Avoid use of scented lotions and cosmetics
    - Administer antihistamines as necessary to relieve itching

11. Headache
    - Assist with position for patient comfort
    - Provide calm, quiet environment for the patient
    - Administer pain control methods, such as relaxation techniques, massage, imaging, and pain medications as prescribed by physician
    - Encourage patient to avoid eye strain
    - Encourage patient to rest as necessary
    - Monitor phone calls and visitors to promote rest
    - Provide indirect lighting in patient room
    - Dim lights in event of photophobia

Human immuno-deficiency virus (HIV) – virus that causes acquired immune deficiency syndrome (AIDS)

12. Diarrhea
   - Monitor number, amount, and consistency of stools
   - Monitor intake and output to avoid dehydration
   - Monitor serum electrolytes
   - Provide meticulous skin care, especially if incontinent
   - Monitor for presence of hemorrhoids
   - Monitor for rectal discomfort and offer Sitz baths, warm soaks, and topical ointments or suppositories
   - Administer antidiarrheal medications as prescribed by physician
   - Provide frequent skin care, especially to anal area to prevent skin breakdown
   - Monitor for presence of blood (*Hemoccult®*)
   - Offer reassurance to patient
   - Avoid foods that are too hot or too cold as they increase peristalsis

DIAGNOSIS

In addition to the specific tests to diagnose hepatitis, serum liver function tests are also performed to determine the extent of liver damage.

1. *SGOT (Aspartate aminotransferase)*—elevated
2. *SGPT (Alanine aminotransferase)*—elevated
3. *Bilirubin*—elevated
4. *Lactate dehydrogenase (LDH)*—elevated
5. *Creatinine phosphokinase (CPK)*—normal
6. *Alkaline phosphatase*—elevated
7. *Albumin*
8. *Prothrombin time*

Patients with Hepatitis B are often tested for **human immunodeficiency virus (HIV)** since it is transmitted in the same manner.

GENERAL METHODS OF TREATMENT

1. Bed rest
2. Adequate fluid intake
3. Nutrition, e.g. high-carbohydrate, low-fat, and high-fiber
   - High-carbohydrate foods include fruits, vegetables, and whole grains.
   - Items that are high in saturated fats and cholesterol should be avoided or eaten in moderate amounts, including egg yolks, butter, cheese, and red meats
   - Foods that are high in fiber include fruits, vegetables, whole grains, prunes, and beans

COMPLICATIONS

1. Cirrhosis
2. Liver failure
3. Liver cancer

4. Chronic hepatitis, which is defined as viral hepatitis; lasts longer than 6 months

5. Fulminant hepatitis

6. Bleeding disorders

CONSIDERATIONS FOR CARE

1. Universal precautions are necessary whenever contact with blood or body fluids is possible. (See Appendix C.)

2. Educate patient and family regarding disease process.

3. Educate patient and family regarding forms of treatment as well as side effects of medications.

4. Educate family members, friends, and sexual partners regarding the need to be checked for the presence of hepatitis.

5. Provide emotional support for the patient and family.

6. Monitor for complications.

7. Educate patient to consult physician prior to consuming alcohol because alcohol is metabolized primarily by the liver.

8. Educate patient to consult physician regarding need to avoid medications that are metabolized by the liver.

9. Encourage frequent rest periods as needed by patient.

10. Enteric isolation is necessary for Hepatitis A and Hepatitis E.

   - Hands should be washed before and after entering the patient room, and if soiling occurs

   - Gown and gloves should be worn if contamination with blood or body fluids is possible

   - Any object that is contaminated with blood or body fluids, especially feces, should be thrown away or double bagged and sterilized

11. Hepatitis must be reported to the state public health department.

12. Educate patient, family and visitors regarding need for meticulous handwashing.

13. Educate patient that he will be unable to donate blood.

14. Educate patient and family regarding the importance of follow-up care.

15. Monitor prothrombin time; injections of Vitamin K may be necessary.

FOR MORE INFORMATION

Department of Public Health and Human Services
Centers for Disease Control
Atlanta, GA 30333

American Liver Foundation
998 Pompton Avenue
Cedar Grove NJ 07009
(201) 857-2626
(800) 223-0179

National Digestive Diseases Clearinghouse
Box NDDIC
Bethesda, MD 20892
(301) 468-6344

ASSIGNMENT SHEET: HEPATITIS

Short Answer

1. Write a brief definition for the terms listed throughout the chapter.

2. Describe the normal physiology of the liver.

3. List the seven (7) functions of the liver.

4. Write a brief definition for hepatitis.

5. List additional names for each of the specific types of hepatitis.

6. Describe the route of transmission for each of the specific types of hepatitis.

7. Describe the vaccinations available to aid in the prevention of hepatitis.

8. Describe the specific form of treatment for each of the types of hepatitis.

9. Describe the nonmedication forms of treatment used for hepatitis.

10. Describe the incubation period for each of the specific types of hepatitis.

11. Describe the method of diagnosis for each of the specific types of hepatitis.

12. Describe eight (8) additional tests that are commonly performed to diagnose hepatitis.

13. Describe the prognosis associated with each of the specific types of hepatitis.

14. Describe the incidence of each of the specific types of hepatitis.

15. List twelve (12) signs and symptoms associated with hepatitis and associated care for these symptoms.

16. List six (6) specific complications often associated with hepatitis.

17. List methods of prevention for each of the specific types of hepatitis.

18. List fifteen (15) considerations for caring for a patient with hepatitis.

19. Describe what is meant by universal precautions, and describe the importance of it as associated with hepatitis. (See Appendix C.)

20. Describe what is meant by enteric precautions.

21. List ten (10) symptoms of dehydration.

22. List the normal ranges for each of the following laboratory values.

    a. Bilirubin
    b. Aspartate aminotransferase (SGOT)
    c. Alanine aminotransferase (SGPT)
    d. Lactate dehydrogenase (LDH)
    e. Creatinine phosphokinase (CPK)
    f. Prothrombin time
    g. Sodium
    h. Potassium
    i. Chloride
    j. Albumin
    k. Alkaline phosphatase
    l. Vitamin A
    m. Vitamin B_{12}
    n. Vitamin D
    o. Iron

KNOWLEDGE INTO ACTION

1. Fluids and nutrition are a very important part of the recovery for a patient with hepatitis. What type of diet could you possibly expect the physician to order for Ms. Lin, a 46-year-old counselor with hepatitis?

2. After Ms. Lin has been in your facility for several days, she has developed arthralgia. She is quite adamant about *not* wanting to take medications. Describe two nonmedication methods of pain control for Ms. Lin. Also write a brief definition for arthralgia.

3. Ms. Lin's urine is quite concentrated in color. You are visiting with a new nursing assistant about Ms. Lin care in her care conference when she says to you, "How do we know if her urine is getting to be more normal in color?" What will your response be?

4. During the care conference for Ms. Lin, the charge nurse reminds everyone to use universal precautions for all patients. Describe what is meant by universal precautions and why it might be especially important when caring for Ms. Lin. (Universal precautions should be used for all patients regardless of their diagnosis.)

5. During Ms. Lin's hospital stay, you are visiting with her about long-term changes she may need to make. Describe two (2) long-term changes that would be important for Ms. Lin to make due to her specific diagnosis.

6. If Ms. Lin had a different type of hepatitis than what she did, she may have been put on enteric precautions. Write a brief definition for enteric precautions, and describe what is included in enteric precautions.

OBJECTIVES

Upon completion of this chapter, the student should be able to:

- Define the key terms listed throughout the chapter
- Describe the physiology of the gastrointestinal system
- State a specific definition for ulcerative colitis
- Describe the incidence of ulcerative colitis
- List the risk factors for ulcerative colitis
- List signs and symptoms associated with ulcerative colitis and associated care for these symptoms
- List the causes of the symptoms associated with ulcerative colitis
- Identify specific methods for diagnosis of ulcerative colitis
- Identify specific methods for treatment of ulcerative colitis
- Describe specific considerations for caring for a patient with ulcerative colitis
- List complications associated with ulcerative colitis

KEY TERMS

Stool – solid waste material excreted from the bowels; bowel movement

Enzyme – proteins that can change another substance chemically without themselves being changed or destroyed

Chyme – semisolid, partially digested food in the stomach and small intestine

Villi – fingerlike projections in the small intestine that absorb nutrients and fluids from food

Liver – organ of the body located in the upper right quadrant of the abdomen

Pancreas – organ located in the upper left quadrant of the abdomen that secretes insulin and digestive enzymes

INTRODUCTION

Ulcerative colitis is a chronic inflammatory disease of the colon or large intestine. (See Figure 32-1.) The disease is characterized by periods of remission and exacerbations of the inflammation and other symptoms. The inflammation generally begins in the rectum and progresses upward until the entire colon is involved. Occasionally the ileum will also be affected.

PHYSIOLOGY OF THE DIGESTIVE SYSTEM

The gastrointestinal tract, or digestive system, begins at the mouth and ends at the anal opening. The function of the digestive system is to digest food, absorb nutrients, and excrete solid wastes (feces or **stool**). The organs of the digestive system include the mouth, esophagus, stomach, small intestine (which is divided into the duodenum, jejunum, and ileum), large intestine, rectum, and anus. The large intestine is divided into the cecum, ascending colon, transverse colon, descending colon, and sigmoid colon. Food is taken into the mouth where teeth begin the mechanical breakdown and saliva begins the chemical breakdown of the food. The partially broken down food travels through the esophagus to the stomach where digestive **enzymes** and the churning of the stomach turn the food into a thick liquid called **chyme**. This process takes approximately 3 to 5 hours. The next step in the process is for the food to travel into the small intestine. The small intestine contains blood-rich projections, called **villi**, which absorb nutrients from the food. The food that has not been absorbed then travels into the large intestine where water is absorbed from the waste product into the circulatory system. The solid waste is held in the rectum until expelled from the body in the form of feces or stool. The **liver**, gallbladder, and **pancreas** are accessory organs for the digestive system. These organs are responsible for secretion and storage of bile and

Crohn's disease – chronic inflammatory disease of the ileum

Bacteria – microorganisms present almost everywhere; divided into three classifications: rod-shaped (bacilli), spiral-shaped, and spherical. Spherical may appear in pairs (diplococci), chains (streptococci), or clusters (staphylococci)

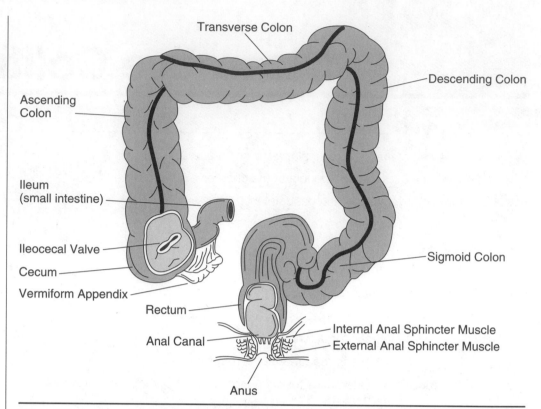

Figure 32-1   Large intestine (From Keir et al., *Medical Assisting: Administrative and Clinical Competencies, 2nd edition,* copyright © 1989, Delmar Publishers)

other digestive enzymes, which are necessary for the breakdown of food. (See Figure 32-2.)

STATISTICS

There are more than 2 million people affected by inflammatory bowel disease (IBD), a term which includes the specific diseases of ulcerative colitis as well as **Crohn's disease** (see Chapter 33). Ulcerative colitis affects males and females equally, though people of Jewish descent are affected more than non-Jews and whites are affected more often than blacks. Nearly 75% of all cases of ulcerative colitis in the United States develop prior to 40 years of age. The frequency of ulcerative colitis has increased in the past decades. It has been estimated that currently 1 out of 1,000 people in the United States is affected by the disease.

RISK FACTORS

There are certain predisposing factors to the disease.

1. Jewish ancestry
2. Infection from **bacteria** or virus
3. Food sensitivities
4. Emotional stress
5. Autoimmune response
6. Heredity (25% have relatives also affected by the disease)
7. Excessive production of enzymes in the digestive tract
8. Allergic reaction

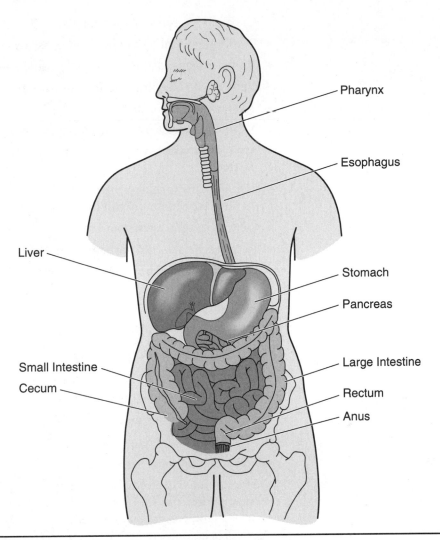

Figure 32-2   Digestive system (From Shapiro, *Basic Maternal/Pediatric Nursing*, copyright © 1994, Delmar Publishers)

SIGNS, SYMPTOMS, AND ASSOCIATED CARE

1. Abdominal cramps due to irritation of the lining of the intestinal wall and cramps associated with diarrhea

    - Assist with position for patient comfort

    - Administer medications to control cramping as prescribed by physician

    - Provide methods to promote comfort, such as relaxation techniques, imaging, massage, and warm baths

    - Avoid constrictive garments and undergarments

    - Avoid foods that increase abdominal cramping

    - Monitor for level of pain and offer comfort measures as necessary

    - Encourage patient to request pain relief methods before pain becomes too severe

2. Bloody diarrhea due to irritation of the intestinal wall

    - Monitor stools for amount of bleeding

    - Offer reassurance to patient

    - Monitor for anemia in the presence of bloody diarrhea

- Check for presence of blood in stools (*Hemoccult*®)
- Monitor amount, frequency, and consistency of stools
- Provide meticulous skin care to the anal area

3. Anemia due to bleeding and malabsorption of nutrients
- Treat anemia according to cause
- Monitor *hemoglobin* and *hematocrit* to check for anemia
- Monitor physical symptoms of anemia such as pallor, weakness, and vertigo

4. Weight loss due to malabsorption of nutrients and decreased appetite due to abdominal pain, cramps, and diarrhea
- Obtain baseline weight and monitor weight on routine basis
- Encourage patient to participate in dietary choices
- Offer nutritional supplements and vitamins as necessary
- Encourage family and friends to bring in food that is appealing to patient as dietary restrictions allow
- Administer parenteral fluids as necessary
- Monitor intake and output (I and O)
- Encourage rest periods before and after meals
- Avoid unpleasant sights and odors in room to make meals more appealing
- Provide meticulous mouth care
- Monitor for skin breakdown due to loss of body tissue
- Encourage clothing styles that do not draw attention to weight loss
- Monitor for symptoms of dehydration, e.g. decreased urine output, constipation, dry skin, tenting of skin, dry mouth, dry eyes, concentrated urine, hypotension, and confusion

5. Rectal bleeding due to irritation of the intestinal mucosa
- Monitor for presence of rectal bleeding
- Monitor for anemia in the presence of rectal bleeding
- Offer reassurance to patient
- Check for the presence of blood in stools (*Hemoccult*®)
- Monitor amount, frequency, and consistency of stools
- Provide meticulous skin care to the anal area

6. Fever due to inflammation of the intestinal mucosa
- Monitor temperature at routine intervals
- Provide comfort measures for patient with elevated temperature, such as cool cloth to forehead, partial or complete bath as needed, clothing and bedding changed frequently due to diaphoresis, and encourage fluids to prevent dehydration
- Avoid exposing patient to a draft
- Cover with blankets as necessary
- Monitor intake and output (I and O)
- Maintain comfortable room temperature for patient
- Avoid plastic mattresses and plastic bed protectors as they increase perspiration
- Use of antiperspirant or deodorant to minimize sweating and odor

Tenesmus – spasms of the anal sphincter or urinary sphincter that gives the feeling of needing to empty the bowel or bladder; may cause pain with defecation or urination

Anal – refers to the anus (external opening of the rectum)

Defecation – bowel movement

Urination – process of eliminating urine from the body

7. Anorexia due to abdominal pain, cramping, and diarrhea associated with eating
    - Obtain baseline weight and monitor on routine basis
    - Encourage patient to participate in dietary choices
    - Offer nutritional supplements and vitamins
    - Monitor for signs of dehydration such as decreased urine output, concentrated urine, dry skin, tenting of skin, dry mucous membranes, dry mouth, dry eyes, confusion, and constipation
    - Encourage family and friends to bring in food that is appealing to patient as dietary restrictions allow
    - Encourage frequent, small meals as tolerated
    - Administer parenteral fluids as necessary
    - Monitor intake and output (I and O)
    - Encourage fluids to prevent dehydration
    - Avoid unpleasant sights and odors in room to make meals more appealing
    - Provide meticulous mouth care
    - Maintain social atmosphere for mealtimes to encourage the patient to eat
    - Encourage clothing that enhances patient appearance
    - Encourage exercise program as tolerated to increase appetite

8. Mucus or pus in bowel movements due to inflammation of the intestinal mucosa
    - Monitor stools for the presence of mucous or pus

9. **Tenesmus**, which is spasms of the **anal** sphincter or urinary sphincter, giving the feeling of needing to empty the bowel or bladder. This may cause pain with **defecation** or **urination** due to diarrhea stools and irritation of intestinal mucosa.
    - Assist with position for patient comfort
    - Assist patient to bathroom as necessary at the urge to defecate
    - Respond to patient call promptly
    - Provide method for patient to call for assistance when needing to get to bathroom
    - Provide bedside commode for patient who has frequent urge to defecate

10. Abdominal distention due to irritation of the intestinal mucosa and increased flatulence
    - Monitor for abdominal distention
    - Measure abdominal girth on routine basis, with area marked so same area measured each time for accuracy
    - Encourage nonconstrictive clothing and undergarments
    - Assist with position for patient comfort
    - Avoid foods that increase formation of intestinal gas

11. Dehydration due to diarrhea and decreased fluid intake
    - Monitor for symptoms of dehydration, e.g. constipation, decreased urinary output, concentrated urine, hypotension, dry skin, dry mouth, tenting of skin, confusion, and dry mucous membranes
    - Monitor intake and output (I and O)
    - Encourage fluid intake according to patient preference
    - Avoid caffeine, which acts as a diuretic

Peritonitis – inflammation of the peritoneum (membrane that lines the abdominal cavity)

Abscess – accumulation of fluid within an enclosed sac; generally due to infection

Fistula – abnormal passageway from one organ to another or from an internal organ to the exterior of the body

Toxic megacolon – extreme dilation of the colon that predisposes the colon to rupturing

Ova and parasites – test done on feces to check for the presence of parasites

Total parenteral nutrition (TPN) – total nutritional requirements provided through intravenous method; used for patients who are unable to take nutrition by mouth

Hyperalimentation – introduction of solution into the body that is high enough in necessary nutrients to sustain life; may by introduced through either a parenteral route or enteral route

12. Hypokalemia due to diarrhea and dehydration
    - Monitor for symptoms of hypokalemia. Symptoms of hypokalemia include muscle weakness or spasms and hypotension.
    - Monitor *serum potassium* levels
    - Provide foods high in potassium, such as bananas, yellow vegetables, dried fruits and citrus fruits, and potatoes
    - Administer potassium supplements as ordered by physician

CAUSE OF SYMPTOMS AND COMPLICATIONS

1. Inflammation of the mucous membrane of the colon
2. Malabsorption of nutrients due to irritation
3. Malnutrition due to malabsorption of nutrients and increase in symptoms associated with eating
4. Narrowing of the lumen of the colon

COMPLICATIONS

Complications of ulcerative colitis may involve almost any organ of the body, specifically the skin, gallbladder, joints, liver, eyes, blood, and blood vessels. Approximately 10 to 20% of patients with ulcerative colitis experience complications in some form. The more-specific complications follow.

1. Stunted growth and delayed development in children due to malabsorption and malnutrition
2. Perforation of the bowel
3. **Peritonitis**
4. Increased chance of colon cancer
5. Formation of **abscess** or **fistula**
6. Malnutrition
7. Electrolyte imbalance (*sodium, potassium,* and *chloride*)
8. **Toxic megacolon**

DIAGNOSIS

Diagnosis is based on the following methods.

1. Signs and symptoms
2. Physical examination
3. *Proctoscopy*
4. *Colonoscopy*
5. Serum laboratory tests, which include a decreased *potassium*, decreased *albumin*, decreased h*emoglobin*, increased *WBC*, and increased *prothrombin time*
6. *Barium enema*
7. Stool analysis to rule out infection or infestation of ***ova and parasites***

TREATMENT

1. Bed rest
2. Fluid replacement therapy—intravenous (IVs), **total parenteral nutrition (TPN), hyperalimentation**

Antibacterial – substance used to destroy bacteria

Antidiarrheal – substance that prevents or treats diarrhea

Pepsin – enzyme secreted by the stomach that is responsible for the breakdown of proteins

3. Medications

- Corticosteroids—used to decrease inflammation
- Sulfasalazine—used to decrease inflammation and **antibacterial**
- **Antidiarrheal** medications
- Antispasmodic medications
- Antibiotics in the presence of secondary infection

4. Diet has not been shown to worsen the course of the disease but has been shown to increase severity or frequency of symptoms associated with ulcerative colitis.

- Low fiber. Fiber is defined as anything that is undigested when it reaches the large intestine; fiber is irritating to the already inflamed mucous membrane and should be taken in limited amounts.
- Cold foods and beverages are restricted as they increase bowel activity
- Tobacco should be avoided as it increases intestinal peristalsis
- Caffeine should be avoided as it stimulates gastric acid and **pepsin** secretion
- Any food that has previously been irritating and has caused pain should be avoided
- Approximately 20% of patients with ulcerative colitis do not have the enzyme necessary to digest milk and milk products, and therefore milk products should be avoided

5. Surgery, curative for ulcerative colitis, is required in approximately 30% of patients

- Proctocolectomy, the removal of the colon and rectum, requires an ileum to be brought out through the abdominal wall (stoma) for excretion of waste products from the body. The external opening is called an ileostomy.
- Continent ileostomy, creation of a pouch from the ileum, is located in the lower abdomen. The pouch contains a valve open to the outside, which is used to drain the waste products from the body on a routine basis.
- Ileoanal anastomosis, the removal of the diseased portion of rectum and colon, leaves the muscle portion of the rectum intact. The ileum is attached to the muscular portion of the rectum, and the patient is able to pass stool normally.

6. Treat anemia depending on cause, e.g. blood transfusion or iron supplement therapy

CONSIDERATIONS FOR CARE

1. Educate patient and family regarding the disease process.
2. Educate patient and family regarding forms of treatment as well as side effects of medications.
3. Provide emotional support to patient and family.
4. Provide nonjudgmental acceptance of emotions and behavior of patient and family.
5. Facilitate finding a support group for patient and family.
6. Educate patient and family regarding the importance of follow-up care.
7. Educate patient and family regarding methods to reduce or eliminate stressors as stress has been shown to exacerbate symptoms due to diminished blood supply to the colon.

8. Dietary instructions to include foods that are appealing and foods that don't exacerbate symptoms; monitor need for dietary and vitamin supplements; provide adequate fluid intake and adequate calories and nutritional requirements.

9. Provide meticulous skin care, especially in the case of incontinence.

10. Respond to patient promptly when needing to go to bathroom due to urgency.

11. Position commode at bedside for patient accessibility due to urgency.

12. Provide bed protectors in the event of incontinence.

13. Monitor for symptoms of complications.

14. Encourage smoking cessation due to increased peristalsis from nicotine.

15. Obtain baseline weight and monitor at frequent intervals.

16. Monitor intake and output (I and O).

17. Monitor serum laboratory results for deviations from normal ranges.

18. Monitor for symptoms of dehydration, such as decreased urine output, constipation, dry skin, tenting of skin, dry mouth, dry eyes, concentrated urine, hypotension, and confusion.

19. Instruct patient and family to watch for symptoms of complications and to report any symptoms promptly to physician.

FOR MORE INFORMATION

American Digestive Disease Society
420 Lexington Avenue
New York, NY 10017

National Foundation for Ileitis and Colitis, Inc.
295 Madison Avenue
New York, NY 10017

United Ostomy Association
1111 Wilshire Boulevard
Los Angeles, CA 90017

Gastrointestinal Research Foundation
205 West Wacker Drive
Chicago, IL 60606

Crohn's and Colitis Foundation of America, Inc.
National Headquarters
444 Park Avenue South
New York, NY 10016-7374

United Ostomy Association Inc.
Suite 120
36 Executive Park
Irvine, CA 92714-6744

ASSIGNMENT SHEET: ULCERATIVE COLITIS

Short Answer

1. Write a brief definition for the terms listed throughout the chapter.

2. Describe the physiology of the gastrointestinal system.

3. Write a brief definition for ulcerative colitis.

4. Describe the incidence of ulcerative colitis.

5. List eight (8) risk factors often associated with ulcerative colitis.

6. List twelve (12) signs and symptoms associated with ulcerative colitis and the rationale and associated care for each of these symptoms.

7. List the four (4) main causes of the symptoms associated with ulcerative colitis.

8. List eight (8) complications associated with ulcerative colitis.

9. List seven (7) specific methods used in the diagnosis of ulcerative colitis.

10. List six (6) specific methods used for the treatment of ulcerative colitis.

11. List nineteen (19) specific considerations for caring for a patient with ulcerative colitis.

12. Describe what is meant by dietary fiber.

13. List the normal range for an oral temperature. (See Appendix D.)

14. Write the normal range for each of the following laboratory tests.
    a. Hemoglobin (Hg)
    b. Hematocrit (Hct)
    c. Albumin
    d. White blood count (WBC)
    e. Prothrombin time
    f. Electrolytes
       • Sodium
       • Potassium
       • Chloride

15. Describe the following procedures used in the diagnosis or treatment of ulcerative colitis.
    a. Hemoccult® stools
    b. Proctoscopy
    c. Colonoscopy
    d. Stool for ova and parasites (O and P)

16. Describe three (3) specific types of surgery used in the treatment of ulcerative colitis.

KNOWLEDGE INTO ACTION

1. Kevin Steinberg, a 34-year-old car salesman, has been told that he was at a higher risk of developing ulcerative colitis due to his Jewish ancestry. Describe three (3) other risk factors that could increase a person's chances of developing ulcerative colitis.

2. Mr. Steinberg initially went to see his physician due to the following symptoms: abdominal cramps, bloody diarrhea, weight loss of 18 pounds, fever, and anorexia. Describe the rationale for each of these symptoms as well as three (3) methods of associated care that should be kept in mind when providing care to Mr. Steinberg.

3. In addition to the symptoms listed in question 2, you are also aware that you need to monitor for dehydration and hypokalemia. Describe what symptoms could indicate each of the mentioned symptoms.

4. In the past, patients admitted to the hospital with ulcerative colitis have had one or more of the following procedures done to aid in the diagnosis of the disease: proctoscopy, colonoscopy, and/or barium enema. Write a brief definition that could be used to aid in the understanding for a patient about to undergo one of the procedures.

5. The dietitian has been asked to consult for a diet recommendation and education for Mr. Steinberg. Describe four (4) recommendations or considerations that could be suggested for Mr. Steinberg to keep in mind when choosing his foods at home.

6. For Mr. Steinberg's treatment, the physician has ordered bed rest, corticosteroids (to decrease

inflammation), and intravenous (IV) fluid replacement therapy. You are aware that if these forms of treatment do not help treat Mr. Steinberg, he may need surgery. Describe two methods of surgery that could be recommended for Mr. Steinberg if nonsurgical forms of treatment are not helpful.

7. Mr. Steinberg's wife, Kathleen, frequently is at her husband's bedside. Prior to discharge, you have been asked by the physician to go over some symptoms that could indicate complications due to the ulcerative colitis. List four (4) symptoms you would need to tell the family that could indicate the presence of complications.

Crohn's Disease

OBJECTIVES

Upon completion of this chapter, the student should be able to:

- Define the key terms listed throughout the chapter
- State a specific definition for Crohn's disease
- Describe the physiology of the gastrointestinal system
- List the risk factors for Crohn's disease
- List signs and symptoms for Crohn's disease and associated care for these symptoms
- Identify specific methods for diagnosis of Crohn's disease
- Describe specific surgical interventions in the treatment of Crohn's disease
- Identify specific nonsurgical methods of treatment for Crohn's disease
- Describe specific complications associated with Crohn's disease and list symptoms of each
- Describe specific considerations for caring for a patient with Crohn's disease

KEY TERMS

Appendix – small appendage located at the junction between the ileum of the small intestine and the opening into the large intestine

Saliva – liquid secreted by the salivary glands to aid in the digestion of food

INTRODUCTION

Crohn's disease is chronic inflammation of the entire mucous membrane of the lower portion of the small intestine (ileum) and frequently the colon. Approximately 50% of people with Crohn's disease have involvement of the ileum and colon (ileocolitis), while 20% of people have involvement of the colon only. The remaining 30% have involvement of one or more segments of the small intestine. Inflammation may also involve the mouth, stomach, esophagus, **appendix**, or anus. The symptoms may be insidious or abrupt.

PHYSIOLOGY OF THE DIGESTIVE SYSTEM

The gastrointestinal tract, or digestive system, begins at the mouth and ends at the anal opening. The function of the digestive system is to digest food, absorb nutrients, and excrete solid wastes (feces or stool). The organs of the digestive system include the mouth, esophagus, stomach, small intestine (which is divided into the duodenum, jejunum, and ileum), large intestine, rectum, and anus. The large intestine is divided into the cecum, ascending colon, transverse colon, descending colon, and sigmoid colon. Food is taken into the mouth where teeth begin the mechanical breakdown and **saliva** begins the chemical breakdown of the food. The partially broken down food travels through the esophagus to the stomach where digestive enzymes and the churning of the stomach turn the food into a thick liquid called chyme. This process takes approximately 3 to 5 hours. The next step in the process is for the food to travel into the small intestine. The small intestine contains blood-rich projections, called villi, which absorb nutrients from the food. (See Figure 33-1.) The food that has not been absorbed then travels into the large intestine where water is absorbed from the waste product into the circulatory system. The solid waste is held in the rectum until expelled from the body in the form of feces or stool. The liver, gallbladder, and pancreas are accessory organs for the digestive system. These organs are responsible for secretion and storage

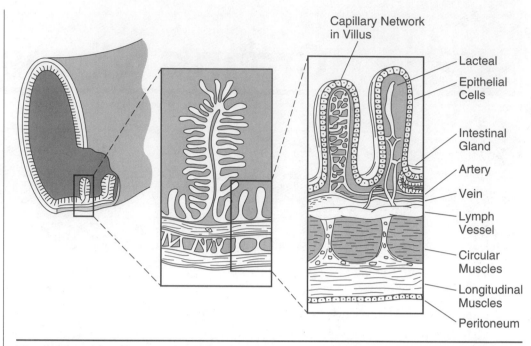

Figure 33-1 Villi of the small intestine (From Burke, *Human Anatomy and Physiology in Health and Disease, 3rd edition,* copyright © 1992, Delmar Publishers)

of bile and other digestive enzymes, which are necessary for the breakdown of food. (See Figure 32-2.)

STATISTICS

Approximately 10 to 70 people in the United States per 100,000 will be diagnosed with Crohn's disease in their lifetime. The average age at onset of symptoms of the disease is 15 to 30 years old.

RISK FACTORS

There is no specifically known cause for Crohn's disease, though emotional stress can cause exacerbations of symptoms. Several of the theories of causes are as follows.

1. Autoimmune response
2. Viral or bacterial infection
3. Jewish ancestry
4. Heredity (25% have relative also affected by the disease)

SIGNS, SYMPTOMS, AND ASSOCIATED CARE

Symptoms of Crohn's disease commonly include the following.

1. Diarrhea due to inflammation of the intestinal mucosa
   - Monitor number, amount, and consistency of stools
   - Monitor intake and output (I and O) to avoid dehydration, e.g. decreased urine output, constipation, dry skin, tenting of skin, dry mouth, dry eyes, concentrated urine, hypotension, and confusion
   - Monitor serum electrolytes (*sodium*, *potassium*, and *chloride*)
   - Provide meticulous skin care, especially if incontinent
   - Monitor for presence of hemorrhoids

- Monitor for rectal discomfort and offer Sitz baths, warm soaks, and topical ointments or suppositories
- Administer antidiarrheal medications as prescribed by physician
- Provide frequent skin care, especially to anal area to prevent skin breakdown
- Monitor for presence of blood (*Hemoccult*®)
- Offer reassurance to patient
- Avoid foods that are too hot or too cold as they increase peristalsis

2. Abdominal pain due to inflammation of the intestinal mucosa
   - Assist with position for patient comfort
   - Administer medications to control cramping as prescribed by physician
   - Offer methods to promote comfort, such as relaxation techniques, imaging, massage, and warm baths
   - Avoid constrictive clothing and undergarments
   - Monitor for level of pain and offer comfort measures as necessary
   - Encourage patient to request pain relief methods before pain becomes too severe

3. Rectal bleeding due to inflammation of the intestinal mucosa
   - Monitor for presence of rectal bleeding
   - Monitor for anemia in the presence of rectal bleeding
   - Offer reassurance to patient

4. Fever due to inflammation of the intestinal mucosa
   - Monitor temperature at routine intervals
   - Provide comfort measures for patient with elevated temperature, such as cool cloth to forehead, partial or complete bath as needed, clothing and bedding changed frequently due to diaphoresis, and encourage fluids to prevent dehydration
   - Avoid exposing patient to a draft
   - Cover with blankets as necessary
   - Monitor intake and output (I and O)
   - Maintain comfortable room temperature for patient
   - Avoid plastic mattresses and plastic bed protectors as they increase perspiration
   - Use of antiperspirant or deodorant to minimize sweating and odor

5. Anorexia due to abdominal pain, cramps, and diarrhea associated with eating
   - Obtain baseline weight and monitor on routine basis
   - Encourage patient to participate in dietary choices
   - Provide nutritional supplements and vitamins
   - Monitor for signs of dehydration, such as decreased urine output, concentrated urine, dry skin, tenting of skin, dry mucous membranes, dry mouth, dry eyes, confusion, hypotension, and constipation
   - Encourage family and friends to bring in food that is appealing to patient as dietary restrictions allow
   - Encourage frequent, small meals as tolerated
   - Administer parenteral fluids as necessary
   - Monitor intake and output (I and O)
   - Encourage fluids to prevent dehydration

- Avoid unpleasant sights and odors in room to make meals more appealing
- Provide meticulous mouth care
- Maintain social atmosphere for mealtimes to encourage the patient to eat
- Encourage clothing that enhances patient appearance
- Exercise program as tolerated to increase appetite

6. Weight loss due to malabsorption of nutrients and loss of appetite due to abdominal pain, cramps, and diarrhea associated with eating
    - Obtain baseline weight and monitor weight on routine basis
    - Encourage patient to participate in dietary choices
    - Provide nutritional supplements and vitamins
    - Encourage family and friends to bring in food that is appealing to patient as dietary restrictions allow
    - Administer parenteral fluids as necessary
    - Monitor intake and output (I and O)
    - Encourage rest periods before and after meals
    - Avoid unpleasant sights and odors in room to make meals more appealing
    - Provide meticulous mouth care
    - Monitor for skin breakdown due to loss of body tissue
    - Encourage clothing styles that do not draw attention to weight loss
    - Monitor for symptoms of dehydration, e.g. decreased urine output, constipation, dry skin, tenting of skin, dry mouth, dry eyes, concentrated urine, hypotension, and confusion

7. Anemia due to bleeding of intestinal mucosa and malabsorption of nutrients
    - Treat anemia according to cause
    - Monitor *hemoglobin* and *hematocrit* to monitor for anemia
    - Monitor physical symptoms of anemia such as pallor, weakness, and vertigo

8. Cramping pain after eating due to irritation of the intestinal mucosa
    - Assist with position for patient comfort
    - Administer medications to control cramping as prescribed by physician
    - Offer methods to promote comfort, such as relaxation techniques, imaging, massage, and warm baths
    - Avoid constrictive clothing and undergarments
    - Avoid foods that increase abdominal cramping
    - Offer small, frequent feeding as tolerated

DIAGNOSIS

1. Signs and symptoms
2. Physical examination
3. *Barium enema*
4. *Sigmoidoscopy*
5. *Colonoscopy*
6. *Upper gastrointestinal series (UGI)*
7. Serum laboratory tests show increased *WBC*, increased *ESR*, decreased *hemoglobin* (anemia), and decreased *calcium*

Perforation – creation of a hole or opening

Stricture – narrowing of an opening or lumen of a passageway in the body due to formation of scar tissue; strictures may also be congenital

COMPLICATIONS

Surgery will be necessary for 65 to 75% of all patients with Crohn's disease. Indications for surgery generally are due to complications and include:

1. Hemorrhage

   Definition: extreme bleeding or blood loss; may be internal or external

   Symptoms: extreme blood loss from an external opening in the body, hypotension, pallor; weakness, loss of consciousness, and weak, rapid pulse

2. Bowel **perforation**

   Definition: creation of a hole or an opening from the colon into the abdominal cavity

   Symptoms: abdominal pain, distention, and fever

3. Intestinal obstruction

   Definition: blockage of the intestinal tract either with stool or from a tumor

   Symptoms: cessation of bowel movements, diarrhea, abdominal pain, and distention

4. Formation of abscess

   Definition: accumulation of fluid within a sac in or around the colon, generally caused by infection

   Symptoms: abdominal pain, distention, and fever

5. Toxic megacolon

   Definition: extreme dilation of the colon, which predisposes the colon to rupturing

   Symptoms: abdominal pain, distention, and fever

6. Formation of fistula

   Definition: abnormal passageway from the colon to another organ of the body or to the exterior of the body

   Symptoms: presence of feces in the urine or vaginal secretion, abdominal pain, fever, and abdominal distention

7. Colorectal cancer

   Definition: cancer of the colon and/or rectum

   Symptoms: abdominal pain and distention, blood in stools, weight loss, and anemia

8. Ineffectiveness of medical treatment to control symptoms

   Definition: inability of treatment to reduce or eliminate symptoms

   Symptoms: continuing or exacerbating symptoms

TREATMENT

Even though surgery is necessary in a majority of patients with Crohn's disease, it must be stressed that surgery is *not* a cure for Crohn's disease. As many as 50% of patients will have an exacerbation of the symptoms within 5 years after surgery, due to recurrence of the disease at the site of the anastomosis. Of the patients who have an exacerbation of symptoms, 40 to 50% will require a second surgery. Several types of surgery have been used for Crohn's disease and include:

1. Resection—removal of the diseased portion of the bowel only, with anastomosis of the healthy tissues

2. Strictureplasty—areas of **stricture** caused by scar tissue formation are widened without resection of the bowel. This is accomplished by longitudinal incisions

Anti-inflammatory –
substance used to treat or
reduce inflammation

Gastric – stomach

in the diseased bowel and application of traction to the bowel after which the incisions are sutured transversely, which widens the strictured area.

3. Dilation of the strictured areas with a balloon catheter, which is inflated inside the strictured lumen to dilate the stricture area

Other methods of treatment for Crohn's disease include:

1. Total parenteral nutrition (TPN) to rest the bowel

2. Medications

   - Sulfasalazine—**anti-inflammatory** medication frequently used post-operatively to prevent exacerbation of symptoms

   - Mesalamine used to prevent exacerbations during periods of remissions and may also facilitate remission during periods of acute exacerbation

   - Corticosteroids—anti-inflammatory, e.g. Prednisone

   - Azathioprine—immunosuppressive to reduce symptoms by decreasing response to antigens

   - Metronidazole—antibiotic used in the treatment of fistulas or fissures

   - Antidiarrheal medications

   - Antispasmodic medications

3. Diet

   - Low fiber. Fiber is defined as anything that is undigested when it reaches the large intestine; fiber, therefore, is irritating to the already inflamed mucous membrane and is restricted.

   - Restrict cold foods and beverages as they increase bowel activity (peristalsis)

   - Avoid tobacco as it increases intestinal peristalsis

   - Avoid caffeine as it stimulates **gastric** acid and pepsin secretion

   - Provide a diet high in calories, protein, and carbohydrates. High-carbohydrate foods include fruits, vegetables, and whole grains. Foods high in protein include meats, fish, milk, cheese, soybeans, and eggs.

   - Provide nutritional and vitamin supplements

   - Avoid any food that has previously been irritating and has caused pain

CONSIDERATIONS FOR CARE

1. Educate patient and family regarding the disease process.

2. Educate patient and family regarding forms of treatment as well as side effects of medications.

3. Provide emotional support to patient and family.

4. Provide nonjudgmental acceptance of emotions and behavior of patient and family.

5. Facilitate finding a support group for patient and family.

6. Educate patient and family regarding the importance of follow-up care.

7. Educate patient and family regarding methods to reduce or eliminate stressors as stress has been shown to exacerbate symptoms by diminishing blood supply to the intestinal tract.

8. Dietary instructions to include foods that are appealing, foods that don't exacerbate symptoms, monitor need for dietary and vitamin supplements, adequate fluid intake, and adequate calories and nutritional requirements.

9. Provide meticulous skin care, especially in the case of incontinence.

10.   Monitor for symptoms of complications.

11.   Encourage smoking cessation due to increased peristalsis from nicotine.

12.   Obtain baseline weight and monitor at frequent intervals.

13.   Monitor intake and output (I and O).

14.   Monitor serum laboratory results for deviations from normal ranges.

15.   Instruct patient and family to watch for symptoms of complications and to report any symptoms promptly to physician.

FOR MORE INFORMATION

Crohn's and Colitis Foundation of America, Inc.
National Headquarters
444 Park Avenue South
New York, NY 10016-7374

United Ostomy Association Inc.
Suite 120
36 Executive Park
Irvine, CA 92714-6744

American Digestive Disease Society
420 Lexington Avenue
New York, NY 10017

National Foundation for Ileitis and Colitis, Inc.
295 Madison Avenue
New York, NY 10017

United Ostomy Association
1111 Wilshire Boulevard
Los Angeles, CA 90017

Gastrointestinal Research Foundation
205 West Wacker Drive
Chicago, IL 60606

ASSIGNMENT SHEET: CROHN'S DISEASE

Short Answer

1. Write a brief definition for the terms listed throughout the chapter.

2. Write a brief definition for Crohn's disease.

3. Describe the physiology of the gastrointestinal system.

4. List four (4) risk factors associated with Crohn's disease.

5. List eight (8) signs and symptoms associated with Crohn's disease and the rationale and associated care for each of these symptoms.

6. List seven (7) specific methods used in the diagnosis of Crohn's disease.

7. List three (3) specific surgical procedures used in the treatment of Crohn's disease.

8. Describe three (3) specific nonsurgical methods of treatment for Crohn's disease.

9. List eight (8) complications associated with Crohn's disease, and list the symptoms of each.

10. List fifteen (15) specific considerations for caring for a patient with Crohn's disease.

11. List nine (9) symptoms of dehydration.

12. Describe the following procedures used in the diagnosis or treatment of Crohn's disease.
    a. Hemoccult® stools
    b. Barium enema
    c. Sigmoidoscopy
    d. Colonoscopy
    e. Upper gastrointestinal series (UGI)

13. Write the normal range for each of the following laboratory tests.
    a. Hemoglobin (Hg)
    b. Hematocrit (Hct)
    c. WBC
    d. ESR
    e. Calcium
    f. Electrolytes
       • Sodium
       • Potassium
       • Chloride

KNOWLEDGE INTO ACTION

1. Latisha Jensen, a 29-year-old department store clerk, has been admitted to your facility with an initial diagnosis of Crohn's disease. She has been admitted with the following symptoms: diarrhea, abdominal pain, anorexia, weight loss, and low-grade fever. For each of the symptoms listed, describe the rationale for the symptom and three (3) methods of associated care to keep in mind when caring for a patient, such as Ms. Jensen, with Crohn's disease.

2. You are aware that there are specific complications that could be associated with Crohn's disease. For each of the following complications, describe specific symptoms that could indicate the presence of that complication.
   a. Hemorrhage
   b. Bowel perforation
   c. Intestinal obstruction
   d. Formation of abscess
   e. Toxic megacolon
   f. Formation of fistula
   g. Colorectal cancer

3. Patients who have been in the hospital to rule out a diagnosis of Crohn's disease have had specific tests done to aid in that diagnosis. List and describe three (3) specific tests that could be done to aid in the diagnosis of Crohn's disease.

4. After undergoing testing, Ms. Jensen is found to have extensive Crohn's disease. The physician mentions to her that surgery may need to be performed if her other forms of treatment are not effective. She says to the physician, "Why can't we just do it now and get it over with? Surgery would cure this disease, right?" What will the physician's response be?

5. As a dietitian, you have been consulted to give diet instructions to Ms. Jensen in regard to her Crohn's disease. Describe what specific guidelines could be included in Ms. Jensen's instructions. (List 5.)

UNIT 9

SEXUALLY TRANSMITTED DISEASES

Acquired Immune Deficiency Syndrome (AIDS)

OBJECTIVES

Upon completion of this chapter, the student should be able to:

- Define the key terms listed throughout the chapter
- Describe the physiology of the immune system
- Differentiate between the specific types of T-cells in the immune system
- State a definition for AIDS
- Differentiate between asymptomatic HIV infection, ARC, and AIDS
- List opportunistic infections and diseases associated with AIDS and describe each
- Describe the incidence and statistics associated with the HIV virus
- List signs and symptoms associated with ARC and AIDS and associated care for each of these symptoms
- Identify specific methods for diagnosis of the HIV virus
- Describe the epidemiology of the HIV virus
- Describe the major routes of transmission of the HIV virus
- Describe myths associated with the transmission of the HIV virus
- List blood and body fluids that require universal precautions to prevent the spread of the HIV virus
- List body fluids that do not require universal precautions to prevent the spread of the HIV virus unless they contain visible blood
- Describe recommendations for the general public regarding the prevention of AIDS
- Describe recommendations for persons at increased risk of infection with HTLV-III virus regarding the prevention of AIDS
- Describe recommendations for persons with a positive HTLV-III antibody test regarding the prevention of AIDS
- List the goals of treatment as associated with the HIV virus
- Identify specific methods of treatment for AIDS
- Describe the correct use of a condom as associated with the prevention of AIDS
- Describe specific considerations for caring for a patient with AIDS
- Describe the prognosis of a person infected with the HIV virus

KEY TERMS

Opportunistic illness – illness or infection that occurs during a time when the immune system is depressed or defective

INTRODUCTION

AIDS is a disease caused by the human immunodeficiency virus (HIV). (See Figure 34-1.) The disease causes the body's immune system to become ineffective to fight off infections. The virus attacks the T-4 lymphocytes, which leaves the person susceptible to wide varieties of **opportunistic illness**. The body responds to the presence of this virus by forming antibodies to attack the virus. The virus has also been referred to as the following.

1. Human t-lymphocytic virus, type III (HTLV-III)
2. Lymphadenopathy-associated virus (LAV)
3. AIDS-related virus (ARV)

Asymptomatic –
exhibiting no symptoms

Tuberculosis –
respiratory disease
caused by the organism
*Mycobacterium
tuberculosis*; this disease
may also infect the central
nervous system, gastro-
intestinal system, skeletal
system, immune system,
integumentary system, or
genitourinary system

**Pneumocystis carinii
pneumonia** – type of
pneumonia caused by the
Pneumocystis carinii
organism; commonly seen
with AIDS

Kaposi's sarcoma – type
of cancer that frequently
involves the skin; may
involve other sites of the
body as well; frequently
found in patients with AIDS

Burkitt's lymphoma – a
type of lymphoma that
commonly involves the
lymph nodes, although it
may involve other parts of
the body; commonly
associated with
Epstein-Barr virus, which
causes mononucleosis

Candida albicans –
fungal infection found
primarily in the mouth and
digestive tract,
characterized by white,
painful lesions

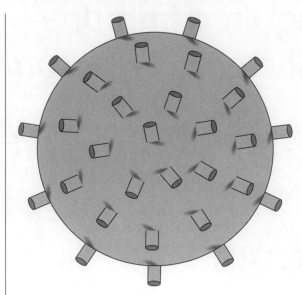

Figure 34-1   Human immunodeficiency virus

AIDS is categorized into three groups according to the symptoms present and the severity of the disease as follows.

1. **Asymptomatic** HIV infection—defined as a person who is HIV positive and remains asymptomatic. The patient is considered able to spread the disease even though he is without symptoms.

2. AIDS-related complex (ARC)—defined as a person who is HIV positive and has specific symptoms. (See section entitled Symptoms of ARC and AIDS.) The symptoms during this phase are often less severe than in a person who has what is referred to as full-blown AIDS.

3. AIDS is diagnosed when a person is HIV positive and also has a T-helper cell (T-4) count under 200, cervical cancer, pulmonary **tuberculosis**, recurrent pneumonia, and/or the following diseases.

   - **Pneumocystis carinii pneumonia** is the most common opportunistic infection for AIDS patients, with 60 to 90% of patients getting the infection. It is the leading cause of death among AIDS patients and is the type of pneumonia caused by the *Pneumocystis carinii* organism.

   - **Kaposi's sarcoma** is the second leading cause of death among AIDS patients. It is a type of cancer that frequently involves the skin and may involve other sites of the body as well.

   - Central nervous system (CNS) involvement is characterized by symptoms of depression, forgetfulness, lack of concentration, decreased alertness, confusion, lack of interest in work and social life, loss of libido, seizures, and/or coma.

   - Toxoplasmosis is an infection due to the *Toxoplasma gondii* organism, which can cause infections of the lungs, liver, immune system, and central nervous system.

   - **Burkitt's lymphoma** is a type of lymphoma that commonly involves the lymph nodes although it may involve other parts of the body; commonly associated with the Epstein-Barr virus, which causes mononucleosis.

   - Herpes simplex virus is responsible for blisters on the mouth or face; Herpes simplex virus type 2 is responsible for sexually transmitted infections of the genital area.

   - **Candida albicans** is a fungal infection found primarily in the mouth and digestive tract and is characterized by white, painful lesions.

Condyloma – growth resembling a wart found on the genital area that is caused by the human papilloma virus

Mycosis fungoides – malignant cancerous growth located on the skin of the body and scalp that has the potential of becoming ulcerated and infected

Mycobacterium – families of organisms that cause leprosy and tuberculosis

Genitourinary – organs contained in the genital and urinary systems of the body

Cryptococcosis – fungal infection; most frequently involves the central nervous system

Cytomegalovirus – virus that most frequently involves the salivary glands

Salivary gland – glands located in the oral cavity that secrete saliva

Cryptosporidiosis – disease caused by the organism *Cryptosporidium parvum*; characterized by diarrhea and abdominal cramps

Gland – organ within the body that secretes a certain substance or hormone; endocrine and exocrine

- **Condyloma** is a growth resembling a wart found on the genital area and is caused by the human papilloma virus.
- **Mycosis fungoides** are malignant cancerous growths located on the skin of the body and scalp that have the potential of becoming ulcerated and infected.
- **Mycobacterium** are groups of organisms that include the organisms that cause leprosy and tuberculosis.
- Tuberculosis is a respiratory disease caused by the organism *Mycobacterium tuberculosis*; this disease may also infect the central nervous system, gastrointestinal system, skeletal system, immune system, integumentary system, or **genitourinary** system.
- **Cryptococcosis** is a fungal infection that most frequently involves the central nervous system.
- **Cytomegalovirus** is a virus that most frequently involves the **salivary glands**.
- **Cryptosporidiosis** is a disease caused by the organism *Cryptosporidium parvum* and is characterized by diarrhea and abdominal cramps.

PHYSIOLOGY OF THE IMMUNE (LYMPH) SYSTEM

The immune system is responsible for fighting diseases and illness caused by viruses, bacteria, and parasites. The main functioning units of the lymph system (immune system) are the specific white blood cells called the lymphocytes. The normal immune system is composed of approximately one trillion lymphocytes. The two main types of lymphocytes are the B-cells and the T-cells. Both of these cells are formed in the bone marrow. The B-cells mature in the red bone marrow, while the T-cells mature in the thymus **gland**. B lymphocytes are responsible for producing antibodies in response to pathogens in the body. T-cells are divided into three groups: "Helper" T-cells (also known as T-4 lymphocytes), which stimulate B-cells to produce antibodies; T "effector" cells, which fight pathogens; and "suppressor" T-cells, which stimulate B-cells to stop producing antibodies after the invading pathogens have been destroyed.

Organs included in the lymph system include thymus gland, lymph nodes, bone marrow, tonsils, appendix, Peyer's patches, and spleen.

STATISTICS

The following statistics give a general view of the severity of the disease as well as statistics regarding population affected, financial statistics, and social statistics.

1. Approximately 90% of people with AIDS are between the ages of 20 and 49.
2. An average of 70% of people diagnosed with AIDS die within 2 years from the time of diagnosis.
3. Some of the losses associated with a diagnosis of AIDS may include but are not limited to the following.
   - Loss of physical strength
   - Loss of social roles
   - Loss of income and savings
   - Loss of mental ability
   - Loss of employment
   - Loss of self-sufficiency
   - Loss of emotional support from family and friends
   - Loss of self-esteem

4. AIDS is the sixth leading cause of death for females between the ages of 25 and 44 in the United States.

5. AIDS is the second leading cause of death for males between the ages of 25 and 44 in the United States.

6. Of the 253,448 reported AIDS cases through December 1992, males accounted for 223,971 (88%) and females accounted for 29,477 (12%). Of the 253,448 patients infected with the HIV virus, 68%, or 171,890 have died.

7. Currently it is estimated that 1.5 million people in the United States are infected with the AIDS virus.

8. Less than 1% of health care workers who were exposed to contaminated blood either through a needle stick or through skin or mucous membranes became infected with the HIV virus.

9. There have been no documented cases of spread of the HIV virus through mouth-to-mouth resuscitation.

10. The HIV virus is a fragile virus and cannot reproduce outside the human body and cannot survive outside the human body for more than a few seconds.

SYMPTOMS OF AIDS-RELATED COMPLEX (ARC) AND ASSOCIATED CARE

Symptoms of ARC may occur anytime between 6 months to 5 years or more after exposure to the virus. Symptoms of ARC include the following.

1. Fatigue is frequently seen in combination with headaches
   - Assist patient with activities of daily living (ADLs) as necessary
   - Schedule care, activities, and treatment around patient's rest schedule
   - Monitor phone calls and visitors around patient's energy level and rest schedule
   - Encourage frequent rest periods
   - Provide assistance as needed to prevent injury due to weakness
   - Provide method for patient to call for assistance
   - Encourage patient to set realistic goals of activities
   - Allow adequate time to do activities and procedures to avoid frustration or possible injury
   - Encourage exercise to maintain muscle strength
   - Provide cane or walker for ambulation and transfer
   - Provide private room to promote rest periods

2. Anorexia
   - Obtain baseline weight and monitor on routine basis
   - Provide nutritional supplements and vitamins
   - Monitor for signs of dehydration, such as decreased urine output, concentrated urine, dry skin, tenting of skin, dry mucous membranes, dry mouth, dry eyes, confusion, hypotension, and constipation
   - Encourage family and friends to bring in food that is appealing to patient as dietary restrictions allow
   - Encourage frequent, small meals as tolerated
   - Offer menu choices according to patient preference
   - Administer parenteral fluids as necessary

- Monitor intake and output (I and O)
- Encourage fluids to prevent dehydration
- Avoid unpleasant sights and odors in room to make meals more appealing
- Provide meticulous mouth care
- Maintain social atmosphere for mealtimes to encourage the patient to eat
- Encourage clothing that enhances patient appearance
- Encourage exercise program as tolerated to increase appetite

3. Weight loss
   - Obtain baseline weight and monitor weight on routine basis
   - Encourage patient to participate in dietary choices
   - Provide nutritional supplements and vitamins
   - Encourage family and friends to bring in food that is appealing to patient as dietary restrictions allow
   - Administer parenteral fluids as necessary
   - Monitor intake and output (I and O)
   - Encourage rest periods before and after meals
   - Avoid unpleasant sights and odors in room to make meals more appealing
   - Provide meticulous mouth care
   - Monitor for skin breakdown due to loss of body tissue
   - Encourage clothing styles that do not draw attention to weight loss
   - Monitor for symptoms of dehydration, e.g. decreased urine output, constipation, dry skin, tenting of skin, dry mouth, dry eyes, concentrated urine, hypotension, and confusion

4. Diarrhea
   - Monitor number, amount, and consistency of stools
   - Monitor intake and output to avoid dehydration
   - Monitor serum electrolytes (*sodium*, *potassium*, and *chloride*)
   - Provide meticulous skin care, especially if incontinent
   - Monitor for presence of hemorrhoids
   - Monitor for rectal discomfort and offer Sitz baths, warm soaks, and topical ointments or suppositories
   - Administer antidiarrheal medications as prescribed by physician
   - Provide frequent skin care, especially to anal area to prevent skin breakdown
   - Monitor for presence of blood (*Hemoccult*®)
   - Offer reassurance to patient
   - Avoid foods that are too hot or too cold as they increase peristalsis
   - Employ enteric precautions

5. Night sweats
   - Offer cool baths in the presence of fever and sweating
   - Avoid plastic mattresses and plastic bed protectors as they increase perspiration
   - Maintain room temperature that is comfortable for the patient
   - Encourage fluid intake to avoid dehydration
   - Monitor temperature at regular intervals

- Offer comfort measures for patient with elevated temperature, such as cool cloth to forehead, partial or complete bath as needed, clothing and bedding changed frequently due to diaphoresis, and encourage fluids to prevent dehydration
- Avoid exposing patient to a draft
- Cover with blankets as necessary
- Monitor intake and output (I and O)
- Use of antiperspirant or deodorant to minimize sweating and odor

6. Lymphadenopathy, especially in the neck, armpits, or groin
   - Monitor for lymphadenopathy
   - Provide comfort measures as necessary due to lymphadenopathy
   - Assist with position for patient comfort

7. Fever
   - Monitor temperature at regular intervals
   - Offer comfort measures for patient with elevated temperature, such as cool cloth to forehead, partial or complete bath as needed, and clothing and bedding changed frequently due to diaphoresis
   - Encourage fluids to prevent dehydration
   - Monitor intake and output (I and O)

8. Arthralgia
   - Assist with position for patient comfort
   - Encourage patient to be as active as possible
   - Protect joints, immobilize joints, and decrease weight-bearing as necessary
   - Provide heat or other methods of pain control, such as massage, relaxation, and imaging
   - Administer medications as prescribed by physician for pain control
   - Monitor level of comfort
   - Assist with ADLs as necessary due to pain
   - Allow adequate time to do as much as possible for themselves, even though it may take longer

9. Myalgia
   - Assist with position for patient comfort
   - Allow adequate time to do activities and procedures to avoid frustration and possible injury
   - Encourage patient to do as much as possible, even though it may take longer
   - Assist with ADLs as necessary
   - Encourage frequent rest periods as needed

10. Mental deterioration
    - Provide calm, quiet environment for patient
    - Avoid startling patient
    - Reorient patient as necessary
    - Allow family members or friends to stay with patient as much as needed if this is reassuring to patient
    - Monitor for level of orientation and changes in mental status
    - Provide protection from injury if the patient is confused

- Offer emotional support to patient and family in the event of confusion
- Assist patient with ADLs in the presence of decreased mental status

11. Persistent cough
    - Encourage fluids to thin mucous secretions to cough up more easily
    - Administer expectorants to aid in coughing up secretions
    - Splint chest to assist patient to cough more effectively
    - Provide container for patient to cough secretions into
    - Dispose of tissues and sputum properly
    - Administer frequent mouth care
    - Meticulous handwashing by patient, visitors, and staff members
    - Employ postural drainage technique to facilitate drainage of mucous from lungs
    - Encourage patient to cover mouth when coughing
    - Observe sputum for signs of hemoptysis or infection
    - Educate regarding effective coughing techniques to facilitate productiveness of cough
    - Humidify air as necessary
    - Utilize universal precautions when handling any blood or body fluids (See Appendix C)

12. Visual disturbances
    - Evaluate for ability to drive safely
    - Avoid eye strain
    - Dim lights in room according to patient preference
    - Avoid injury due to visual disturbances
    - Promote adequate lighting when reading, watching TV, or other activities
    - Remove environmental hazards such as throw rugs, cluttered hallways, and excess furniture

13. Intestinal inflammation
    - Observe color, amount, and consistency of stools
    - Monitor for abdominal pain and abdominal distention
    - Avoid foods that increase intestinal gas formation
    - Encourage fluids
    - Control odors in patient room with ventilation and room deodorizers
    - Provide private room as necessary
    - Prevent embarrassment for the patient due to odors
    - Assist with position for patient comfort
    - Measure abdominal girth on routine basis, with area marked so same area measured each time for accuracy
    - Avoid constrictive clothing and undergarments

14. Thick, white crust covering inside of mouth
    - Provide meticulous mouth care
    - Offer foods and fluids that are nonirritating to the mouth
    - Administer nasogastric (NG) or parenteral fluids as necessary
    - Administer medications as prescribed by physician to treat the infection
    - Observe for sores in mouth
    - Offer foods that are easy to chew

15. Sores in the mouth, anus, or nose
    - Monitor for sores in the mouth, anus, or nose
    - Provide meticulous skin care with mild, unscented soap
    - Avoid use of tapes and other adhesives on skin as able
    - Apply medications or creams to prevent itching
    - Provide protective mittens for confused patients to prevent scratching and damage to skin
    - Encourage fluid intake
    - Pat skin gently dry
    - Avoid harsh soaps or bleach in clothing and linens
    - Avoid clothing and bedding that is irritating
    - Assess skin redness and irritation on routine basis
    - Observe for open areas and signs of infection. Symptoms of infection include redness, swelling, pain, discharge, area is hot to touch, loss of function, or fever.
    - Avoid use of scented lotions and cosmetics
    - Administer antihistamines to relieve itching
    - Provide meticulous mouth care at frequent intervals through day
    - Offer food and beverages that are nonabrasive, e.g. avoid spicy foods, acidic fruits and juices, carbonated beverages, highly salted foods, and foods that are extremely hot or cold
    - Offer ice chips and fluids frequently according to patient preference
    - Use humidifier at bedside to humidify air
    - Monitor intake and output (I and O)
    - Elevate head while sleeping
    - Administer antacids as necessary
    - Administer nasogastric (NG) or parenteral fluids as necessary
    - Administer medications as prescribed by physician to treat any accompanying infection
    - Offer foods that are easy to chew and swallow
    - Utilize antiseptic mouthwash and soft bristled toothbrush
    - Maintain proper fit of dentures
    - Provide moisture to lips with lip balm, mineral oil, or petroleum jelly
    - Avoid use of harsh toothpaste
16. Dyspnea
    - Assist with position for patient comfort
    - Administer oxygen as needed and as directed by physician
    - Avoid constrictive garments and undergarments
    - Use fan in room to circulate air and assist in making breathing easier
    - Encourage frequent rest periods to conserve energy
    - Arrange schedule of activities around patient rest periods
    - Assist with ADLs as necessary
    - Assess breath sounds on routine basis
    - Observe for signs of hypoxia, e.g. cyanosis, diaphoresis, decreased level of consciousness, and confusion
    - Monitor ease of respirations and respiratory rate

Exposure – process of having come in contact with an infectious person or an infectious agent; process of coming in contact with or being subjected to radiation

Epidemiology – study of the cause of disease and disease transmission and methods to control disease

Homosexual – sexual preference or attraction for persons of the same sex

Bisexual – sexual preference for a person of either sex

Heterosexual – sexual preference or attraction for persons of the opposite sex

Hemophilia – hereditary disorder in which there is an abnormality in the clotting mechanism of the blood and prolonged bleeding time

Coagulation – refers to the clotting of the blood

- Encourage as many activities as possible in a sitting position, e.g. dressing, bathing, cooking, and cleaning
- Humidify air as needed
- Provide reassurance to patient

DIAGNOSIS

Diagnosis is based on the following methods. Note that a patient's blood may not develop antibodies for several weeks to several months.

1. Symptoms
2. ELISA test (enzyme-linked immunosorbent assay test)—used to detect the presence of antibodies to HIV; this test is also used in the screening of blood and blood products
3. Western Blot test—used to detect antibodies to HIV; this test is more specific than the ELISA test and also more expensive
4. Presence of characteristic opportunistic infections
   - ELISA tests and Western Blot tests are available through the state health departments as well as many local clinics, laboratories, and health care facilities
   - Psychological counseling should be done both before and after the performance of tests to diagnose AIDS
   - If the blood tests are negative, and if the client has participated in behaviors that may have infected him, the possibility of retesting in 6 months will be discussed. The majority of individuals will develop antibodies within 2 to 12 weeks after **exposure** to the virus; however, a small percentage may take up to 6 months to develop antibodies to the virus.
   - If the ELISA test is positive, it will be retested. If it is positive a second time, the Western Blot test will be performed. The tests combined provide 99.9% accuracy.

EPIDEMIOLOGY OF AIDS

According to the U.S. Department of Health and Human Services,* the following is the **epidemiology** of AIDS, according to the groups of people affected.

1. Sexually active **homosexual** and **bisexual** men, 73%, some of whom also used intravenous drugs
2. **Heterosexual** men or women who presently abuse or formerly abused intravenous drugs, 17%
3. Person with **hemophilia** or other **coagulation** disorders, 1%
4. Heterosexual contacts of someone with AIDS or at risk for AIDS, 1%
5. Persons who have had transfusions of blood or blood products, 2%
6. Infants born to infected mothers, 1%
7. Some 5% of the patients do not fall into any of these groups, but researchers believe that transmission occurred in similar ways

* Source: *Coping With AIDS: Psychological and Social Considerations in Helping People with HTLV-III Infection.* Published by the U.S. Department of Health and Human Services, 1986.

Amniotic fluid – fluid within the amniotic sac that cushions the developing fetus and protects the fetus from injury

Pleural fluid – the fluid that accumulates with pleural effusion

Pericardial fluid – fluid in the sac (cavity) surrounding the heart

Peritoneal fluid – fluid located in the peritoneum that cushions the organs from one another and prevents friction between the organs

TRANSMISSION OF AIDS

The AIDS virus has been known to be transmitted or is capable of transmission through the following modes.

1. Sexual intercourse with an infected person (vaginal, anal, or oral)
2. Using drug needles or syringes previously used by an infected person
3. Mother to infant before, during, or after birth; AIDS may be spread through the breast milk of an infected mother
4. Receiving blood or blood products; blood has been routinely tested for the AIDS virus since 1985, and the possibility of transmission in this manner is extremely low. The person may donate blood prior to the onset of the body making antibodies against the virus and prior to the onset of symptoms.
   - Even though there is a remote possibility of transmitting the AIDS virus through "French kissing," there have been no documented cases of transmission in this manner.

MYTHS REGARDING TRANSMISSION OF AIDS

Many myths have been circulating through the United States regarding methods of transmission of AIDS. The following methods *cannot* transmit the AIDS virus.

1. Casual contact with a person infected with the AIDS virus
2. Mosquito bites or other insects
3. Eating utensils and drinking glasses
4. Eating food that a person infected with the AIDS virus has prepared
5. Toilet seats, telephones, or showers
6. Hugging, shaking hands with, or touching a person who is infected with the AIDS virus
7. Coughing or sneezing by the person infected with the AIDS virus
8. Donating blood
9. Swimming pools

UNIVERSAL PRECAUTIONS

The following blood and body fluids require the use of universal precautions any time you come in contact with them or are likely to come in contact with them.
   - Blood
   - Semen
   - **Amniotic fluid**
   - Vaginal fluids
   - **Pleural fluid**
   - **Pericardial fluid**
   - **Peritoneal fluid**
   - Synovial fluid
   - Cerebrospinal fluid

Body fluids that do not require universal precautions for the spread of the HIV virus (unless they contain visible blood).
   - Tears
   - Urine

- Vomit
- Feces
- Saliva
- Nasal drainage
- Sputum
- Sweat

These body fluids and waste products have not been documented to spread the HIV virus, but they are capable of spreading other illness and diseases.

PREVENTION OF AIDS

The U.S. Public Health Service recommends that the following steps be taken to prevent spread of HTLV-III infection and AIDS.

Recommendations for the General Public

- Don't have sex with multiple partners or with persons who have had multiple partners (including prostitutes). The more partners you have, the greater your risk of contracting AIDS.
- Obviously, avoiding sex with people with AIDS, members of the risk groups, or people who have had a positive result on the HTLV-III antibody test would eliminate the risk of sexually transmitted infection by the virus. However, if you do have sex with a person you think is infected, protect yourself by taking appropriate precautions to prevent contact with the person's body fluids. ("Body fluids" include blood, semen, urine, feces, saliva, and women's genital secretions.)
  — Use condoms, which may reduce the possibility of transmitting the virus.
  — Avoid practices that may injure body tissues (e.g. anal intercourse).
  — Avoid oral-genital contact.
  — Avoid open-mouthed, intimate kissing.
- Don't use intravenous drugs. If you do, don't share needles or syringes.

People at increased risk of HTLV-III infection include homosexual and bisexual men; present or past intravenous drug users; people with clinical or laboratory evidence of infection, such as signs or symptoms compatible with AIDS or AIDS-related illness; people born in countries where heterosexual transmission is thought to play a major role in the spread of HTLV-III (e.g. Haiti and Central African countries); male or female prostitutes and their sex partners; sex partners of infected persons or persons at increased risk; persons with hemophilia who have received clotting factor products; and newborn infants of high-risk or infected mothers.

Recommendations for Persons at Increased Risk of Infection with HTLV-III

Those at increased risk of infection should follow the preceding recommendations given for the general public. In addition, because it is possible to carry HTLV-III without knowing it and thus transmit it to others, the following recommendations should also be heeded.

- Consult your physician for counseling. Consider asking for the HTLV-III antibody test, which would enable you to know your status and take appropriate actions.
- During sexual intercourse, protect your partner from contact with your body fluids (blood, semen, urine, feces, saliva, and women's genital secretions).

- Don't donate blood, plasma, body organs, other body tissue, or sperm.
- If you are a woman at increased risk, consider the risk to your baby before becoming pregnant as AIDS can be transmitted from infected mother to infant. Before becoming pregnant, you should take the HTLV-III antibody test. If you choose to become pregnant, you should be tested during the term of the pregnancy.

Recommendations for Persons with a Positive HTLV-III Antibody Test*

- Seek regular medical evaluation and follow-up.
- Either avoid sexual activity or inform your prospective partner of your antibody test results and protect him or her from contact with your body fluids during sex. Body fluids include blood, semen, urine, feces, saliva, and women's genital secretions. Use a condom, and avoid practices that may injure body tissues (e.g. anal intercourse). Avoid oral-genital contact and open-mouthed, intimate kissing.
- Inform your present and previous sex partners, and any persons with whom needles may have been shared, of their potential exposure to HTLV-III and encourage them to seek counseling and antibody testing from their physician or at appropriate health clinics.
- Don't share toothbrushes, razors, or other items that could become contaminated with blood.
- If you use drugs, enroll in a drug treatment program. Needles and other drug equipment must never be shared.
- Don't donate blood, plasma, body organs, other body tissue, or sperm.
- Clean blood or other body fluid spills on household or other surfaces with freshly diluted household bleach—1 part bleach to 10 parts water. Don't use bleach on wounds.
- Inform your doctor, dentist, and eye doctor of your positive HTLV-III status so proper precautions can be taken to protect you and others.
- Women with a positive antibody test should avoid pregnancy until more is known about the risks of transmitting HTLV-III from mother to infant.
- In addition to these recommendations for the public, health workers are reminded to follow normal enteric procedures. Be especially careful when handling or disposing of hypodermic needles. Do not resheath or break needles.

TREATMENT

The treatment of AIDS has two main goals:

1. Prevention of complications
2. Treatment of symptoms

Specific methods of treatment for AIDS include the following.

1. Medications:
   - AZT (also known as azidothymidine, zidovudine, or Retrovir). The purpose of this medication is to block the reproduction of the AIDS virus; AZT is recommended when the T-4 count falls below 500 (a normal T-4 count is greater than 1,000).
   - ddC (Zalcitabine)
   - ddL (Dideoxyinosine)

---

* Source: *Coping With AIDS: Psychological and Social Considerations in Helping People with HTLV-III Infection.* Published by the U.S. Department of Health and Human Services, 1986.

Antifungal – substance used to destroy fungus

Spermicide – material or solution that destroys sperm

Sexually transmitted disease (STD) – disease that is transmitted as a result of sexual activity with an infected person

2. **Antifungal** medications to treat fungal infections

3. Radiation and chemotherapy for treatment of the malignancies associated with the HIV virus

4. Antidiarrheal medications and antiemetics

5. Antidepressant medications as necessary

6. Pentam or pentamidine for the treatment of *Pneumocystis carinii pneumonia*

7. Treatment for cytomegalovirus eye infections includes Foscarnet or Ganciclovir

8. Yeast infections and fungal infections are treated with Fluconazole

9. Chemotherapy, radiation, or alpha interferon are often necessary for the treatment of Kaposi's sarcoma

CORRECT USE OF A CONDOM

1. Always use a condom that is made of latex rubber.

2. The package should specify that the condom is to prevent disease.

3. The condom should cover the entire penis.

4. Condoms are more likely to break during anal intercourse due to the greater amount of friction involved.

5. A **spermicide** containing nonoxynol-9 has been shown to kill germs that transmit **sexually transmitted disease (STDs)** and should be used in conjunction with condoms.

6. Check the expiration date on the condom package.

7. Use a water-based lubricant if one is needed when using a condom.

8. Condoms should be stored in a cool, dry place. Direct sunlight should be avoided. Do not store condoms in an area that is exposed to extreme temperatures.

9. Use caution when opening a condom package to prevent damage to the condom.

10. A condom should never be used more than one time.

11. Apply the condom when the penis is erect prior to any contact between the penis and the partner's body.

12. Dispose of condoms where no one else will handle them.

13. Wash hands thoroughly after any contact with a used condom.

CONSIDERATIONS FOR CARE

1. Educate patient and family regarding the disease process.

2. Educate patient and family regarding forms of treatment as well as side effects of medications.

3. Provide emotional support to patient and family.

4. Provide nonjudgmental acceptance of emotions and behavior of patient and family.

5. Facilitate finding a support group for patient and family.

6. Counseling may be necessary for patient and family to work through emotions associated with the disease.

7. Depression may develop as a result of the patient being unable to provide financially, contribute to responsibilities in the home, other responsibilities

Hospice – supportive care that is directed at meeting the social, spiritual, physical, psychological, and safety needs of a dying person and his or her family

Pneumococcal – caused by pneumococci

previously held by the patient, as well as the financial burden imposed by medical care.

8. Educate patient and family regarding the importance of taking medications at the scheduled time.

9. Educate patient and family regarding the importance of follow-up care.

10. Monitor neurological function and muscle strength.

11. Encourage patient to perform activities and care around periods of peak energy.

12. Keep in mind feelings the patient may have accompanying the disease, such as anger, fear of discrimination, fear of death, and fear of loss of network of family and friends.

13. Keep in mind the strain put on family relationships if the family is unaware of gay life style or drug abuse prior to the diagnosis of AIDS.

14. Refer to social workers to assist with financial difficulties.

15. Refer to physical therapist and occupational therapist to assist patient in methods of maintaining or improving strength and methods of compensating for losses in muscles strength and coordination.

16. Educate patient and family regarding methods to prevent the spread of the HIV virus.

17. Refer to Home Health Care Agency, **Hospice** care agency, Public Health Nurse Agency, or similar regarding care in the home.

18. Refer to a home meal delivery system.

19. Allow patient to ventilate feelings, and take threats of suicide seriously; threats of suicide should be dealt with promptly with referrals made to counselors, physician, and therapists.

20. Refer for therapy for intravenous drug abusers.

21. Counsel patients of child-bearing age regarding the risks involved with becoming pregnant and the chances involved regarding passing the disease on to children before, during, or after birth. There is a 30 to 50% chance that the child of an infected mother will also be infected.

22. Refer for legal assistance for patients wishing to complete living wills, wills, and/or legal guardianships.

23. Refer for assistance with funeral arrangements for patient and family as necessary.

24. Patients infected with the HIV virus should be encouraged to alert past sexual partners, intravenous drug use partners, as well as health care professionals who are or have been involved in their care. Notification of health care professionals has been a controversial issue due to the issue of confidentiality.

25. Health care professionals should be knowledgeable about and feel comfortable discussing homosexual practices and intravenous drug use in order to relate to patients and assist them in coping and making decisions.

26. Educate patient that condoms are not 100% effective in the prevention of AIDS and other STDs.

27. Educate patient that forms of birth control are not effective in the prevention of AIDS and STDs and should be used in conjunction with condoms.

28. Be aware that the stress of being infected with the AIDS virus may be less stressful than not knowing whether or not you are infected.

29. Educate patient regarding the availability of influenza vaccine and **pneumococcal** vaccine, according to recommendation of the physician.

30. Facilitate dietary consult to assist patient and family in meal planning to meet nutritional needs.
31. Refer to social service worker or clergy when the family is deciding what to tell other family members and friends regarding the diagnosis of AIDS.
32. Encourage care givers to take a break from routine cares of the patient as able.
33. Monitor for oral and skin lesions.
34. Educate patient to avoid people with illness and infections due to compromised immune system.
35. Meticulous handwashing on the part of the staff, patient, and visitors.

PROGNOSIS

Greater than 50% of people with the AIDS virus will develop an AIDS-related illness within 10 years after exposure if no treatment is initiated. It is estimated that 20 to 30% of people infected with the AIDS virus will develop an AIDS-related illness within 5 years. At this point, no person diagnosed with "full-blown" AIDS has been known to survive. Death does not come from the HIV virus itself, but from the opportunistic infections that are able to take over the body due to the compromised immune system.

FOR MORE INFORMATION

National AIDS Hotline (1-800-342-AIDS)
(1-800-342-2437)

CDC National AIDS Clearinghouse
P.O. Box 6003
Rockville, MD 20849-6003

U.S. Public Health Service
Public Affairs Office
Room 725-H
Hubert H. Humphrey Building
200 Independence Avenue, SW
Washington, DC 20201
(202) 245-6867

American Red Cross AIDS Education Office
1730 D Street, NW
Washington, DC 20006
(202) 737-8300

ASSIGNMENT SHEET: AIDS

Short Answer

1. Write a brief definition for the terms listed throughout the chapter.

2. Describe the physiology of the immune system.

3. Differentiate between the three (3) specific types of T-cells.

4. Write a brief definition for AIDS.

5. Differentiate between the definition for each of the following.

   a. Asymptomatic HIV infection
   b. AIDS-related complex (ARC)
   c. AIDS

6. List fourteen (14) opportunistic infections or diseases associated with AIDS, and write a brief definition for each.

7. List ten (10) statistics that refer to the incidence of AIDS and other pertinent information regarding AIDS.

8. List sixteen (16) signs and symptoms associated with ARC and AIDS and associated care for each of these symptoms.

9. Identify four (4) specific methods used to aid in the diagnosis of AIDS.

10. Describe seven (7) statistics relating to the epidemiology of the HIV virus.

11. Describe the four (4) possible routes of transmission for the AIDS virus.

12. Describe nine (9) myths regarding the routes of transmission for the AIDS virus.

13. List nine (9) body fluids that require universal precautions to prevent the spread of the HIV virus.

14. List eight (8) body fluids that do not require universal precautions to prevent the spread of the HIV virus, unless they contain visible blood.

15. Describe three (3) recommendations for the general public regarding prevention of AIDS.

16. Describe four (4) recommendations for persons at increased risk of infection with HTLV-III regarding prevention of AIDS.

17. Describe ten (10) recommendations for persons with a positive HTLV-III antibody test regarding prevention of AIDS.

18. List the two (2) main goals associated with treating AIDS.

19. Identify nine (9) specific methods of treatment for AIDS.

20. Describe thirteen (13) specific items necessary for the correct use of a condom in prevention of the spread of the HIV virus (and other STDs).

21. List thirty-five (35) considerations for caring for a patient with AIDS.

22. Describe the prognosis for the person infected with the HIV virus.

23. Describe the losses a patient may suffer with AIDS.

24. List ten (10) symptoms associated with dehydration.

25. Write the normal range for each of the following laboratory tests.

    a. T-4 lymphocyte count
    b. Sodium (Na)
    c. Potassium (K)
    d. Chloride (Cl)

KNOWLEDGE INTO ACTION

1. You have been asked to give a presentation on AIDS at a community meeting. You want to tell them the facts about AIDS as well as the myths. You want to start with the methods that have been known to transmit the AIDS virus. (List 4.)

2. You also want to list methods that *cannot* transmit the AIDS virus. (List 7.)

3. Several of the members of the group are concerned about themselves and their children regarding transmission of the AIDS virus. Describe what you would tell them about steps that could be taken to prevent the spread of the AIDS virus.

4. Currently there is no cure for the AIDS virus, and a vaccination has not been approved. There are treatments, however, that have been shown to prevent, treat, or delay complications, as well as treatment for the symptoms that often accompany AIDS. Describe five (5) specific methods of treatment that can be used for the treatment of symptoms or to prevent, treat, or delay the onset of complications.

5. You are going to finish your presentation with information regarding the correct use of a condom in the protection of transmission of the AIDS virus. Describe seven (7) pieces of information you would include in your presentation regarding the correct use of a condom.

6. Katie Frey, a 29-year-old female with a long history of AIDS, is being discharged from the hospital. She says to you, "I realize I'm getting weaker and I probably don't have long to live." What will your response be?

7. In your conversation with Katie, she asks you about resources that would be able to assist her once she gets home. What will your response be?

8. Katie's parents arrive to take her home from the hospital. They say to you, "Katie never really has said much about this cancer that she has. Can you tell us a little bit more about it?" What will your response be?

9. You are working in a family health clinic that centers around pregnancy testing and family care. Linda Drake, a 31-year-old female who is HIV positive, comes to your clinic for counseling. She is talking to you about becoming pregnant "before my biological clock runs out." She also admits she is concerned the child could also be infected with the HIV virus. What will your response be?

10. Describe the importance of utilizing universal precautions when caring for a patient who is HIV positive.

CHAPTER 35
Syphilis

INTRODUCTION

Syphilis is a sexually transmitted disease (STD) that is spread through contact with a person who has syphilis.

STATISTICS

Approximately 130,000 new cases of syphilis are reported annually in the United States.

CAUSE

Syphilis is caused by the bacterium *Treponema pallidum*. The bacterium can spread throughout the body causing damage to many organs.

TRANSMISSION

Syphilis is spread through contact with a person who has syphilis during sexual intercourse, oral sex, or anal sex. The bacterium spreads via the sores of an infected person to the mucous membranes of the sexual partner's anus, genital area, or mouth. Infection by an inanimate object is rare due to the fact that the *Treponema pallidum* bacterium is very fragile. The bacterium can be transmitted to an unborn child from the infected mother.

KEY TERMS

Chancre – skin lesion that is present during syphilis; generally appearing two to three weeks after exposure to *Treponema pallidum*

Vulva – external female reproductive parts or genitalia

SIGNS, SYMPTOMS, AND ASSOCIATED CARE

Syphilis has been divided into four stages—primary, secondary, latent, and late (or tertiary).

Stage 1: The symptom in the primary stage is a **chancre**.
- Appears 10 days to 3 months after exposure
- Generally painless and often goes undetected
- Appears on cervix, penis, **vulva**, vagina, tongue, lips, or other parts of the body
- Disappears within a few weeks whether treated or not

Syphilis is very contagious during this stage.

Stage 2: If treatment is not obtained during the primary stage, the disease progresses to the secondary stage with the following signs and symptoms.
  a. Skin rash
- Appears 3 to 6 weeks after the appearance of the chancre
- Rash may cover the entire body or only on the hands or feet
- Any physical contact during this stage may spread the disease
- Heals whether treated or not in several weeks to several months

  b. Headache
- Dim lights in event of photophobia accompanying headache
- Administer medications or other methods of pain relief, such as relaxation techniques, imaging, and massage
- Assist with position for patient comfort
- Provide calm, quiet environment for the patient
- Provide pain control methods, such as relaxation techniques, massage, imaging, and pain medications, as prescribed by physician
- Encourage patient to avoid eye strain during periods of headache
- Encourage frequent rest periods as necessary
- Monitor phone calls and visitors to promote rest periods

  c. Fever
- Monitor temperature at routine intervals
- Provide comfort measures for patient with elevated temperature, such as cool cloth to forehead, partial or complete bath as needed, clothing and bedding changed frequently due to diaphoresis, and encourage fluids to prevent dehydration
- Avoid exposing patient to a draft
- Cover with blankets as necessary
- Monitor intake and output (I and O)
- Maintain comfortable room temperature for patient
- Avoid plastic mattresses and plastic bed protectors as they increase perspiration
- Use antiperspirant or deodorant to minimize sweating and odor

  d. Sore throat
- Provide meticulous mouth care at frequent intervals through day
- Offer food and beverages that are nonabrasive, e.g. avoid spicy foods, acidic fruits and juices, carbonated beverages, highly salted foods, and foods that are extremely hot or cold

- Offer ice chips and fluids often according to patient preference
- Place humidifier at bedside to humidify air
- Monitor intake and output (I and O)
- Administer nasogastric (NG) or parenteral fluids as necessary
- Administer medications as prescribed by physician to treat any accompanying infection
- Offer foods that are easy to chew and swallow
- Utilize antiseptic mouthwash

e. Fatigue

- Assist patient with activities of daily living (ADLs) as necessary
- Schedule care, activities, and treatment around patient's rest schedule
- Monitor phone calls and visitors around patient's energy level and rest schedule
- Encourage frequent rest periods
- Encourage activity as able
- Provide assistance as needed to prevent injury due to weakness
- Provide method for patient to call for assistance
- Encourage patient to set realistic goals of activities
- Allow adequate time to do activities and procedures to avoid frustration or possible injury
- Encourage exercise to maintain muscle strength
- Provide cane or walker for ambulation and transfer
- Provide private room to promote rest periods

f. Alopecia

- Offer emotional support for patient
- Assist in obtaining wigs, scarves, or head covering as patient desires
- Avoid use of white linens as this may make hair loss more noticeable and distressing to the patient
- Avoid use of harsh shampoos, chemicals, colors, or permanents in hair
- Avoid using blowdriers or curling irons in hair
- Cut hair in a style that is easy to maintain

g. Generalized lymphadenopathy

- Monitor for lymphadenopathy
- Provide comfort measures as necessary due to lymphadenopathy

h. Anorexia

- Obtain baseline weight and monitor on routine basis
- Encourage patient to participate in dietary choices
- Provide nutritional supplements and vitamins
- Monitor for signs of dehydration, such as decreased urine output, concentrated urine, dry skin, tenting of skin, dry mucous membranes, dry mouth, dry eyes, confusion, hypotension, and constipation
- Encourage family and friends to bring in food that is appealing to patient as dietary restrictions allow
- Encourage frequent, small meals as tolerated
- Administer parenteral fluids as necessary
- Monitor intake and output (I and O)
- Encourage fluids to prevent dehydration

- Avoid unpleasant sights and odors in room to make meals more appealing
- Provide meticulous mouth care
- Maintain social atmosphere for mealtimes to encourage the patient to eat
- Encourage clothing that enhances patient appearance
- Encourage exercise program as tolerated to increase appetite

Syphilis is very contagious during this stage. Symptoms of this stage may last up to two (2) years.

Stage 3: If treatment is not obtained during the secondary stage, the disease progresses to the latent stage during which there are no symptoms and the individual is no longer contagious.

Stage 4: Two-thirds of those untreated will have no further symptoms of the disease; however, if untreated, one-third will go on to develop late (tertiary) syphilis with complications. Complications are due to the bacteria invading the specific organs and tissues of the body.

COMPLICATIONS

Complications of untreated syphilis include the following:

1. Neurosyphilis occurs when the syphilis bacterium invades the nervous system
   - Occurs in 3 to 7% of untreated syphilis
   - Symptoms include headache, stiff neck, fever, seizures, numbness, weakness, or visual complaints
   - May take up to 20 years for the symptoms to manifest
2. Blindness
3. Mental illness
4. Heart disease
5. Bone damage
6. Joint damage
7. Death

DIAGNOSIS

The early symptoms of syphilis are similar to other diseases, thus the disease is termed "the great imitator." Diagnosis of syphilis is made in one or more of the following methods.

1. Presence of symptoms
2. Syphilis bacteria isolated from specimen of chancre
3. Blood tests, such as the *venereal disease research laboratory (VDRL)* or *rapid plasma reagin (RPR)* tests. Both of these blood tests can produce false-positive results in individuals with certain viral infections, autoimmune disorders, or other conditions.
4. *Fluorescent treponemal antibody-absorption (FTA-ABS)* test is a serum test that is accurate in 70 to 90% of cases
5. *Treponema pallidum hemagglutination assay (TPHA)* test, which is used to detect syphilis antibodies in the person's blood
6. Lumbar puncture is performed to check for infection of the nervous system. This is especially performed during the latent or late stage.

Stillbirth – fetus that is dead at birth

Condoms – latex or rubber sheathes placed over the penis during sexual intercourse to aid in the prevention of pregnancy or sexually transmitted diseases

TREATMENT

Penicillin is generally used to treat syphilis, and the individual is no longer able to transmit the disease 24 hours after beginning treatment. A blood test is important to check the effectiveness of treatment. Neurosyphilis may need to be retested up to 2 years following treatment. Any organ damage that has already occurred will not respond to the treatment of the disease.

EFFECTS OF SYPHILIS DURING PREGNANCY

1. Approximately 25% of pregnancies occurring in women with active syphilis infection will result in **stillbirth**.
2. Approximately 40 to 70% of pregnancies occurring in women with active syphilis will transmit the disease to the child.
3. Infants with congenital syphilis will generally develop symptoms between 2 weeks and 3 months after birth.
   - Skin sores, which are infectious and require extreme caution when handling
   - Hoarse cry
   - Rash
   - Hepatomegaly
   - Jaundice
   - Anemia
   - Deformities of the bones, skin, eyes, or teeth
4. Symptoms in infants may go undetected, and the child may develop symptoms of late-stage syphilis when older, generally in the teenage years.

PREVENTION OF TRANSMISSION

1. Care must be taken to avoid contact with the chancres associated with syphilis.
2. Use **condoms** during sexual intercourse.
3. Test and treat syphilis in the early phases of pregnancy.

CORRECT USE OF A CONDOM

1. Always use a condom that is made of latex rubber.
2. The package should specify that the condom is to prevent disease.
3. The condom should cover the entire penis.
4. Condoms are more likely to break during anal intercourse due to the greater amount of friction involved.
5. A spermicide containing nonoxynol-9 has been shown to kill germs that transmit STDs and should be used in conjunction with condoms.
6. Check the expiration date on the condom package.
7. Use a water-based lubricant if one is needed when using a condom.
8. Condoms should be stored in a cool, dry place. Direct sunlight should be avoided. Do not store condoms in an area that is exposed to extreme temperatures.
9. Use caution when opening a condom package to prevent damage to the condom.
10. A condom should never be used more than one time.

11. Apply the condom when the penis is erect prior to any contact between the penis and the partner's body.

12. Dispose of condoms where no one else will handle them.

13. Wash hands thoroughly after any contact with a used condom.

CONSIDERATIONS FOR CARE

1. Universal precautions must be taken during any exposure to blood or body fluids. (See Appendix C.)

2. Educate patient regarding preventing transmission of the disease.

3. Educate patient regarding treatment as well as possible side effects of the medications. Educate patient regarding importance of completing medication regimen even though symptoms may be gone.

4. If a woman is pregnant, she should be tested for syphilis if any chance of infection has been present.

5. Follow-up is important to check the effectiveness of the treatment.

6. Notify sexual partners of the disease diagnosis so they can get tested and treated.

7. Keep lesions clean and dry.

8. Health care professionals should use protective devices during any possible contact with blood, body fluids, or lesions drainage.

9. Wound and skin isolation is often used.

FOR MORE INFORMATION

National Institute of Allergy and Infectious Diseases
National Institutes of Health
Bethesda, MD 20892

ASSIGNMENT SHEET: SYPHILIS

Short Answer

1. Write a brief definition for the terms listed throughout the chapter.

2. Write a brief definition for syphilis.

3. Describe the incidence of syphilis.

4. List the cause of syphilis.

5. Describe how syphilis can be transmitted.

6. Describe each of the four (4) stages of syphilis, the symptoms, and associated care with each.

7. Describe seven (7) specific complications that are often associated with syphilis.

8. Describe six (6) specific methods used to aid in the diagnosis of syphilis.

9. Describe the specific method of treatment for syphilis.

10. Describe four (4) effects of syphilis on pregnancy and the newborn.

11. Describe three (3) specific methods used to prevent the transmission of syphilis.

12. Describe nine (9) considerations for caring for a patient with syphilis.

13. Describe thirteen (13) considerations for the correct use of a condom.

KNOWLEDGE INTO ACTION

1. Scott Kinder, a 21-year-old male with a new diagnosis of syphilis, has been admitted to the hospital. His physician feels Mr. Kinder was exposed to the syphilis several years previously. On admission, Mr. Kinder complains of headache, stiff neck, fever, numbness, weakness, and visual changes. During his hospitalization, Mr. Kinder has a seizure. His physician orders a lumbar puncture. Due to the symptoms Mr. Kinder currently has, as well as the order for a lumbar puncture, for what could the physician be checking?

2. You are working at a public health and family care clinic. Lonnie Poller, a 17-year-old high school student, comes to the clinic after her boyfriend has recently been diagnosed with syphilis. Which of the following tests could most likely be ordered to see if Lonnie has also been infected with syphilis? (Choose the best answer.)

   a. Lumbar puncture and electrophoresis
   b. Elisa test and western blot test
   c. Fluorescent treponemal antibody-absorption test (FTA-ABS)
   d. Hemoglobin and hematocrit

3. Lonnie tests positive for syphilis, and the physician wants to initiate treatment for the syphilis immediately. List the treatment of choice for syphilis.

4. During this examination with the physician for the treatment of her syphilis, Lonnie confides that she thinks she may be pregnant as she has missed two menstrual periods, her breasts are tender and swollen, and she has been experiencing what she describes as "morning sickness." What information could the physician share with Lonnie regarding the effects of syphilis during pregnancy?

5. Lonnie and her sexual partner have both been treated for syphilis. Describe what you could tell them about condom use for the prevention of the spread of syphilis in the future or with future partners. (List seven [7] things to remember for correct use of a condom.)

6. You have a nursing student working with you this semester. You are discussing the importance of utilizing universal precautions. Describe how you would describe universal precautions to the student.

Genital Herpes

OBJECTIVES

Upon completion of this chapter, the student should be able to:

■ Define the key terms listed throughout the chapter

■ State a specific definition for genital herpes

■ Describe the incidence of genital herpes

■ List the cause of genital herpes

■ Describe the signs and symptoms of genital herpes and associated care for these symptoms

■ Identify specific methods for diagnosis of genital herpes

■ Identify specific methods for treatment of genital herpes

■ Describe complications that may result from genital herpes

■ Describe specific considerations for caring for a patient with genital herpes

KEY TERMS

Sensory nerves – nerves that transmit sensory impulses to the brain

INTRODUCTION

Genital herpes is a sexually transmitted disease (STD) caused by the herpes simplex virus (HSV). Currently there is no cure for genital herpes, though there are medications available to help control and prevent symptoms.

STATISTICS

Herpes simplex affects an estimated 30 million people in the United States with 500,000 new cases reported annually (1,500 to 2,200 of these occur in newborn babies).

CAUSE

Herpes simplex virus 1 and herpes simplex virus 2 are the two types of herpes simplex virus. Both types of HSV can cause infections either in the genital area or the oral area. "Cold sores" are generally associated with HSV type 1. Infections in the genital area are most frequently associated with HSV type 2 and can involve the anus, penis, upper legs, buttocks, or vagina. Spread of HSV type 2 occurs by sexual contact with an infected person or through contact with the open sores or blisters associated with the infection. The virus is very fragile and is rarely spread through inanimate objects. The virus remains in an inactive state along the **sensory nerves**. Exacerbations of the disease have been known to be caused by illness, fever, menstruation, stress, sexual contact, and sunlight. Exacerbations of the disease are generally short in duration and tend to be less severe than the primary infection.

SIGNS, SYMPTOMS, AND ASSOCIATED CARE

Symptoms of genital herpes (HSV 2) usually appear 2 to 10 days after exposure to the virus. Symptoms last an average of 2 to 3 weeks and include the following.

367

Lesion – infection or injury to the skin

1. **Lesions** (sores) at the site of infection, which may develop into blisters or open sores; the sores eventually become crusted and heal without scarring
   - Provide meticulous skin care with mild, unscented soap
   - Avoid use of tapes and other adhesives on skin
   - Administer medications or creams to prevent itching
   - Provide protective mittens for confused patients to prevent scratching and damage to skin
   - Encourage fluid intake
   - Pat skin gently dry
   - Avoid harsh soaps or bleach in clothing and linens
   - Avoid clothing and bedding that is irritating
   - Assess skin redness and irritation on routine basis
   - Observe for open areas and signs of infection
   - Avoid use of scented lotions and cosmetics
   - Administer antihistamines to relieve itching
   - Utilize universal precautions at all times when coming in contact with blood or body fluids (See Appendix C)

2. Pressure feeling in the abdomen
   - Assist with position for patient comfort
   - Avoid constrictive garments and undergarments
   - Offer methods to promote comfort such as relaxation techniques, imaging, massage, and warm baths
   - Monitor for level of pain and offer comfort measures as necessary
   - Administer medications as necessary and as prescribed by physician for the control of pain
   - Encourage patient to request pain relief methods before pain becomes too severe

3. Pain in genital area, buttocks, or legs
   - Administer pain medications as directed by physician
   - Assist to position patient to relieve or reduce pain as possible
   - Avoid constrictive garments
   - Offer comfort measures, such as heat, massage, relaxation techniques, and medications to relieve pain
   - Encourage patient to report pain before it gets out of control
   - Monitor appetite due to pain
   - Encourage activity as able
   - Assist with activities of daily living (ADLs) as needed due to pain

4. Urethral or vaginal discharge
   - Monitor amount, color, consistency, and odor of vaginal or urethral discharge
   - Provide meticulous skin care to perineal area
   - Monitor discharge for signs of bleeding or infection
   - Utilize universal precautions at all times when coming in contact with blood or body fluids (See Appendix C)
   - Provide sanitary napkins as necessary for patient use
   - Dispose of sanitary napkins in appropriate manner
   - Change clothing and bedding as necessary due to vaginal or urethral discharge

5. Fever
   - Monitor temperature at routine intervals
   - Offer comfort measures for patient with elevated temperature, such as cool cloth to forehead, partial or complete bath as needed, clothing and bedding changed frequently due to diaphoresis, and encourage fluids to prevent dehydration. Symptoms of dehydration include decreased urine output, constipation, dry skin, tenting of skin, dry mouth, dry eyes, concentrated urine, hypotension, and confusion.
   - Avoid exposing patient to a draft
   - Cover with blankets as necessary
   - Monitor intake and output (I and O)
   - Maintain comfortable room temperature for patient
   - Avoid plastic mattresses and plastic bed protectors that increase perspiration
   - Encourage use of antiperspirant or deodorant to minimize sweating and odor

6. Myalgia
   - Offer heat or other methods of pain control such as massage, relaxation, and imaging
   - Administer medications as prescribed by physician for pain control
   - Monitor level of comfort
   - Protect joints, immobilize joints, and decrease weight-bearing as able
   - Assist with ADLs as necessary due to pain
   - Assist with position for patient comfort
   - Encourage patient to keep as active as possible
   - Employ frequent rest periods to provide joint rest and pain relief
   - Offer warm, moist packs for the relief of pain
   - Allow adequate time to do as much as possible, even though it may take longer
   - Use pillows to support extremities

7. Dysuria
   - Offer comfort to patient experiencing pain
   - Encourage fluid intake
   - Placement of urinary catheter if extreme dysuria

8. Headache
   - Provide dim lights or indirect lighting in event of photophobia
   - Administer medications or other methods of pain relief, such as relaxation techniques, imaging, or massage
   - Assist in position for patient comfort
   - Provide calm, quiet environment for the patient
   - Encourage patient to avoid eye strain
   - Encourage frequent rest periods as necessary
   - Monitor phone calls and visitors to promote rest periods

9. Swollen glands in the groin area
   - Monitor for lymphadenopathy
   - Assist in position for patient comfort
   - Use comfort measures as necessary due to lymphadenopathy

Leukocytosis – increased number of leukocytes in the blood

Antiviral – substance used in the treatment of a virus

Cesarean section – surgical removal of a fetus through an incision in the lower abdomen

10. Malaise
    - Assist patient with ADLs as necessary
    - Schedule care, activities, and treatments around patient's rest schedule
    - Monitor phone calls and visitors around patient's energy level and rest schedule
    - Encourage frequent rest periods
    - Encourage activity as able
    - Provide assistance as needed to prevent injury due to weakness
    - Provide method for patient to call for assistance
    - Encourage patient to set realistic goals of activities
    - Allow adequate time to do activities and procedures to avoid frustration or possible injury
    - Encourage exercise to maintain/promote muscle strength
    - Provide cane or walker for ambulation and transfer
    - Provide private room to promote rest periods

DIAGNOSIS

During an inactive stage, there are no visible symptoms of the virus.

1. The primary form of diagnosis includes a scraping of the sore and growing the culture for herpes virus
2. A blood test can be done to indicate the presence of antibodies to the virus to detect if the person is an HSV carrier
3. *Leukocytosis*

TREATMENT

1. Acyclovir—**antiviral** medication taken orally to reduce the course of the episode and limits severity of recurrences if taken within 24 hours of the onset of the symptoms. It may also be taken on a daily basis to suppress the activity of the virus and help prevent recurrences. It needs to be stressed that Acyclovir is not a cure for herpes but can decrease the virus's ability to reproduce itself. Currently there is no cure for herpes. Acyclovir is also available for topical and intravenous (IV) routes.
2. Keep open areas clean and dry. Watch for symptoms of infection to these areas, e.g. redness, swelling, discharge, pain, hot to touch, fever, and loss of function. Avoid contact with open areas.

COMPLICATIONS

1. HSV episodes can be severe and long lasting in a person whose immune system is suppressed
2. A pregnant woman can pass the virus to her fetus. There is a 30% chance of a baby becoming infected if the mother is having her first outbreak at the time of a vaginal birth.
3. Increased risk of premature delivery or miscarriage
4. Newborns who become infected have a 50% chance of dying or suffering neurologic damage. If herpes lesions are detected in or near the birth canal at the time of delivery, the physician will perform a **cesarean section** to deliver

the baby, though approximately 1 in 16 (6%) will develop herpes even with cesarean delivery.

5. Herpes simplex has been linked with an increased incidence of cervical cancer

CORRECT USE OF A CONDOM

Transmission of genital herpes may be reduced by the following correct use of a condom during sexual intercourse.

1. Always use a condom that is made of latex rubber.
2. The package should specify that the condom is to prevent disease.
3. The condom should cover the entire penis.
4. Condoms are more likely to break during anal intercourse due to the greater amount of friction involved.
5. A spermicide containing nonoxynol-9 has been shown to kill germs that transmit STDs and should be used in conjunction with condoms.
6. Check the expiration date on the condom package.
7. Use a water-based lubricant if one is needed when using a condom.
8. Condoms should be stored in a cool, dry place. Direct sunlight should be avoided. Do not store condoms in an area that is exposed to extreme temperatures.
9. Use caution when opening a condom package to prevent damage to the condom.
10. A condom should never be used more than one time.
11. Apply the condom when the penis is erect prior to any contact between the penis and the partner's body.
12. Dispose of condoms where no one else will handle them.
13. Wash hands thoroughly after any contact with a used condom.

CONSIDERATIONS FOR CARE

1. Universal precautions must be used any time there is contact with blood or body fluids. (See Appendix C.)
2. Women with a history of genital herpes should consult their physician prior to becoming pregnant if possible, or inform the physician of their history of genital herpes early in the pregnancy.
3. Educate the patient to avoid coming in contact with the sores as much as possible and to wash hands thoroughly after any contact with the sores.
4. Health care workers need to wear gloves if contact with the sores is possible.
5. The infected areas need to be kept clean and dry to prevent spread of the infection.
6. Educate patient to avoid sexual contact from the onset of symptoms until the sores are completely healed.
7. Educate patient to be aware of early symptoms of an infection so they can initiate treatment promptly.
8. Sexual partners of the affected person need to be notified to warn them of the disease.
9. The male should wear a condom during intercourse to help prevent the spread of the herpes virus. A spermicidal agent containing nonoxynol-9 has been shown to be effective also in preventing the spread and is suggested in addition to a condom as opposed to a substitution for a condom. (See previous section, "Correct Use of a Condom.")

10. Counseling is recommended for couples, as 18% of people attribute a divorce or relationship breakup to the disease.

11. Approximately 35% of people affected by the disease suffer from impotence or a form of reduced sexual drive and should have counseling made available to them.

12. Genital herpes has been associated with a form of meningitis or encephalitis, and the patient needs to be made aware of possible symptoms.

13. Genital herpes can be transmitted to the eye causing herpes keratitis if the virus is transferred to the eyes after touching an infected area.

14. *PAP smear* should be done annually or as directed by physician due to increased risk of cervical cancer.

FOR MORE INFORMATION

American Social Health Association Herpes Hotline
(919) 361-8488

Herpes Resource Center
P.O. Box 13827
Research Triangle Park, NC 27709

ASSIGNMENT SHEET: GENITAL HERPES

Short Answer

1. Write a brief definition for the terms listed throughout the chapter.

2. Write a brief definition for genital herpes.

3. Describe the incidence of genital herpes.

4. Describe the cause of genital herpes.

5. Describe the transmission of genital herpes.

6. Distinguish between Herpes Simplex type 1 and type 2.

7. List ten (10) symptoms associated with genital herpes and associated care for each of the symptoms.

8. Describe three (3) specific methods of diagnosis for genital herpes.

9. Describe the treatment method for genital herpes.

10. Describe five (5) complications often associated with genital herpes.

11. Describe fourteen (14) considerations for caring for a patient with genital herpes.

12. Describe thirteen (13) important considerations to keep in mind for correct use of a condom.

13. Write the normal levels for a white blood cell count (WBC) laboratory test.

14. Describe the PAP smear procedure used in the diagnosis of complications associated with genital herpes.

KNOWLEDGE INTO ACTION

1. Dianna Wheeler, a 22-year-old college student, comes to your facility with a history of exposure to the herpes simplex virus from a boyfriend. She says to you that she has sores in her perineal area. What would you expect the lesions to look like?

2. In addition to the lesions, you find out that Ms. Wheeler has had complaints of vaginal discharge, fever, dysuria, myalgia, and malaise. Describe three (3) methods of associated care for Ms. Wheeler to keep in mind that can reduce or eliminate each of the symptoms she is describing.

3. Describe any special precautions you would want to take when coming in contact with Ms. Wheeler's lesions.

4. Ms. Wheeler asks you how they will be able to tell if she has become infected with the herpes simplex virus. What will your response be?

5. Ms. Wheeler's tests come back positive for herpes simplex virus. She is quite concerned about the diagnosis and asks you about treatment for the infection. What will your response be?

6. Ms. Wheeler's physician has recommended that she have a yearly PAP smear due to the herpes simplex virus. Describe why this would be a recommendation for Ms. Wheeler. Also describe what is meant by a PAP smear.

7. Ms. Wheeler asks her physician about sexual activity in the presence of her herpes simplex virus. What could be some recommendations the physician could make regarding sexual activity for Ms. Wheeler with her herpes simplex virus? (List 3.)

Chlamydia

OBJECTIVES

Upon completion of this chapter, the student should be able to:

- Define the key terms listed throughout the chapter
- State a specific definition for chlamydia
- Describe the incidence of chlamydial infections
- Describe the signs and symptoms of chlamydial infections
- Describe the route of transmission of chlamydial infections
- Describe the complications associated with chlamydial infections
- Identify specific methods for diagnosis of chlamydial infections
- Identify specific methods for treatment of chlamydial infections
- Describe the effect of chlamydial infections in newborns
- Identify specific methods to prevent the spread of chlamydial infections
- List specific considerations for caring for a patient with chlamydia

KEY TERMS

Contagious – able to be transmitted either by direct or indirect contact; also known as communicable

Epididymitis – inflammation of the epididymis, which is a place of storage and maturation for sperm

Proctitis – inflammation of the anus, rectum, and surrounding tissues

Conjunctivitis – inflammation of the mucous membrane lining the eyelid

INTRODUCTION

Chlamydia is the most common sexually transmitted disease (STD) in the United States. The infection is caused by the bacterium *Chlamydia trachomatis*. Chlamydia is highly **contagious**.

STATISTICS

In the United States, there are approximately 4 million cases of chlamydia diagnosed annually with a total cost of more than $2 billion.

SIGNS, SYMPTOMS, AND ASSOCIATED CARE

Symptoms initially may be absent or very mild, usually appearing 1 to 3 weeks after exposure. In 50 to 75% of women and 25% of men no symptoms appear until complications occur. Initial symptoms, when present, include the following.

Males:
- Discharge from the penis
- Itching or burning around opening of penis
- Dysuria
- Frequent urination
- Pain and swelling in testicles (**epididymitis**)
- **Proctitis**
- **Conjunctivitis**

Dyspareunia – pain occurring in the genital area during or after sexual intercourse

Pelvic inflammatory disease (PID) – infection involving the internal female reproductive organs

Fallopian tube – tube located between the ovary and the uterus; transports the ovum

Ectopic pregnancy – fertilized ovum that attaches frequently in the fallopian tubes or elsewhere outside of the endometrium of the uterus

Prostatitis – inflammation of the prostate gland

Females:

- Vaginal discharge
- Vaginal itching
- Lower abdominal pain
- Slight fever
- Bleeding between menstrual periods
- Dysuria
- Nausea
- Painful intercourse (**dyspareunia**)
- Proctitis
- Conjunctivitis

The signs and symptoms of this disease are signals that chlamydia should be considered as a diagnosis. Associated care for these signs and symptoms is aimed at patient comfort measures and staff protection measures.

TRANSMISSION

Chlamydia is transmitted through contact with the urethra, vagina, mouth, eyes, or rectum of an infected person.

COMPLICATIONS

1. **Pelvic inflammatory disease (PID)** can cause infertility due to the scarring on the **fallopian tubes**, which prevents the egg from being fertilized. It can also cause **ectopic pregnancy** due to the fertilized egg growing in the fallopian tube as opposed to the uterus. Approximately 1 million new cases of PID are reported annually in the United States; of these, approximately 100,000 will become infertile. (See Figure 37-1.)
2. Premature labor
3. Epididymitis
4. Infertility
5. Proctitis
6. Conjunctivitis
7. Throat inflammation
8. Lymphadenopathy in groin area
9. Urethral strictures
10. **Prostatitis**

DIAGNOSIS

Chlamydial infections have similar symptoms to that of gonorrhea, and the two are often confused. Since symptoms may be mild or absent initially, diagnosis often is not made until complications of the infection occur. A diagnosis is made by examining a small amount of fluid from an infected site. Diagnosis is also aided with presence of symptoms.

TREATMENT

Chlamydia is treated with a 7- to 10-day course of antibiotics, such as tetracycline or doxycycline. Penicillin is not effective against chlamydia.

Monogamy – sexual relationships with one person exclusively; generally refers to married couples remaining faithful to one another

Diaphragm – (a) primary muscle used for breathing, located at the base of the lungs; (b) a method of contraception that places a rubber cup over the cervix during sexual intercourse

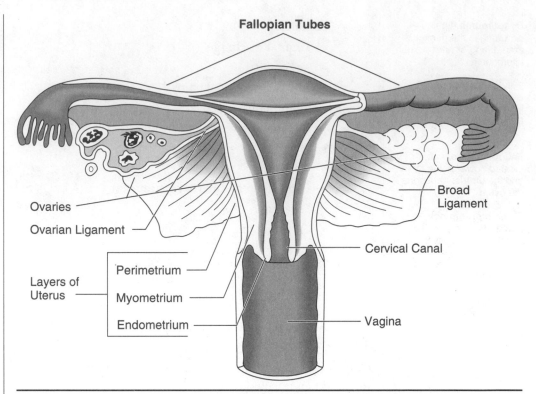

Figure 37-1   Female reproductive system (From Anderson, *Basic Maternal/Newborn Nursing, 6th edition*, copyright © 1994, Delmar Publishers)

EFFECTS OF CHLAMYDIA IN NEWBORNS

Babies can be exposed to the chlamydial bacteria in the birth canal during delivery. These children can develop conjunctivitis (discharge and swollen eyelids), usually within the first 10 days of life. They may also develop pneumonia (progressively worsening cough and congestion), which would manifest itself within 3 to 6 weeks after birth. Both of these conditions are treated with antibiotics.

PREVENTION OF CHLAMYDIAL INFECTIONS

1. Abstain from sexual activity.
2. Practice mutual **monogamy** with an uninfected partner.
3. Many physicians recommend that persons who have more than one sex partner should be tested routinely, even though they have no symptoms.
4. The use of latex condoms or **diaphragms** during sexual intercourse may reduce the transmission of the chlamydia bacteria. Condoms provide the best protection, especially when used in conjunction with a spermicide containing nonoxynol-9.
5. Know your sexual partners well and ask whether they have ever had an STD.
6. Use a spermicide that contains the chemical nonoxynol-9 in addition to a condom or diaphragm.
7. Be aware of the symptoms of an STD and discuss possible symptoms with your partner prior to becoming sexually active with them.
8. Washing before and immediately after sexual contact to wash away germs may help to decrease the risk of STD.
9. Urinating after sexual contact, especially for men, may flush out germs and decrease the risk of STD.
10. Avoid sexual contact until treatment is completed and partner(s) is also treated.

CONSIDERATIONS FOR CARE

1. Instruct the person who is infected with the chlamydia bacteria that sex partners need to be notified to obtain testing and possible treatment. Otherwise, reinfection could occur and the disease could spread.

2. Instruct the person who is infected with the chlamydia bacteria to complete the regimen of antibiotics since chlamydia could recur if treatment is stopped before the infection is completely gone.

3. Females at risk should be tested for chlamydia prior to becoming pregnant.

4. Instruct patient regarding the correct way to take medications as well as possible side effects of the medications.

5. Return to physician 4 to 7 days (or as directed) upon completion of medication to check the effectiveness of the treatment and to ensure that the disease is cured.

6. Instruct regarding specific ways to avoid the spread of chlamydia and other STDs.

7. Provide emotional support to the patient.

8. Assess level of pain and offer pain control methods as available.

CORRECT USE OF A CONDOM

1. Always use a condom that is made of latex rubber.

2. The package label should specify that the condom is to prevent disease.

3. The condom should cover the entire penis.

4. Condoms are more likely to break during anal intercourse due to the greater amount of friction involved.

5. A spermicide containing nonoxynol-9 has been shown to kill germs that transmit STDs and should be used in conjunction with condoms.

6. Check the expiration date on the condom package.

7. Use a water-based lubricant if one is needed when using a condom.

8. Condoms should be stored in a cool, dry place. Direct sunlight should be avoided. Do not store condoms in an area that is exposed to extreme temperatures.

9. Use caution when opening a condom package to prevent damage to the condom.

10. A condom should never be used more than one time.

11. Apply the condom when the penis is erect prior to any contact between the penis and the partner's body.

12. Dispose of condoms where no one else will need to handle them.

13. Wash hands thoroughly after any contact with a used condom.

FOR MORE INFORMATION

National STD Hotline
1-800-227-8922

American Social Health Association
P.O. Box 13827
Research Triangle Park, NC 27709

ASSIGNMENT SHEET: CHLAMYDIA

Short Answer

1. Write a brief definition for the terms listed throughout the chapter.

2. Write a brief definition for chlamydia.

3. Describe the incidence of chlamydial infections.

4. Describe the frequency of symptoms in males and females.

5. List symptoms associated with chlamydial infections in males and females.

6. Describe the transmission of chlamydial infections.

7. Describe ten (10) possible complications associated with chlamydial infections.

8. Describe the specific method for diagnosis of chlamydial infections.

9. Describe the specific method for treatment of chlamydial infections.

10. Describe the effects of chlamydial infections in newborns.

11. Describe ten (10) specific methods of prevention of chlamydial infections.

12. Describe eight (8) considerations for caring for a patient with a chlamydial infection.

13. Describe thirteen (13) measures for the correct use of a condom.

KNOWLEDGE INTO ACTION

1. Marianne Mogard, a 17-year-old student, comes to your clinic with symptoms of possible chlamydia after sexual intercourse with an infected person. In addition to the presence of symptoms, describe another method to aid in the diagnosis of chlamydia.

2. Ms. Mogard's test for chlamydia is positive. Describe the treatment, if any, that would be recommended for an infection with chlamydia.

3. As a precaution, Ms. Mogard's physician orders a pregnancy test. The reason for the pregnancy test is due to the effects of chlamydia in newborns. Describe what those effects could include.

4. Your position in the clinic is to counsel people who have tested positive for chlamydia regarding methods to prevent future infections. Describe six (6) of the methods you could discuss with Ms. Mogard and other patients to prevent future infections of chlamydia.

5. Ms. Mogard's physician requests a return visit in 3 weeks. Describe what the purpose of this return visit could accomplish.

UNIT 10

ENDOCRINE DISORDERS

- **CHAPTER 38** Diabetes Mellitus

Diabetes Mellitus

OBJECTIVES

Upon completion of this chapter, the student should be able to:

■ Define the key terms listed throughout the chapter

■ Describe the physiology of the endocrine system

■ Describe the function of the alpha, beta, and delta cells within the pancreas

■ Write a brief definition for diabetes mellitus

■ Describe the incidence of diabetes

■ List and describe the types of diabetes

■ List the signs and symptoms associated with diabetes as well as the rationale for each of the symptoms

■ List the risk factors associated with the development of diabetes

■ Identify specific methods for diagnosis of diabetes

■ List specific complications associated with diabetes

■ List methods to reduce the risk of developing complications or methods to monitor for complications

■ Describe the goals of treatment for Type I and Type II diabetes

■ Identify specific methods for treatment of Type I diabetes

■ Identify specific methods for treatment of Type II diabetes

■ Classify insulin types according to their onset, peak, and duration

■ Describe the use of insulin in the treatment of diabetes

■ Describe the importance of diet in the treatment of diabetes

■ List and describe the exchange lists used in the diabetic diet

■ Identify signs and symptoms of hypoglycemia as well as specific methods of treatment for hypoglycemia

■ Identify signs and symptoms of hyperglycemia as well as specific methods of treatment for hyperglycemia

■ Describe the advantages and drawbacks regarding the use of home blood glucose monitoring

■ Describe specific considerations for caring for a patient with diabetes

INTRODUCTION

Whenever a person eats, food is broken down into substances the body needs to sustain life. One of these substances, sugar (also known as glucose), leaves the stomach through the bloodstream. It travels throughout the bloodstream thereby triggering the pancreas to secrete insulin, which is needed by the body's cells to use the glucose for energy. Insulin also is needed in order for the liver to store excess glucose in the form of glycogen for times when the needed level of glucose for energy in the body falls too low.

When a person has diabetes, there is either complete lack of insulin, inadequate amounts of insulin, or the body's cells are not able to use the insulin efficiently.

PHYSIOLOGY OF THE ENDOCRINE SYSTEM

The endocrine system consists of endocrine glands and exocrine glands. Endocrine glands are glands in which secretions from the gland are released directly into the bloodstream. Exocrine glands are glands in which secretions from the glands are released into a duct system and on to the bloodstream. (See Figure 38-1.)

The pancreas (see Figure 38-2) is a gland within the endocrine system that has endocrine (**insulin** production) and exocrine functions (production of enzymes used in the digestion of food).

Within the pancreas are the Islets of Langerhans, which contain alpha, beta, and delta cells.

1. Alpha cells make and secrete **glucagon**, which stimulates the liver to release stored glycogen.
2. Beta cells make and secrete insulin.
3. Delta cells make and secrete **somatostatin**, which equalizes the level of glucose in the bloodstream by controlling the secretion of insulin and glucagon.

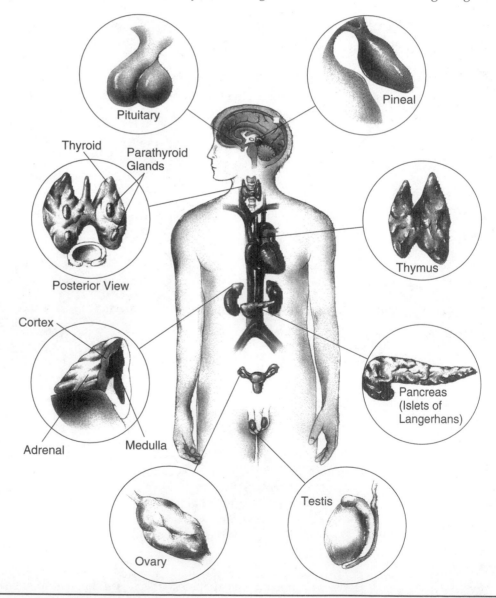

Figure 38-1   The endocrine system (From Delmar, *Anatomy and Physiology Plates*, copyright © 1993, Delmar Publishers)

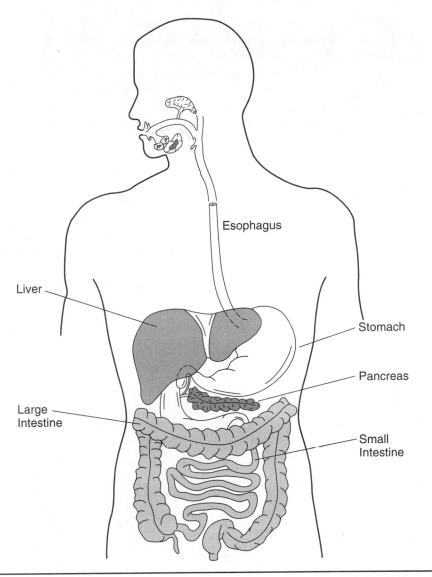

Figure 38-2   Pancreas and surrounding organs (Adapted from Townsend, *Nutrition and Diet Therapy, 6th edition*, copyright © 1994, Delmar Publishers)

STATISTICS

Between 10 and 11 million people in the United States are affected with diabetes. Between 500,000 and 700,000 people are diagnosed with diabetes annually in the United States. With more than 150,000 people dying annually in the United States due to the complications of diabetes, it is considered the seventh leading cause of death. This number is considered to be understated due to the number of people who die annually with undiagnosed diabetes. Approximately 50% of people in the United States with diabetes are unaware that they have this disease. The annual cost of care associated with diabetes is greater than $20.4 billion in the United States.

TYPES OF DIABETES

There are four types of diabetes. This chapter will deal with Type I and Type II diabetes.

- *Type I diabetes*—also referred to as juvenile onset or insulin-dependent diabetes (IDDM). There are approximately 300,000 people in the United States with Type I diabetes. This type of diabetes is thought to be an autoimmune disease whereby

Gestational – occurring during the period of development of the fetus from conception to birth

the body destroys the insulin producing cells in the pancreas (the Islets of Langerhans). With this type of diabetes, the body either ceases production of insulin or it is produced in only small amounts. In either case, the body does not have adequate insulin to utilize glucose for energy. The disease accounts for approximately 5 to 10% of the total population with diabetes and is diagnosed primarily in children. Symptoms of Type I diabetes usually develop suddenly. People with this type of diabetes have an increased incidence of thyroid disease.

- *Type II diabetes*—also referred to as adult onset or noninsulin-dependent diabetes (NIDDM). There are approximately 13 million people in the United States with Type II diabetes. With this type of diabetes, the cells produce insufficient amounts of insulin or the body's cells are not able to use the insulin efficiently or are not sensitive to the insulin. This type of diabetes accounts for 90 to 95% of the total diabetic population. People with this type of diabetes are generally over the age of 45. Symptoms of Type II diabetes develop insidiously.

- *Type III diabetes*—also referred to as **gestational** diabetes, occurs during pregnancy with a small population of women. Generally the symptoms of diabetes disappear once the pregnancy is over (95% of the time); however, women with a history of gestational diabetes have a higher chance of developing Type II diabetes later in life.

- *Type IV diabetes*—refers to diabetes associated with hormonal changes, diseases of the pancreas, or effects of drugs.

Impaired glucose tolerance (IGT) class refers to people with elevated blood glucose levels though not elevated sufficiently enough to be termed true diabetics.

RISK FACTORS

There are a multitude of things that will increase a person's predisposition to diabetes. They are as follows.

1. Obesity—studies have shown that 60 to 90% of patients with Type II diabetes are overweight. One of the theories is that pancreatic cell exhaustion, due to prolonged intake of excess calories, causes the pancreas to secrete larger than normal amounts of insulin, thereby leading to beta cell exhaustion.

2. Aging—as the body ages, the pancreatic cells no longer produce insulin as efficiently as they once did, and the body's cells are no longer able to utilize the insulin as it once did.

3. Heredity
   - When a parent has Type II diabetes, the child is twice as likely to develop diabetes also.
   - If both parents have Type II diabetes, the child is four times more likely to also develop diabetes.
   - If an identical twin has diabetes, the other twin has approximately a 90% chance of also developing diabetes.

4. African-Americans have a 1.5 times higher frequency of diabetes than the general population

5. Hispanic- and Asian-Americans have two times higher frequency of diabetes than the general population

6. Pima Indian tribe (located in southwestern United States)—approximately half of their adult population has or will develop Type II diabetes

Polyuria – extreme amounts of urine produced and discharged from the urethra; a common symptom of diabetes

Polydipsia – extreme thirst; common sign of diabetes mellitus

Polyphagia – increased appetite and consumption of food; common symptom of diabetes

Ketone – end product of the metabolism of fat in the body

SIGNS AND SYMPTOMS

Signs and symptoms for Type I diabetes generally appear suddenly. The symptoms for Type II diabetes appear insidiously but are the same as those for Type I. They are as follows.

1. **Polyuria** is due to the body's attempt to rid itself of excess sugar by increasing the amount of fluids leaving the body in the form of urine.
2. **Polydipsia** is due to the dehydration caused by the increased amount of urine.
3. **Polyphagia**—even though there is an ample energy source (glucose) within the body, the body is not able to use the glucose and, therefore, triggers the response so the person feels hungry.
4. Weight loss—the body is not able to use the glucose for the energy it needs, so instead it turns to stored fats and protein. This depletes the store of fats and protein within the body, causing the person to lose weight.
5. Weakness is due to the lack of glucose being metabolized for energy and the use of the body's store of fats and proteins being used up for energy.
6. Blurred vision is due to the fluctuation of blood glucose levels causing swelling of the blood vessels that nourish the eye.

DIAGNOSIS

Type I diabetes is generally diagnosed due to the signs and symptoms associated with diabetes, whereas Type II diabetes is often diagnosed as a result of complications of undiagnosed diabetes or during routine blood analysis for a physical examination. Methods of diagnosis for both types are as follows.

1. Symptoms
2. Physical examination
3. Elevated *blood glucose levels*—blood glucose levels will be elevated as the body is unable to use glucose for energy thereby increasing the level in the bloodstream. Several tests are done to check blood glucose levels.
   - *Fasting blood sugar (FBS)*—method of checking the blood glucose level of a person who has not recently eaten; often done prior to eating breakfast in the morning
   - *Oral glucose tolerance test*—blood glucose levels are checked before and after the patient drinks a specific amount of liquid that contains large amounts of sugar
   - *2 hour postprandial test*—blood glucose level checked two hours after a meal
4. Presence of glucose in the urine—the body attempts to get rid of the excess glucose in the blood by filtering the glucose out of the blood and sending it out of the body via urine (See Figure 38-3)
5. Presence of **ketones** in the urine—when the body uses fat for energy, the breakdown of the fats (ketones) accumulates in the bloodstream and is filtered out of the body through the kidneys and therefore is present in the urine
6. Presence of complications associated with diabetes (See next section, Complications)
7. Family history of diabetes or risk factors associated with diabetes
8. *Gly-Hb test (glycosylated hemoglobins)*—when there is a consistent increase in the normal glucose levels in the blood, the glucose binds itself to the *hemoglobin* in the blood. The life span of the red blood cells that contain the hemoglobin is 120 days, upon which time they are destroyed. This test gives a picture of the glucose control levels over the 4-month period prior to the test being done. The life span of the *RBCs* is approximately 4 months.

Amputation – removal of limb or other body part; generally a surgical procedure but may occur due to an accident or trauma

Retinopathy – refers to disease of the retina

Retina – portion at the posterior of the eye that receives the visual image from the lens

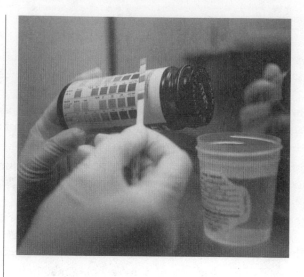

Figure 38-3 Urine testing for presence of glucose and ketones (From Hegner, *Nursing Assistant: A Nursing Process Approach, 7th edition,* copyright © 1995, Delmar Publishers)

COMPLICATIONS

There are many serious complications associated with diabetes, many of which can be prevented with control of blood sugar and other risk factors. The main complications associated with diabetes are as follows.

1. Heart attack—patients with diabetes have more than double the risk of the general population of having a heart attack.
2. Stroke—patients with diabetes have more than double the risk of the general population of having a stroke.
3. Diabetic neuropathy—patients with diabetes often complain of numbness and tingling to the extremities. They are less able to feel heat, cold, pain, and pressure, most often to the feet and lower legs.
4. Decreased circulation—the fluctuation of the blood glucose levels causes swelling of the blood vessels, which causes scar tissue to form and eventual loss of elasticity and narrowing of the lumen of the blood vessel and can involve any organ of the body. More than 4,000 cases of renal failure occur annually due to diabetic complications.
5. Increased incidence of sores (ulcerations) due to decreased sensation to the extremities as well as decreased circulation. Injuries that would heal quickly in the nondiabetic patient heal slowly in the diabetic patient and frequently turn into severe ulcers and infections that often lead to amputation. More than 20,000 people annually in the United States with diabetes have an **amputation** due to diabetic related complications.
6. Increased susceptibility to infection due to hyperglycemia delaying the response of *WBCs* to the site of the infection as well as allowing bacteria to destroy the WBCs.
7. Diabetic **retinopathy** refers to complications associated with the **retina** of the eye due to diabetes. The damage is due to decreased circulation to the retina. Approximately 5,000 people lose their eyesight annually in the United States due to complications associated with diabetes.
8. Coma may result when the brain is not supplied with the glucose it needs to function.

METHODS TO MONITOR OR REDUCE RISK OF COMPLICATIONS

There are many things a diabetic patient can do to reduce the risk of developing the complications often associated with diabetes. There are also many things the diabetic patient should do to monitor for the development of these complications. Following is a list of methods for both.

1. Monitor blood glucose levels.
2. Regulate diet, exercise, and medications as instructed by physician to maintain blood glucose levels within a normal range.
3. Maintain weight at normal or near normal range.
4. Reduce other risk factors associated with complications such as avoiding high-fat, high-cholesterol diets, smoking cessation, weight reduction, alcohol in moderation or not at all, and controlling hypertension.
5. Inspect feet and lower legs daily for signs of infection or skin breakdown.
6. Wash feet daily with warm water and soap. Pat feet dry.
7. Wear shoes that offer support without being too tight.
8. Avoid injury to the lower legs and feet.
9. Caution with cutting toenails to avoid injury. Toenails should be filed straight across rather than at an angle or curve.
10. Report sores to physician promptly for treatment.
11. Avoid use of heating pads or hot water bottles to legs and feet due to decreased sensation to heat and pain.
12. Educate patient to monitor extremities for color, temperature, and sensation.
13. Conduct an annual eye examination to monitor for diabetic retinopathy or other problems.
14. Educate patient to report symptoms of any complication promptly to physician.
15. Avoid garments that are tight and restrict circulation to the extremities.
16. Avoid crossing the legs.
17. Avoid sitting for long periods of time or remaining in any position for a prolonged period of time.
18. Conduct an annual dental examination to monitor for symptoms of gum disease or infections.
19. Apply lotions to hands and feet to avoid cracking of dry skin.
20. Use cotton stockings to help absorb perspiration from the feet and to help prevent complications.
21. Avoid going barefooted.
22. Use sunscreen to avoid sunburn.

TREATMENT FOR TYPE I DIABETES MELLITUS

The goal for treatment for either of the two main types of diabetes is two-fold.

1. Maintain blood glucose levels within normal ranges.
2. Prevent long-term complications.

Treatment for Type I diabetes falls into three main categories: diet, exercise, and insulin.

1. Diet (see section, Diet)
2. Exercise
   - Exercise helps to reduce the blood glucose levels
   - Exercise can make the body's cells more sensitive to the circulating insulin
   - Exercise, in combination with reducing other risk factors, decreases the risk of complications often associated with diabetes, such as heart attack and stroke
   - Exercise promotes a feeling of well-being as well as increasing a person's level of energy.

Sulfonylureas – medications that stimulate insulin production by the pancreas and increase the body cells' sensitivity to the insulin; used for the control of diabetes mellitus

3. Insulin (see section, Insulin)

4. Another form of treatment for diabetes is a pancreas transplant and beta-cell transplantation. This form of treatment requires the patient to take large amounts of medication to reduce the risk of rejection by the body.

TREATMENT FOR TYPE II DIABETES MELLITUS

The goal for treatment for either of the two main types of diabetes is two-fold.

1. Maintain blood glucose levels within normal ranges.

2. Prevent long-term complications.

Treatment for Type II diabetes falls into two main categories: diet and exercise.

1. Diet (see section, Diet)

   • Many times if Type II diabetics bring their weight to normal or near normal, their body's sensitivity to insulin increases, and they no longer have symptoms of diabetes.

2. Exercise

   • Exercise helps to reduce the blood glucose levels

   • Exercise can make the body's cells more sensitive to the circulating insulin

   • Exercise, in combination with reducing other risk factors, decreases the risk of complications often associated with diabetes, such as heart attack and stroke

   • Exercise aids a person to lose weight, which may in turn cause the person with Type II diabetes to control blood glucose levels more easily as well as the possibility of controlling the disease entirely

   • Exercise promotes a sense of well-being and increases a person's energy level

If the blood glucose levels are unable to be controlled with diet and exercise, a third regimen of treatment is added.

3. Medication

   • Oral hypoglycemics, which are a class of medications called **sulfonylureas**. These medications stimulate insulin production by the pancreas and increase the body cells' sensitivity to the insulin, e.g. Chlorpropamide (Diabinese), Acetohexamide (Dymelor), Tolbutamide (Orinase), Glyburide (Diabeta, Micronase), Glipizide (Glucotrol), and Tolazamide (Tolinase).

     — Side effects of oral hypoglycemics can include skin rashes, headache, nausea, and increased sensitivity to sunlight (photophobia)

   • Insulin—prescribed if the combination of diet, exercise, and oral hypoglycemics does not keep blood glucose levels within a normal range (See section, Insulin)

INSULIN

Insulin is a necessary part of treatment for all Type I diabetics and for Type II diabetics who are unable to control their blood glucose levels with diet, exercise, and oral hypoglycemics. It is also used for Type II diabetics who are pregnant or are having surgery.

Insulin is divided into categories according to their onset, peak, and duration. Onset is defined as the length of time it takes for the insulin to begin working in the bloodstream and lower blood glucose levels. Peak is defined as the length of time it takes for the

Table 38-1 Categories of Insulin

Type	Onset	Peak	Duration
Regular	½–1 hour	2–5 hours	6–8 hours
Semilente	1–2 hours	2–10 hours	10–16 hours
NPH	1–2 hours	4–14 hours	18–26 hours
Lente	1–3 hours	6–15 hours	18–26 hours
PZI	4–6 hours	14–24 hours	8–26 hours
Ultralente	4–6 hours	8–26 hours	24–36 hours

insulin to reach its maximum effectiveness, and duration is described as the length of time the insulin continues to lower blood glucose levels. (See Table 38-1.)

Insulin had always in the past been obtained from the pancreas of cows and pigs. More recently, human insulin has been developed. Two forms of human insulin have been developed.

1. Semisynthetic insulin—pork insulin is converted to a form similar to that of human insulin
2. Biosynthetic insulin—also known as recombinant insulin; manufactured using genetic engineering

The preference for human insulin results from human insulin requiring a smaller dose than animal insulin, and there are fewer instances of allergic reactions to human insulin. The drawback to human insulin is based on being more expensive than animal insulin.

Insulin injection sites include the following.

1. Upper arms
2. Abdomen
3. Buttocks
4. Thighs

These sites should be rotated to avoid injury to the tissue from the continuous use of one site. The site rotation should be charted so the patient has a record of previous sites used. (See Figure 38-4.)

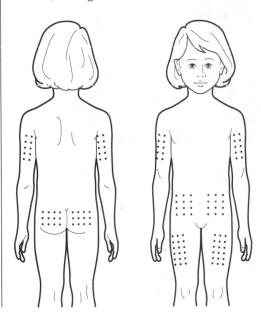

Figure 38-4 Insulin injection sites (From Shapiro, *Basic Maternal/Pediatric Nursing,* copyright © 1994, Delmar Publishers)

Subcutaneous – below the skin

Bolus – large dosage of a substance or medication given in one administration; also refers to a mass of food that has been chewed and is ready to be swallowed

Polyunsaturated – fats that become liquid at room temperature

Complex carbohydrates – starches

A new method of delivering insulin is the **subcutaneous** insulin infusion pump. The pump delivers a constant infusion of insulin and can be programmed to deliver a **bolus** of insulin at mealtime. The pump can also be regulated by the patient according to the level of blood glucose.

DIET

The American Diabetic Association (ADA) recommends a diet that includes 20 to 30% of calories from fats (**polyunsaturated**), 12 to 20% from proteins (sources that are low in fat), and 50 to 60% from carbohydrates (**complex carbohydrates**). Also recommended is up to 40 grams of fiber daily, less than 3000 milligrams of sodium daily, and cholesterol intake not to exceed 300 mg daily.

The basis of the diabetic diet is the exchange list. This list groups food according to similarities in the number of calories per serving as well as amounts of protein (4 calories per gram), fat (9 calories per gram), and carbohydrates (4 calories per gram). The foods on each of the lists can be exchanged with the foods on the same list due to their similarities. The six exchange lists include:

1. Meats and meat substitutes
   - Protein—7 grams
   - Fat—3–8 grams (according to fat content of meat)
   - Calories—55–100 (according to fat content of meat)
   - Serving size example: 1 ounce of meat
2. Starches and breads
   - Carbohydrates—15 grams
   - Protein—3 grams
   - Fat—trace
   - Calories—80
   - Serving size example: 1 slice bread, ½ cup cooked pasta, 1 small baked potato
3. Vegetables
   - Carbohydrates—5 grams
   - Protein—2 grams
   - Calories—25
   - Serving size example: ½ cup cooked vegetables, 1 cup raw vegetables
4. Milk and dairy
   - Carbohydrates—12 grams
   - Protein—8 grams
   - Fat—trace to 8 grams
   - Calories—90 to 150 (according to fat content of product)
   - Serving size example: 1 cup milk, 1 cup plain nonfat yogurt
5. Fruits
   - Carbohydrates—15 grams
   - Calories—60
   - Serving size example: ½ cup fresh fruit, ¼ cup dried fruit
6. Fats
   - Fat—5 grams
   - Calories—45
   - Serving size example: 1 tsp. butter, 1 slice bacon, 2 tsp. mayonnaise

Hypoglycemia –
decreased amounts of
glucose in the blood

Convulsion – seizure;
involuntary contraction
and relaxation of muscles

Table 38-2   Diabetic Exchange Diet

Calories	Exchanges					
	Fruit	Bread	Meat	Milk/Dairy	Vegetable	Fat
1,000	3	3	6	1	2	2
1,200	3	4	5	2	2	3
1,500	3	5½	5	2½	2	4
1,800	4	6	6	3	3	4
2,000	5	7	7	3	3	6
2,200	5	10½	6	3	3	6
2,500	5	10½	7	3	3	11

Note: See your physician and dietary consultant for additional guidelines and menu suggestions.

Also included in the exchange list are foods belonging to the "free food list," which can be used in moderate amounts throughout the day. Examples of these foods include sugar-free soda pop, coffee, celery, lettuce, low-salt seasonings, and sugar-free gums and candies.

The dietitian will work in conjunction with the physician and patient to work out a meal plan according to the age of the patient, weight of the patient, medications, and activity level. The dietitian will help to decide how many servings or "exchanges" the person can have from each of the lists. It is important to keep the patient's ethnic background, life style, and food preferences in mind when planning a diet to increase patient compliance. (See Table 38-2.)

The patient will need to be educated regarding the importance of measuring food exchanges for accuracy until he becomes accustomed to serving sizes.

HYPOGLYCEMIA

Signs and Symptoms

Hypoglycemia (often referred to as insulin reaction) can occur when there is an imbalance of diet, exercise, and medication. Hypoglycemia occurs more frequently in Type I diabetics due to the administration of insulin. Symptoms of hypoglycemia come on suddenly and include:

1. Hunger
2. Lethargy
3. Weakness
4. Diaphoresis
5. Tachycardia
6. Shallow respirations
7. Headache
8. Personality changes
9. Coma and **convulsions** may result in untreated hypoglycemia

Treatment

Treatment for hypoglycemia includes:

1. Sugar in some form. Liquids will leave the stomach sooner than solids and reach the blood circulation faster to return blood glucose levels to normal

Dextrose – sugar

Hyperglycemia – increased amounts of glucose in the blood

Ketoacidosis – accumulation of ketone bodies in the bloodstream that causes a decreased pH level in the body (acidosis)

quicker. Avoid giving oral forms of sugar to patients with a decreased mental status due to the possibility of aspiration. Examples of foods to give are orange juice, soda pop, honey, corn syrup, or candy.

2. Glucagon is a prescription medication that is used when the person is unable to take oral forms of sugar. The medication stimulates the liver to release stored sugar (glycogen) to the bloodstream to increase the blood glucose levels.

   • The patient's family should be aware of administration techniques of glucagon prior to the time of the emergency when they may need to use it.

   • Administration of glucagon may cause nausea and vomiting. Therefore, the patient should be turned on her side after administration to avoid possible aspiration of emesis.

3. Infusion of intravenous (IV) **dextrose**.

4. Monitor blood glucose levels to prevent from going too high.

HYPERGLYCEMIA

Signs and Symptoms

Hyperglycemia can occur when there is an imbalance of diet, exercise, and medication. Symptoms of hyperglycemia generally appear slowly and include:

1. Polyuria
2. Polydipsia
3. Shallow breathing
4. Tachycardia
5. Cool, dry skin
6. Dry mouth and tongue
7. Untreated hyperglycemia may lead to **ketoacidosis**, which can be life-threatening and must be treated immediately.

Treatment

Treatment for hyperglycemia includes:

1. Lowering the blood glucose level with insulin; intravenous (IV) method often used during periods of extreme hyperglycemia
2. Monitor blood glucose levels frequently to prevent from going too low

HOME BLOOD GLUCOSE MONITORING

Blood glucose monitoring is an important part of monitoring the effects of diet, exercise, and medications on the blood glucose level. Blood glucose levels are generally checked before meals and at bedtime. They should also be checked before and after exercise as well as anytime symptoms of hypoglycemia or hyperglycemia occur. (See Figure 38-5.)

Advantages of blood glucose monitoring include the following.

1. Close monitoring of blood glucose levels allows a patient to regulate the amounts of diet, exercise, and medication to maintain blood glucose levels within normal ranges.
2. Close monitoring of blood glucose levels helps to prevent complications associated with diabetes as well as episodes of hypoglycemia and hyperglycemia.
3. Blood glucose monitoring is more accurate to reflect the current status of blood glucose levels than urine testing. Urine testing reflects the blood

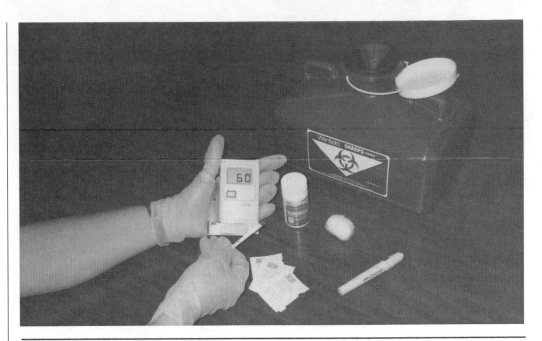

Figure 38-5   Blood glucose monitor

glucose level several hours prior to the test due to the formation of urine. Urine testing also can be altered by kidney glucose threshold differences between patients, pregnancy, dietary changes, Vitamin C supplements, and presence of bladder infections.

Drawbacks of home blood glucose include the following.

1. The initial cost of the blood glucose monitor as well as the ongoing cost of the reagent strips for the monitor.

2. Individuals with poor sight, decreased mental ability and decreased coordination may have difficulty managing the blood glucose monitor.

3. Many individuals are apprehensive of the process of obtaining the blood sample for the blood glucose monitor.

CONSIDERATIONS FOR CARE

1. Educate patient and family regarding the disease process.

2. Educate patient and family regarding forms of treatment as well as side effects of medications.

3. Facilitate dietary consult to educate patient and family regarding dietary restrictions and choices.

4. Educate patient and family regarding complications associated with diabetes as well as methods to monitor or control the onset of these complications.

5. Provide emotional support for patient and family.

6. Provide nonjudgmental acceptance of emotions and behavior of patient and family.

7. Facilitate finding a support group for patient and family.

8. Educate patient and family that diabetes is a lifelong disease that can be controlled but not cured.

9. Provide information regarding newsletters and other educational materials that may be obtained.

Endocrinologist – physician specializing in the area of endocrinology (study of the endocrine system)

Diabetologist – physician specializing in the care of patients with diabetes

10. Educate patient and family regarding the importance of following the medication schedule and dietary instructions recommended for the best control of blood glucose levels.

11. Provide information regarding obtaining a medical alert bracelet or necklace for the patient as well as a medical alert notification to be carried in the purse or wallet with pertinent information.

12. Educate patient and family regarding the importance of follow-up care.

13. Educate patient regarding the need to quit smoking due to the risk factors posed, e.g. increased heart attack, strokes, and skin breakdown.

14. Educate regarding the need to eliminate alcohol or take only in moderation according to dietary and physician recommendations due to the fact that alcohol is high in calories and contains low amount of nutrients. Stress also that alcohol is metabolized by the liver and can eventually cause liver cell destruction. Alcohol has also been shown to cause side effects when the person is taking Tolbutamide (Orinase) or Chlorpropamide (Diabinese).

15. Educate patients who take insulin injections that they should avoid sites in areas that are affected during an exercise workout, e.g. a person who walks or jogs should avoid injecting insulin into the thigh.

16. Educate patients regarding the importance of checking blood glucose levels prior to, during, and after exercise to monitor the effects of exercise on their blood glucose levels and to monitor for symptoms of hypoglycemia.

17. Educate patient and family to record the blood glucose levels, dietary information, amount and level of exercise, as well as reactions or symptoms of problems.

18. Educate patient and family regarding the use of blood glucose monitor and/or urine glucose and ketone monitoring.

19. Educate patient and family regarding the correct procedure for insulin injection as well as the importance of site rotation.

20. Provide a referral to a physician who specializes in the treatment of diabetes, either an **endocrinologist** or **diabetologist**.

21. Realize that the diagnosis of diabetes carries with it adjustments that the patient and the family need to make regarding new responsibilities and new restrictions. The patient and family may also respond to the diagnosis with fear due to their previous experience with the disease as well as their level of knowledge regarding the disease.

22. Educate patient and family regarding the importance of establishing a routine and sticking with the routine as closely as possible once home.

23. Obtain baseline weight and monitor weight on routine basis in the hospital as well as at home.

24. For patients on insulin, educate regarding the importance of knowing the onset, peak, and duration of their insulin to monitor for symptoms of hypoglycemia or hyperglycemia.

25. If a patient has an episode of hypoglycemia or hyperglycemia, encourage to determine the cause of the episode, e.g. exercise, diet, or medication balance, to prevent further occurrences.

26. If flying, stress importance of carrying diabetic supplies onto the plane with the patient.

FOR MORE INFORMATION

American Association of Diabetes Educators
Suite 1240
444 N. Michigan Avenue
Chicago, IL 60611
(312) 644-2233 or 1-800-338-3633

Juvenile Diabetes Foundation International
432 Park Avenue South
New York, NY 10016-8013
(212) 889-7575 or 1-800-223-1138

American Diabetes Association
National Service Center
1660 Duke Street
P.O. Box 25757
Alexandria, VA 22313
(703) 549-1500 or 1-800-232-3472

National Diabetes Information Clearinghouse
Box NDIC
Bethesda, MD 20892
(301) 468-2162

ASSIGNMENT SHEET: DIABETES MELLITUS

Short Answer

1. Write a brief definition for the terms listed throughout the chapter.

2. Describe the physiology of the endocrine system.

3. Describe the function of the alpha, beta, and delta cells of the pancreas.

4. Write a brief definition for diabetes mellitus.

5. Describe the incidence of diabetes.

6. List and describe the four (4) types or classifications of diabetes.

7. List six (6) signs and symptoms associated with Type I and Type II diabetes and the rationale for each of the symptoms.

8. List six (6) risk factors that predispose a person to the development of diabetes.

9. List eight (8) specific methods used to aid in the diagnosis of diabetes.

10. List and describe eight (8) complications associated with diabetes.

11. List twenty-two (22) methods to monitor and reduce the risk of developing complications associated with diabetes.

12. Identify four (4) specific methods used for the treatment of Type I diabetes.

13. Describe the two (2) main goals of treatment for Type I and Type II diabetes.

14. Identify three (3) specific methods used for the treatment of Type II diabetes.

15. Classify the types of insulin according to their onset, peak, and duration.

Type	Onset	Peak	Duration
Regular			
Semilente			
NPH			
Lente			
PZI			
Ultralente			

16. Describe the importance of the use of insulin in the treatment of diabetes.

17. Describe the importance of diet in the treatment of diabetes.

18. List and describe the six (6) exchange lists used in the diabetic diet.

19. List nine (9) signs and symptoms associated with hypoglycemia.

20. Identify four (4) specific methods used in the treatment of hypoglycemia.

21. Identify seven (7) specific signs and symptoms associated with hyperglycemia.

22. Identify two (2) specific methods used in the treatment of hyperglycemia.

23. Describe three (3) advantages to the use of home blood glucose monitoring.

24. Describe three (3) drawbacks to the use of home blood glucose monitoring.

25. List twenty-six (26) considerations for caring for a patient with diabetes.

26. Write the normal range for each of the following laboratory tests.
    a. Blood glucose level (Blood sugar—BS)
    b. Oral glucose tolerance test
    c. Two-hour postprandial test
    d. Glycosylated hemoglobin

27. Describe what is meant by the terms onset, peak, and duration in relationship to the use of insulin.

28. List four (4) insulin injection sites.

KNOWLEDGE INTO ACTION

1. Andre Lightfield, a 12-year-old, has been admitted to your facility with a new diagnosis of diabetes. He will be sent home on regular and NPH insulin. Describe what is meant by the onset, peak, and duration of insulin. Describe the importance for a patient to know this information.

2. You are discussing possible sites for Andre to give himself his insulin injections. List the four (4) possible insulin injection sites Andre could use.

3. During your teaching, Andre says to you, "Why do I need to know all these places? Why can't I just use the same spot every day?" What will your response be?

4. Write a sample menu for Andre to follow using the guidelines of an 1,800-calorie diabetic exchange diet. Include the following in the diet:

   4 Fruit exchanges
   6 Bread exchanges
   6 Meat exchanges
   3 Milk/Dairy exchanges
   3 Vegetable exchanges
   4 Fat exchanges

5. Due to the fact that Andre is a new diabetic and is very active, you are concerned he may easily develop hypoglycemia. Describe five (5) possible symptoms of hypoglycemia and the initial treatment for hypoglycemia.

6. In visiting with Andre and his parents, you encourage them to purchase a home blood glucose monitoring machine. Andre is concerned that he may not be able to "poke myself" to check his blood glucose. Describe why a blood glucose monitor would be a more accurate reflection of glucose levels in the body than checking urine for sugar.

7. List four (4) additional considerations for care that could make the adjustment of Andre's diabetes easier on Andre as well as his family.

APPENDICES

APPENDIX A

Laboratory Values

GUIDE TO ABBREVIATIONS

g or gm	gram
mg	milligram
µg	microgram
ng	nanogram
dl	deciliter
L	liter
ml	milliliter
mm	millimeter
µ	micron or micrometer
mm Hg	millimeters of mercury
U	unit
mEq	milliequivalent

Acid phosphatase—enzyme present in the prostate gland, red blood cells, and platelets
  Normal range: 0 to 0.8 U/L
  Elevation: indicates cancer of the prostate, prostatitis, thrombophlebitis, bone cancer, breast cancer, cirrhosis, renal failure

Alanine aminotransferase (SGPT)—enzyme present in the liver, brain, and muscles
  Normal range: 4 to 35 U/L
  Elevation: indicates tissue destruction in the brain, muscles, or liver

Albumin—protein present in the blood; produced in the liver; maintains fluid level within the tissues
  Normal range: 4.0 to 6.0 g/dL
  Elevation: indicates dehydration
  Decrease: indicates kidney disease, inflammatory process in the body, severe burns

Alkaline phosphatase—enzyme present in the liver, bones, teeth, kidneys, intestines, and plasma
  Normal range: 30 to 120 U/L
  Elevation: indicates tissue destruction in the liver, lung, bone, and pancreas, malignant diseases; also elevated during the first month after birth and during pregnancy
  Decrease: indicates malnutrition, hypothyroidism

Amylase—enzyme necessary for the breakdown of starches in the digestive tract; produced by the pancreas, salivary glands, and liver
  Normal range: 111 to 296 U/L
  Elevation: indicates pancreatitis, pancreatic cancer, diabetes mellitus, acute alcohol intoxication
  Decrease: indicates fibrosis of the pancreas, cirrhosis, chronic alcoholism, severe burns

Anti-HAV IgM
  Normal range: positive in the presence of hepatitis A virus antigens

Anti-HCV
  Normal range: positive in the presence of hepatitis C virus antigens

Anti-HDV
  Normal range: positive in the presence of hepatitis D virus antigens

Antinuclear antibodies (ANA)—present during certain immunologic diseases, e.g. rheumatoid arthritis, cirrhosis, mononucleosis, myasthenia gravis
  Normal range: negative

Arterial blood gases (ABGs)
  Normal range (pCO_2): 35 to 45 mm Hg
  Normal range (pH): 7.35 to 7.45 pH units (pH greater than 7.45 indicates alkalosis; pH lower than 7.35 indicates acidosis)
  Normal range (pO_2): 75 to 100 mm Hg
  Normal range (HCO_3): 24 to 28 mEq/L

Aspartate aminotransferase (SGOT)—enzyme necessary for the metabolism of carbohydrates and amino acids; present in brain, liver, and muscle
  Normal range: 8 to 42 U/L
  Elevation: indicates tissue destruction in the brain, liver, or muscle
  Decrease: indicates chronic liver disease, pregnancy, diabetic ketoacidosis

Basophil—(*See* White blood cell)

Bilirubin (total)—produced by the breakdown of hemoglobin in the liver and gives bile the yellow coloration; accumulation causes jaundice
  Normal range: 0.1 to 1.0 mg/dL
  Elevation: indicates hepatitis, newborn hemolytic dysfunction (elevation greater than 20 mg/dL may cause brain damage in the newborn), cirrhosis, infectious mononucleosis
  Decrease: indicates iron deficiency anemia

Blood sugar—(*See* Glucose)

Blood urea nitrogen (BUN)—nitrogen, which is normally present in the blood; end product of protein metabolism; excreted by the kidneys

Normal range: 8 to 18 mg/dL

Elevation: indicates abnormal kidney function, CHF, gastrointestinal bleeding, dehydration, gastrointestinal bleeding, diabetes mellitus

Decrease: indicates liver failure, overhydration, malnutrition

Calcium—element present in the body necessary for the growth of bones and teeth; 98% stored in teeth and bones

Normal range (male): 8.8 to 10.3 mg/dL

Normal range (female): 8.8 to 10.0 mg/dL

Elevation: parathyroid disease, immobilization, hyperthyroidism (elevation greater than 13.5 mg/dL causes symptoms of toxicity), cancer of the bone, breast, kidney, lung, or bladder

Decrease: indicates diarrhea, pancreatitis, celiac disease, Vitamin D deficiency, hypoparathyroidism (levels below 7.0 mg/dL would have symptoms of tetany)

Carcinoembryonic antigen (CEA)—antigens that occur in the presence of malignant growth of tissues

Normal range: < 3.0 ng/mL

Elevation: indicates original tumor growth, return of tumor growth or metastasis, pancreatitis, renal failure

Chloride—salt compound of hydrochloric acid; important for maintaining fluid balance within the body

Normal range: 95 to 105 mEq/L

Elevation: indicates tissue destruction of the kidneys or heart, anemia, dehydration, stomach cancer

Decrease: indicates diarrhea, pneumonia, fever, burns, overhydration

Cholesterol—forms bile salts for digestion of fat and is necessary for hormone formation by testes, ovaries, and adrenal glands

Normal range: < 200 mg/dl

Elevation: indicates diabetes; diet includes high-cholesterol intake; increases risk for heart disease and atherosclerosis

Decrease: indicates anemia, infection, cachexia, hepatitic insufficiency

Cholesterol (high density lipoproteins [HDL])

Normal range (male): 30 to 70 mg/dl

Normal range (female): 30 to 90 mg/dl

Decrease: indicates increased risk for heart disease

Cholesterol (low density lipoproteins [LDL])

Normal range: 50 to 190 mg/dl

Elevation: indicates increased risk for heart disease

Complete blood count (CBC)

- **Basophils** (granular or polymorphonuclear granulocytes)—necessary in the presence of inflammation and in the presence of allergy or injury

  Normal range: 1 to 3%

- **Eosinophils** (granular or polymorphonuclear granulocytes)—necessary for the destruction of certain organisms in the body and also in the presence of allergic reactions

  Normal range: 1 to 3%

- **Hematocrit**—percentage by volume of the number of red blood cells in blood

  Normal range (male): 33 to 49%

  Normal range (female): 33 to 43%

  Elevation: indicates dehydration, polycythemia, extreme diuresis, burns

  Decrease: indicates anemia, blood loss

- **Hemoglobin**—pigment in red blood cells that contains iron and is necessary for carrying oxygen to the tissues of the body

  Normal range (male): 13 to 18 g/dl

  Normal range (female): 12.0 to 16.0 g/dl

  Elevation: indicates chronic lung disease, polycythemia, dehydration, diuresis, renal tumors

  Decrease: indicates anemia, blood loss, chemotherapy

- **Lymphocytes** (nongranular or monogranular agranulocytes)—necessary for providing the body with immunity against diseases

  Normal range: 25 to 33%

- **Monocytes** (nongranular or monogranular agranulocytes)—necessary for inflammation in the presence of allergy or injury

  Normal range: 3 to 7%

- **Neutrophils** (granular or polymorphonuclear granulocytes)—protect body against infection through the process of phagocytosis

  Normal range: 54 to 62%

- **Platelet count**—necessary for the coagulation of blood; produced by bone marrow

  Normal range: 150,000 to 400,000 mm^3

  Elevation: cancer, rheumatoid arthritis, polycythemia vera

  Decrease: indicates leukemia, chemotherapy, liver disease

- **Red blood cell (RBC) count** (erythrocyte)—contain hemoglobin; function is to transport oxygen to and carbon dioxide away from the tissues of the body

Normal range (male): 4.3 to $5.9 \times 10^6/mm^3$

Normal range (female): 3.5 to $5.0 \times 10^6/mm^3$

Elevation: dehydration, polycythemia, chronic lung disease

Decrease: indicates anemia, blood loss

- **White blood cell (WBC) count** (leukocyte)—function to protect the body against infection; necessary for inflammatory and allergic response

    Normal range: 5,000 to 10,000 mm^3

    Elevation: indicates infection, leukemia, traumatic injury, myocardial infarction, burns, splenectomy

    Decrease: indicates chemotherapy, splenomegaly

CPK—(*See* Creatinine phosphokinase)

Creatinine—substance found in muscle and blood; waste product of muscle metabolism

Normal range: 0.6 to 1.2 mg/dl

Elevation: kidney infection or disease (elevation above 6.0 mg/dl indicates severe impairment of the kidneys), cancer of the urinary system, myocardial infarction (MI), congestive heart failure (CHF)

Decrease: indicates eclampsia, pregnancy

Creatinine Phosphokinase (CPK or Creatinine Kinase)—enzyme present in brain, skeletal muscles, and cardiac muscle (heart, liver, and skeletal muscles)

Normal range: 55 to 170 U/L

Elevation: indicates myocardial infarction, muscle injury, muscular dystrophy, convulsions, musculoskeletal trauma, delirium tremens

Decrease: indicates prolonged inactivity, muscle atrophy, pregnancy

Electrolytes—(*See* Sodium, Potassium, and Chloride)

ELISA test—Enzyme-linked immunosorbent assay test

Normal range: positive in the presence of human immunodeficiency virus antigen

Eosinophil—(*See* White blood cell)

Erythrocyte sedimentation rate (ESR)—rate at which red blood cells settle to the bottom of serum in a test tube to which an anticoagulant has been added

Normal range (male): 0 to 20 mm/hr

Normal range (female): 0 to 30 mm/hr

Elevation: indicates inflammation in a nonspecific part of the body

Decrease: indicates polycythemia vera, congestive heart failure (CHF)

ESR—(*See* Erythrocyte sedimentation rate)

Fasting blood sugar—(*See* Glucose)

Fluorescent treponemal antibody-absorption (FTA-ABS)

Normal range: positive in the presence of syphilis

FTA-ABS—(*See* Fluorescent treponemal antibody-absorption)

Glucose—glucose normally found in the bloodstream which is available for metabolism for energy; formed from carbohydrates in the diet; stored in the liver and muscles in the form of glycogen

Normal range: 70 to 110 mg/dl

Elevation: indicated diabetes mellitus, hyperthyroidism, tumors of the adrenal gland, acromegaly, hypopituitarism, infections, hypothermia

Decrease: indicates pancreatic cancer, insulin shock, Addison's disease, malnutrition, alcoholism

Glycosylated hemoglobin (Gly-Hb test)—correlation between blood glucose and amino acids; used to determine blood sugar control for the previous 1 to 2 months

Normal range: when there is a consistent increase in the normal glucose levels in the blood, the glucose binds itself to the hemoglobin in the blood. The life span of the red blood cells which contain the hemoglobin is 120 days, upon which time they are destroyed. This test gives a picture of the glucose control levels over the 4-month period prior to the test being done. The life span of the RBCs is approximately 4 months.

Elevation: indicates uncontrolled increase in the blood glucose levels

Gly-Hb test—(*See* Glycosylated hemoglobin)

Granulocytes—(*See* Basophils, Eosinophils, and Neutrophils under Complete blood count)

HBeAg—antigen present in the blood of a person with hepatitis B virus indicating a highly infectious condition

HBsAg (Hepatitis B surface antigen)—Hepatitis B virus antigen

Normal range: positive in the presence of hepatitis B virus antigen

Hematocrit—(*See* Complete blood count)

Hemoglobin—(*See* Complete blood count)

Iron—necessary for the formation of hemoglobin

Normal range: 50 to 140 µg/dl

Lactate dehydrogenase (LDH)
Normal range: 150 to 450 U/ml
Elevation: indicates heart attack, liver disease, congestive heart failure (CHF)

LDH—(*See* Lactate dehydrogenase)

Lymphocytes—(*See* White blood cell)

Monocyte—(*See* White blood cell)

Neutrophil—(*See* White blood cell)

Oral glucose tolerance test—specified amount of glucose is given orally (or intravenously) with blood samples drawn at specific intervals after administration to determine glucose metabolism in the body (See Figure A-1)
Normal range: Fasting < 120
1 hour < 190
2 hours < 140
3 hours < 125
Elevation: indicates diabetes

Partial Thromboblastin Time (PTT)—used to evaluate ability of blood to clot; used to determine heparin dosage in anticoagulant therapy
Normal range: 22 to 40 seconds
Elevation: indicates heparin therapy, liver disease, disseminated intravascular coagulation (DIC)
Decrease: indicates metastatic cancer

Platelet count—(*See* Complete Blood Count)

Potassium—mineral normally present in the body; important for fluid balance within the body as well as muscle contractility; excreted by the kidneys
Normal range: 3.5 to 5.0 mEq/L
Elevation: indicates kidney failure, traumatic injuries, presence of infection, diabetic ketoacidosis, extreme potassium supplements in IV therapy (levels greater than 7.5 mEq/L may cause cardiac arrhythmias)

Decrease: causes symptoms of muscle weakness and diminished level of consciousness; indicates dehydration, diabetic acidosis, metabolic alkalosis

Prostate-specific antigen (PSA)
Normal range: presence indicates a diagnosis of prostatic cancer

Prothrombin time (PT)—used to evaluate ability of blood to clot; used to determine Warfarin (Coumadin) dosage with anticoagulant therapy
Normal range: 9 to 12 seconds
Elevation: indicates liver disease, anticoagulant therapy, liver disease, disseminated intravascular coagulation (DIC)

Red blood cell count (RBC)—(*See* Complete blood count)

Rheumatoid factor—immunoglobulin used to diagnose rheumatoid arthritis as it is present in 50 to 95% of rheumatoid arthritis diagnoses
Normal range: < 80 IU/ml
Elevation: indicates rheumatoid arthritis, lupus erythematosus, hepatitis

Salicylate level—used to measure levels of salicylates during treatment of arthritis or in the case of overdose
Therapeutic range: 15 to 30 mg/dl
Toxic range: greater than 30 mg/dl

Serum IgE (Immunoglobulin E)
Normal range: 5 to 100 IU/ml
Elevation: present in 50% of patients during an allergic reaction

SGOT—(*See* Aspartate aminotransferase)

SGPT—(*See* Alanine aminotransferase)

Sodium—element normally present in the blood; necessary for normal function of heart muscle contraction as well as fluid balance within the body; necessary for the transmission of nervous system impulses
Normal range: 135 to 147 mEq/L

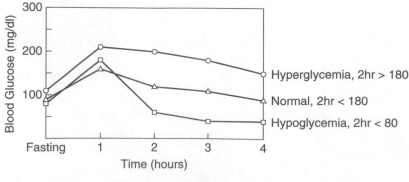

Glucose Tolerance Test (GTT) Graph

Figure A-1 Oral glucose tolerance test graph (From Smith et al., *Medical Terminology: A Programmed Text, 7th edition,* copyright © 1995, Delmar Publishers)

Elevation: indicates kidney infection or disease, dehydration, diabetes insipidus, CNS disorders, congestive heart failure (CHF)
Decrease: diarrhea, burns

T-3 (Triiodothyronine)—hormone secreted by the thyroid gland
Normal range: 75 to 220 mg/dl
Elevation: indicates hyperthyroidism
Decrease: indicates hypothyroidism

T-4 lymphocyte count (also known as CD4 cells)—main fighter of infections for the immune system
Normal range: greater than 1,000 per cubic mm of blood

Thyroxine (T-4)—hormone secreted by the thyroid gland; regulates metabolism within the body
Normal range: 4.0 to 11.0 µg/dl
Elevation: indicates hyperthyroidism, estrogen therapy
Decrease: indicates hypothyroidism, liver disease, malnutrition

TPHA—(*See* T. Pallidum hemagglutination assay test)

Treponema pallidum hemagglutination assay test (TPHA)—*Treponema pallidum* is the bacterium responsible for causing syphilis

TSH (Thyroid-stimulating hormone)—hormone secreted by the pituitary gland which is necessary for the stimulation of the thyroid gland
Normal range: 2 to 11 U/ml
Elevation: indicates hypothyroidism
Decrease: indicates hyperthyroidism

Two-hour postprandial glucose test—used to determine client's ability to metabolize carbohydrates
Normal range: 65 to 140 mg/dl

Urinalysis
Color: light straw to dark amber
Odor: aromatic
Protein: 2 to 8 mg/100 ml
Specific gravity: 1.005 to 1.030
Transparency: clear
Glucose: negative
Ketones: negative
RBC: 1 to 2 per low power field
WBC: 3 to 4
pH: 4.5 to 8 (See Figure A-2)

VDRL—(*See* Venereal disease research laboratory)

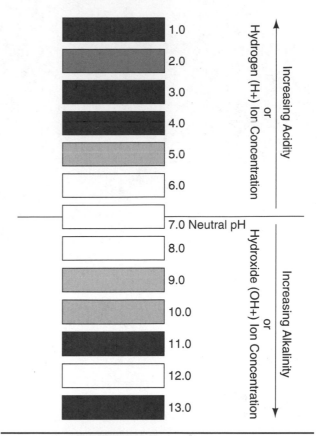

Figure A-2 pH range of body fluids (From Fong et al., *Body Structures and Functions, 8th edition*, copyright © 1993, Delmar Publishers)

Venereal disease research laboratory (VDRL)—used to detect the presence of syphilis
Normal range: negative

Vitamin A—necessary for normal production of skin, teeth, and bone
Normal range: 10 to 50 µg/dl

Vitamin C—necessary for normal production of connective tissue
Normal range: 0.6 to 2.0 mg/dl

Vitamin K—necessary for normal blood clotting
Normal range: 10 µg/ml

Western blot test—used to detect antibodies to HIV; this test is more specific than the ELISA test and also more expensive

White blood cell count—(*See* Complete blood count)

- Basophil
- Eosinophil
- Lymphocyte
- Monocyte
- Neutrophil

Amniocentesis—removal of amniotic fluid through a puncture through the abdominal wall and into the amniotic sac; fluid is aspirated for the purpose of detection of genetic defects and abnormalities as well as determination of sex determination of the fetus and maturity of the fetus; performed after the first trimester

Angioplasty—procedure used to dilate coronary arteries that are narrowed due to disease or accumulation of plaque. Through the use of a special x-ray technique called fluoroscopy, a thin tube (catheter) is guided from the artery in the leg (femoral) or arm (brachial) to the aorta. From there, it is guided to the coronary arteries. A smaller catheter is threaded through the original catheter. The smaller catheter has a balloon tip that is inflated to dilate the area of coronary artery constriction. The balloon is deflated and both catheters are removed. (See Figure B-1.)

Arterial blood gases (ABGs)—test done to determine the amount of oxygen, carbon dioxide, and other gases present in the arterial blood (See Appendix A)

Arthrodesis—surgical fusion of a joint for the purpose of immobilization for the relief of pain

Arthroplasty—surgical repair or replacement of a joint due to disease or trauma; in the replacement of a joint, an artificial joint is used

Arthroscopy—visualization of a joint through the use of an arthroscope (See Figure B-2)

Aspiration curettage—procedure in which tissue samples are suctioned from the endometrium

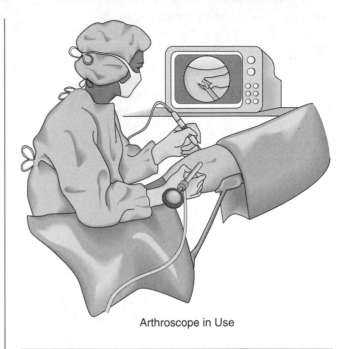

Arthroscope in Use

Figure B-2 Arthroscopy of the knee (From Smith et al., *Medical Terminology: A Programmed Text, 7th edition*, copyright © 1995, Delmar Publishers)

Barium enema—procedure involving the instillation of a liquid barium mixture into the rectum and colon in order for visualization and examination of the colon with x-ray

Biopsy—removal of tissue for examination with a microscope to diagnose or rule out specific diseases; often done to examine for the presence of malignant cells

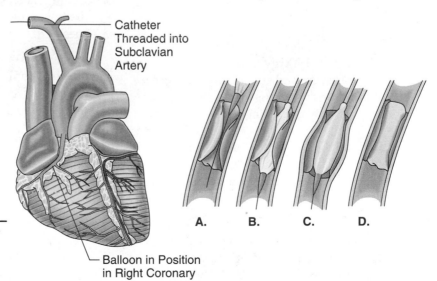

Catheter Threaded into Subclavian Artery

A.   B.   C.   D.

Balloon in Position in Right Coronary

Figure B-1 Steps involved in angioplasty (From Smith et al., *Medical Terminology: A Programmed Text, 7th edition*, copyright © 1995, Delmar Publishers)

Blood transfusion—intravenous infusion of blood or blood products into the patient; generally used as replacement therapy for blood or blood components, e.g. platelets

Bone marrow aspiration (examination)—removal of bone marrow through aspiration for the purpose of examining the bone marrow with a microscope and laboratory testing to diagnose or rule out specific diseases

Bone marrow transplant—transplanting of bone marrow from one person to another; used frequently in the treatment of leukemia; autologous bone marrow transplants may also be done in which the individual's bone marrow is removed, cleansed of impurities or treated for disease, and reinfused back in to the patient; autologous bone marrow transplant is often used for the treatment of specific types of cancer

Bone scan—introduction of radioactive agents into the bloodstream that bind to the bones and allow enhanced x-rays of the bones to be taken

Brain scan—injection of radioactive isotope into the bloodstream that binds to the brain and allows enhanced x-rays of the brain to be taken

Breast self-examination—examination by the individual of the breast tissue and surrounding tissue; best performed within one week after the end of the menstrual cycle and continued monthly; examination should involve visually inspecting the breast tissue as well as palpation of the breast tissue; changes to observe include dimpling of the skin, discharge from the nipples, lumps, pain, tenderness, inequality of size or shape of the breasts or retraction of the nipple; the purpose of breast self-examination is to become familiar with the breasts and surrounding tissues to notice changes in the breast tissue or surrounding tissue, which may be cancerous

- *Procedure*: Step 1 involves manual palpation of the breast tissues and surrounding tissues in an upright position, often in the shower due to the easy gliding of the fingers over the skin; Step 2 involves visual inspection of the breasts using a mirror to monitor for asymmetry; Step 3 involves manual palpation of the breast tissues and surrounding tissues in a supine position, using the opposing hand to examine each breast

Bronchoscopy—visualization of the trachea and bronchi of the lungs through the use of a bronchoscope; often used to detect malignancies as well as other diseases of the lung

Carotid endarterectomy—surgical removal of lesions and buildup within the carotid artery; often used for the treatment of transient ischemic attacks

Chemotherapy—instillation of antineoplastic chemicals for the purpose of treating malignancies; routes of chemotherapy include intravenously (IV), subcutaneously, orally, intramuscularly (IM), continuous IV infusion, intrathecally, intracavitary, intravesically, topically, and intra-arterially

Chest percussion (chest physiotherapy)—refers to the procedure of using the hands or a machine for manually vibrating and thumping the chest wall both anteriorly and posteriorly for the purpose of loosening secretions within the lungs to facilitate expectoration

Chest x-ray—radiographic test of the chest; used to determine lung infections, lung expansion, trauma to the chest, and heart size

Cholecystography—radiographic examination of the gallbladder

Chorionic villus sampling—sample of chorionic villus (vascular early development membrane of the fetus) taken by inserting a catheter through the vagina of the female and into the uterus; performed between the eighth and twelfth week of pregnancy to determine specific birth defects, e.g. Down syndrome

Colectomy—surgical removal of part or all of the colon; often resulting in the need for a colostomy or ileostomy; generally done to treat malignancies of the colon or diseases of the colon

Colonoscopy—visualization of the colon through the use of a colonoscope to detect diseases of the colon as well as malignancies of the colon

Colon resection—removal of the diseased portion of the bowel only, with anastomosis of the healthy tissues

Colostomy—surgical procedure involving creating an opening from the colon to the abdominal wall for the purpose of evacuation of feces; procedure that becomes necessary when a portion of the colon, rectum, and anus is removed due to disease or malignancy of the colon

Colposcopy—visualization of the cervix and vagina through the use of a colposcope; often used for further diagnosis in the event of an abnormal PAP smear and to diagnose malignancies

Computerized axial tomography (CT scan)—x-ray technique that provides a detailed, cross-sectional image of body tissues; a computer is used to record the x-rays as they pass through the tissues of the body

Conization—surgical removal of a cone-shaped portion of the cervical tissue for the purpose of treating a disease of the mucous membrane of the cervix

Coronary artery bypass graft—a large vessel from the leg (saphenous vein) or chest (internal mammary artery) is removed. One end of the vessel is attached to the aorta while the other end is attached to the coronary artery past the obstructed area. This new route for blood flow allows oxygenated blood to travel to the area of the heart that previously had restricted blood flow due to obstruction.

CT scan—(*See* Computerized axial tomography)

Cystectomy—refers to surgical removal of the urinary bladder or the gallbladder for the purpose of treating disease of the involved organ or malignancy of the involved organ

Cystoscopy—visualization of the urinary bladder through the use of a cystoscope

Digital rectal examination—examination of the rectum through the use of manually inspecting the area with a gloved finger for the purpose of locating tumors or growths within the rectum; also used in males for the purpose of determining an enlargement of the prostate gland

Digital subtraction angiography—injection of dye into the vascular system of the body to obtain a computerized visualization of the vessels of the body; generally focusing on the heart

Dilatation and curettage (D and C)—surgical procedure in which the uterus is scraped after expanding the cervical opening: used for treatment purposes for uterine bleeding, tissue biopsy, and removal of tissue shreds postdelivery or postabortion

Doppler ultrasound test—use of instrument that enhances sound waves and records them on a screen to visualize internal organs or determine fetal position and size (See Figure B-3)

Echocardiogram—method of diagnosis through the use of ultrasound; used to determine the presence of cardiac valve disease, the size of each chamber of the heart, and the thickness of the heart wall and the septum

EEG—(*See* Electroencephalogram)

EKG—(*See* Electrocardiogram)

Electrocardiogram (EKG)—graph and record of the electrical activity of the heart by the placement of electrodes over certain parts of the body, mainly on the chest and abdomen; used to determine the rhythm and quality of the contractions of the heart

How the Doppler Probe Works

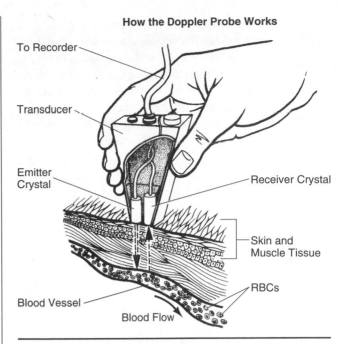

Figure B-3 Doppler ultrasound test (From Keir et al., *Medical Assisting: Administrative and Clinical Competencies*, *3rd edition*, copyright © 1993, Delmar Publishers)

Electroencephalogram (EEG)—graph and record of the electrical activity of the brain by the placement of electrodes over certain parts of the skull; used in the diagnosis of brain lesions and seizure disorders; also used to determine the presence or absence of brain activity after severe head trauma or anoxia

Electromyography—graph and record of muscle contraction when electrical stimulation is introduced

Endarterectomy—procedure that removes or scrapes the lining of an artery; generally done to remove plaque buildup within the intima of the vessel

Esophagoscopy—visualization of the esophagus through the use of an endoscope; used to determine the presence of disease or malignancy of the esophagus as well as to determine the extent of stricture of the esophagus in certain diseases

Excretory urography—(*See* Intravenous pyelography)

Fetal cell transplant—removing the cells obtained from 6- to 11-week old fetuses; these cells are injected into the organ of the patient as a form of treatment for a specific disease

Fiberoptic colonoscopy—(*See* Colonoscopy)

Genetic testing—providing heredity information by studying the genes of an individual or couple; generally is done to determine the risk factor for certain genetically inherited traits or diseases

Hemoccult® stools—procedure involving placing a small smear of a stool (feces) specimen on a slide and applying a reagent to determine the presence of blood in the stool; used to detect the presence of blood, which often accompanies diseases of the intestinal tract as well as malignancies of the intestinal tract, three consecutive bowel movements are generally tested due to the fact that bleeding may be intermittent

Hormonal therapy—treatment of certain diseases and malignancies through the use of regulated dosages of specific hormones

Hysterectomy—surgical removal of the uterus often for the treatment of endometriosis or malignancies; procedure may be accomplished through an incision in the abdominal wall or through the vagina

Hysteroscopy—visualization of the uterus through the use of an endoscope

Ileal conduit—surgical urinary diversion method in which the ureter is connected to a portion of the ileum and an opening is made into the abdominal wall for the purpose of the excretion of urine; procedure done when the bladder is surgically removed for the treatment of malignancy, disease, or trauma

Immunotherapy—method of fighting disease by enhancing the individual's immune system by injection of chemicals into the body; specifically used in the treatment of cancer

Intravenous pyelography (IVP or excretory urography)—injection of iodine into the vascular system of the body is followed by radiographic (x-ray) visualization of the kidneys, ureters, and bladder

Joint aspiration—removal of synovial fluid for examination

Leukapheresis—removal of blood from an individual, removing the white blood cells, and reinjecting the WBCs back into the individual

Liver biopsy—removal of a small piece of liver tissue via a needle inserted into the liver; the tissue is studied for the purpose of diagnosis, e.g. cancer

Liver scan—introduction of radioactive agents into the bloodstream, that bind to the liver and allow enhanced x-rays of the liver to be taken

Lobectomy—surgical removal of a portion (lobe) of an organ, often the lung, for the treatment of disease or malignancy

Lumbar puncture (spinal tap)—aspiration of spinal fluid from the spinal canal through a puncture in the back into the spinal canal for the purpose of diagnosing disease associated with the brain and spinal cord; may also be used for the injection of medications into the spinal canal (See Figure B-4)

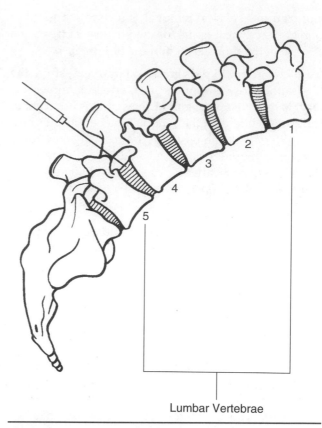

Lumbar Vertebrae

Figure B-4   Lumbar puncture (From Keir et al., *Medical Assisting: Administrative and Clinical Competencies*, 2nd edition, copyright © 1989, Delmar Publishers)

Lumpectomy—surgical removal of a breast tumor without removal of the surrounding tissue, muscle, or lymph nodes

Lung transplant—transplantation of a lung or lungs from a donor into the patient; used in the treatment of long-term lung disease

Lymphadenectomy—surgical removal of a lymph node; generally done in response to an enlarged lymph node or for purposes of biopsy

Lymphangiogram—radiography (x-ray) of the lymph system using an injection of contrast dye into the vasculature of the lymph system; the area of injection is determined by the lymph nodes that need to be visualized

Lymph node biopsy—removal of a small piece of lymph node via a needle inserted into the lymph node; the tissue is studied for the purpose of diagnosis, e.g. cancer

Magnetic resonance imaging (MRI)—techniques that use magnets and radiofrequency to obtain an image of specific tissues and structures located within the body

Mammography—x-ray of the tissue of the breast, often used to diagnose malignancies of the breast and to determine the presence of cystic tissue of the breast

Mastectomy—surgical removal of the breast; often used in the treatment of cancer of the breast

Mediastinoscopy—visualization of the mediastinum through the use of an endoscope

MRI—(*See* Magnetic resonance imaging)

Nephrostomy—surgical creation of an opening into the renal pelvis for the purpose of draining urine

Neurological examination—Basic areas of the neurological examination include the following:

- Check patient level of consciousness (LOC)
- Cranial nerve check
- Check patient orientation to time, place, and person with questions to determine the presence of short-term and long-term memory
- Check muscle strength, movement, and coordination as well as tendon reflexes
- Check sensations to heat, cold, touch, and pain

Occupational therapy—therapist who assists patients in the habilitation or rehabilitation in the area of activities of daily living

Orchiectomy—surgical removal of the testicle(s)

Osteoplasty—surgical repair of a bone due to trauma or disease

Osteotomy—surgical procedure in which a bone is surgically cut into for repair

Oximetry—machine used to measure the oxygen saturation of circulating blood in the body; an electrode is attached to a finger, toe, or earlobe, and the electrode is connected to the machine

Papanicolaou test (Pap test or Pap smear)—scraping of cells from the cervix and surrounding tissues to detect presence of abnormal cells, especially for determining the presence of malignant cells

PAP test—(*See* Papanicolaou test)

Paracentesis—removal of abdominal fluid through a puncture in the abdominal wall and insertion of a tube/needle connected to a syringe or vacuum-sealed sterile container

Peak flow meter—metered instrument to measure the amount of exhaled air with maximum inspiration and exhalation

Pelvic examination—examination of the pelvis region of the female by manually palpating the region

Physical therapy—person who attempts to provide habilitation or rehabilitation to normal function due to disease, trauma, or surgery (See Figure B-5)

Plasmapheresis—removal of blood from a donor and separating the red blood cells from the blood sample with reinjection of the red blood cells into the original donor or another patient

Pneumonectomy—surgical removal of a lung for the treatment of lung disease, malignancy, or trauma

Positron emission tomography (PET)—a radioactive isotope is injected into the bloodstream, and a computerized image is taken of the tissues of the specific area of the body; this test is also able to measure the metabolic activity within a specific area of the body

Positron emission transaxial tomography scan—(*See* Positron emission tomography)

Postural drainage—procedure in which the patient is positioned in alternating positions to facilitate drainage and expectoration of secretions in the lung through the use of gravity (See Figure B-6)

Proctoscopy—visualization of the rectum through the use of a proctoscope for the purpose of diagnosing disease, trauma, or malignancies of the rectum

Proctosigmoidoscopy—visualization of the rectum and sigmoid colon through the use of a proctosigmoidoscope for the purpose of diagnosing disease, trauma, or malignancies of the rectum and sigmoid colon

Prostatectomy—surgical removal of the prostate gland due to disease, trauma, or malignancies of the prostate gland

Pulmonary function studies—tests done to determine the lung capacity as well as ability for exchange of oxygen and carbon dioxide within the lungs

Radiation therapy—therapy for the treatment of malignancies and certain other disorders through the use of specified amounts of radiation directed at the specific location on the body to be treated

Radioisotope scans—scans in which a radioactive isotope is injected directly into the blood and specific tissues of the body are visualized

Radionuclide angiography—radionuclides are injected into the bloodstream and visualized with a scanner that is able to record the visual image as it is distributed to the specific area

Schiller's test—procedure used to determine the presence of cervical cancer by applying iodine to the surface of the cervix; portions of the cervix that do not stain brown in response to the iodine often indicate malignancy

Sigmoidoscopy—visualization of the sigmoid colon through the use of a sigmoidoscope

Speech therapy—person who assists patients to cope with or overcome difficulties with written or verbal

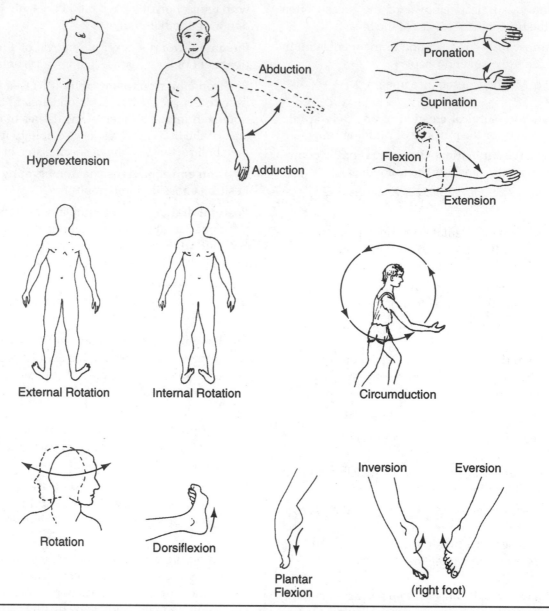

Figure B-5 Therapeutic joint movement (From Burke, *Human Anatomy and Physiology in Health and Disease, 3rd edition*, copyright © 1992, Delmar Publishers)

communication as well as articulation difficulties or swallowing difficulties

Spinal tap—(*See* Lumbar puncture)

Spirometer—machine used to measure the volume a person inhales and exhales to determine the extent of diminished breathing capacity in the presence of lung disease

Spleen biopsy—removal of a small piece of spleen tissue via a needle inserted into the spleen; the tissue is studied for the purpose of diagnosis, e.g. cancer

Splenectomy—surgical removal of the spleen due to disease or trauma

Sputum for culture, sensitivity, and gram stain—growth of microorganisms from a specific surface or

tissue (culture) after which a slide is made of the culture to determine the causative agent of the infection (gram stain) and finally to determine which treatment would be most effective in treating the microorganism (sensitivity)

Sputum specimen—expectoration of a sputum sample from the respiratory tract, which is obtained to diagnose disease, infection, or the presence of malignant cells

Stool for ova and parasites—stool specimen obtained to determine the presence of ova and parasites in the stool

Suprapubic catheter—catheter inserted directly through the abdominal wall and into the bladder for the purpose of draining urine from the bladder

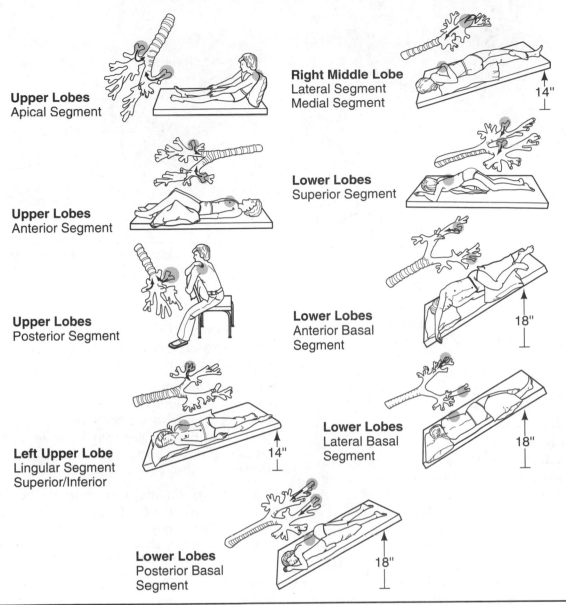

Upper Lobes
Apical Segment

Upper Lobes
Anterior Segment

Upper Lobes
Posterior Segment

Left Upper Lobe
Lingular Segment
Superior/Inferior

Lower Lobes
Posterior Basal
Segment

Right Middle Lobe
Lateral Segment
Medial Segment

Lower Lobes
Superior Segment

Lower Lobes
Anterior Basal
Segment

Lower Lobes
Lateral Basal
Segment

Figure B-6   Positioning for postural drainage (From Shapiro, *Basic Maternal/Pediatric Nursing*, copyright © 1994, Delmar Publishers)

Synovectomy—surgical removal of synovial membrane; generally done to remove damaged synovial membrane in the presence of injury or disease, e.g. arthritis

Tensilon test—Tensilon (edrophonium chloride) is injected intravenously to check for increased muscle strength to aid in the diagnosis of myasthenia gravis

TENS unit—(*See* Transcutaneous electrical nerve stimulation)

Thoracentesis—surgical aspiration of fluids in the chest through a puncture directly into the chest wall for the purpose of removal of fluids, for obtaining a biopsy, or for infusing medication into the chest or lungs (See Figure B-7)

Thymectomy—surgical removal of the thymus gland often for the treatment or reduction of symptoms associated with *Myasthenia Gravis*

Tracheotomy—surgical creation of an opening between the trachea and the external neck to create an artificial airway for the patient to breathe in and out through; often done due to severe trauma to the head, neck, or chest or for the replacement of a long-term endotracheal tube

Transcutaneous electrical nerve stimulation (TENS Unit)—electrical stimulation supplied to the skin through the use of a small unit attached to electrodes directly on the skin, which interferes with neurotransmission of pain; often used post-operatively for the control of pain or with chronic pain associated with illness, injury, or disease

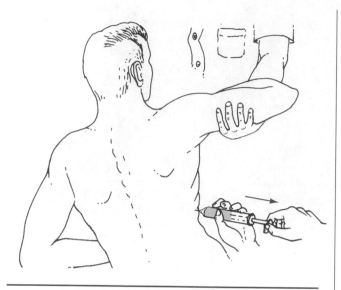

Figure B-7   Fluid being removed from the pleural cavity by thoracentesis (From Burke, *Human Anatomy and Physiology in Health and Disease, 3rd edition,* copyright © 1992, Delmar Publishers)

Transrectal prostatic ultrasonography—visualization of the prostate gland through the use of an ultrasound device placed in the rectum; often used during biopsy of the prostate gland

Transurethral resection of the prostate (TURP)—device inserted into the urethra for the purpose of removing tissue from the prostate; the procedure generally is done to remove an obstruction of the urethra by an enlarged prostate (See Figure B-8)

TURP—(*See* Transurethral resection of the prostate and Figure B-8)

UGI—(*See* Upper gastrointestinal series)

Ultrasound—sound wave visualization of organs and tissues of the body as the sound waves "bounce off" the various tissues and organs of the body and are recorded

Upper gastrointestinal series (UGI)—x-ray examination of the stomach and small intestine after the patient has consumed a specified amount of liquid

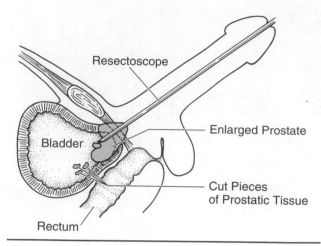

Figure B-8   Transurethral resection of the prostate (TURP) (From Burke, *Human Anatomy and Physiology in Health and Disease, 3rd edition,* copyright © 1992, Delmar Publishers)

contrast medium; UGI is done for the purpose of diagnosing diseases of the stomach and small intestine as well as determining the presence of malignancies

Ureterosigmoidostomy—surgically rerouting the ureter into the sigmoid colon for the purpose of elimination of urine from the body after removal of the bladder and urethra; generally done as a result of malignancy of the bladder or severe trauma to the bladder

Ureterostomy—routing of the ureters to the abdominal wall for the purpose of elimination of urine from the body after removal of the bladder and urethra; generally done as a result of malignancy of the bladder or severe trauma to the bladder

Urinalysis—examination of a urine specimen to aid in the diagnosis of bladder infection, kidney infection, or other diseases of the body or urinary system; urinalysis may also be done to detect the presence of certain legal or illegal substances in the body (See Appendix A)

X-ray—the use of radiography to examine tissues and bony structures of the body

Universal Precautions

Universal precautions refer to the practice of maintaining a barrier between yourself and the potential contact with any blood or body fluids. It is essential to assume that any and all blood or body fluids are contaminated and have the capability of causing disease and illness. Contact with blood or body fluids refers to not only the skin but also mucous membranes and skin punctures. The following precautions must be followed at all times to reduce the risk of the spread of AIDS, hepatitis B, and other infections that are potentially transmitted through blood or body fluids from an infected person. (See Figure C-1.)

1. Gloves must be worn at all times when there is a potential of coming in contact with any blood or body fluid of another person. Gloves must also be worn any time there is direct contact with mucous membranes or open sores or wounds of another person. Gloves must be changed between patients, when they become soiled, or if there is a possibility the gloves have a hole or tear in them.

2. Gowns must be worn at all times when there is a potential of contamination with any blood or body fluid of another person. Examples include procedures in which contamination is possible, a confused or combative patient, or a patient who is vomiting or coughing forcefully.

3. Goggles or face shields must be worn at all times when there is a potential of contamination with any blood or body fluid of another person. Examples include procedures in which contamination is possible, a confused or combative patient, or a patient who is vomiting or coughing forcefully.

4. Extreme caution must be taken to avoid any injury with needles or sharp instruments. A special container must be used for disposal of needles and other sharp instruments. Needles must never be recapped. If recapping should become necessary, a one-handed recapping method is recommended to prevent accidental puncture. Needles and other sharp instruments must never be left on counters or tabletops and must never be thrown away with other disposable items.

5. If contact with blood or body fluids does occur, the skin must be washed immediately with antimicrobial soap, and the incident must be reported.

6. Proper labeling and handling of all specimens are necessary to prevent contamination or accidental contact.

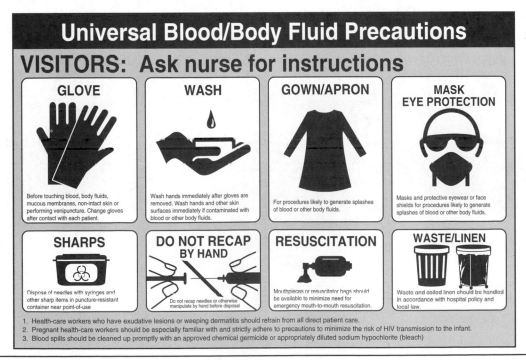

Figure C-1 Universal precautions (From Shapiro, *Basic Maternal/Pediatric Nursing,* copyright © 1994, Delmar Publishers)

Vital Signs

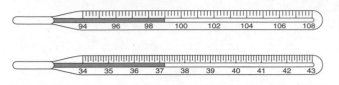

Figure D-1 Thermometer (From Hegner, *Assisting in Long-Term Care, 2nd edition Workbook*, copyright © 1992, Delmar Publishers)

Vital signs normally consist of the following measurements.

1. **Temperature**—measurement of the heat of the body. Temperatures can be measured, using a thermometer (See Figure D-1), through the following sites.

   a. Oral (mouth)—normal 98.6°F

   b. Rectal—normal 99.6°F

   c. Axillary (armpit) or groin—normal 97.6°F (See Figure D-2)

2. **Pulse**—measurement of the number of times the heart beats per minute; a normal pulse range is 60 to 90 beats per minute. Pulses can be felt at the following frequently used sites.

   a. Radial (thumb side of the wrist)

   b. Carotid (neck)

   c. Apical (over the heart, using a stethoscope)

3. **Respirations**—measurement of the number of breaths in (inspiration) and breaths out (expiration) per minute. Normal respiratory rate is 12 to 20 breaths per minute.

4. **Blood pressure**—measurement of the pressure exerted on the arteries of the body as the heart

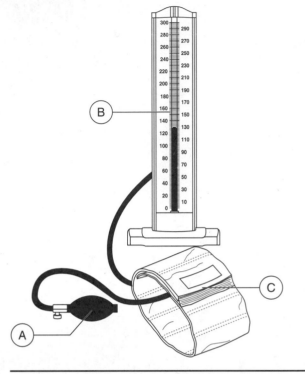

Figure D-3 Blood pressure equipment: (a) bulb, (b) mercury manometer, (c) blood pressure cuff (From Hegner, *Assisting in Long-Term Care, 2nd edition Workbook*, copyright © 1992, Delmar Publishers)

contracts (systole) and relaxes (diastole). Blood pressure is measured using a sphygmomanometer and stethoscope (See Figure D-3). Normal blood pressure readings are as follows.

   a. Systolic—120 (range of 100 to 140)

   b. Diastolic—80 (range of 60 to 90)

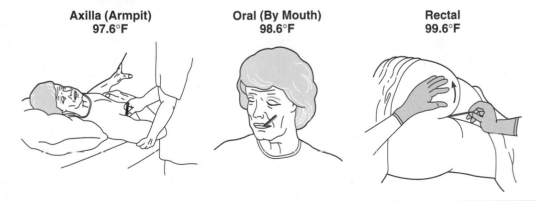

| Axilla (Armpit) 97.6°F | Oral (By Mouth) 98.6°F | Rectal 99.6°F |

Figure D-2 Normal temperatures according to site (From Badasch, *Essentials for the Nursing Assistant in Long-Term Care, 2nd edition,* copyright © 1994, Delmar Publishers)

Glossary

Abruptio placenta—premature separation of the placenta

Abscess—accumulation of fluid within an enclosed sac; generally due to infection

Acetylcholine—compound found in organs and tissues throughout the body; necessary for nerve impulse transmission at the synapses and neuromuscular junctions

Acidosis—excess accumulation of acids within the tissues of the body

Acromegaly—excess production of growth hormones in the pituitary gland

Activities of daily living (ADLs)—personal care activities such as eating, bathing, elimination, ambulation, and dressing

Acute—sudden onset of symptoms with a short duration

Addison's disease—disease resulting from a decreased amount of glucocorticoids from the adrenal gland

Adenocarcinomas—cancerous tumors of a gland

Adipose—fat tissue

Adjacent—situated next to

Adrenal glands—small endocrine glands located on the top portion of each individual kidney; responsible for manufacturing and storing the hormones epinephrine, norepinephrine, sex hormones, aldosterone, and cortisol

Agnosia—inability to understand sensory input (seeing, hearing, and feeling)

Albumin—protein found in the blood that is important for maintaining fluid balance in the body (blood volume)

Alignment—positioning the body, or portions of the body, in a straight line

Alkalosis—decreased acidity of the tissues of the body due to reduction of acids

Allergen—substance an individual is allergic to that causes allergic symptoms (sneeze, cough, watery eyes, and hives)

Alleviating—lessening the severity of symptoms or a disease

Alopecia—hair loss

Alpha 1-antitrypsin—protein that is often deficient in patients with emphysema

Alveolar sacs—(*See* Alveoli)

Alveoli—small air sacks of the lungs in which carbon dioxide and oxygen exchange takes place during the process of respiration

Alzheimer's disease—disease characterized by gradually worsening dementia; generally affects individuals over the age of 60

Amenorrhea—absence of menstruation (menses)

Amino acids—compounds that are the basic structure of proteins

Amniotic fluid—fluid within the amniotic sac that cushions the developing fetus and protects the fetus from injury

Amputation—removal of limb or other body part; generally a surgical procedure but may occur due to an accident or trauma

Amyloid—a protein similar to starch

Anal—refers to the anus (external opening of the rectum)

Analgesic—substance taken to reduce or relieve pain

Anastomosis—joining of two ends together, generally after a portion of the structure has been removed (e.g. colon)

Androgens—hormones that are important in the development of secondary sex characteristics in males

Anemia—decrease in red blood cells (RBCs), hemoglobin, or blood loss

Anesthesia—decreased sensation generally accompanied by complete sedation, generally for the purpose of surgery

Aneurysm—blood-filled sac formed by tearing and separation of the walls of blood vessels, allowing blood to escape into the layers of the vessel

Angina—chest pain caused by decrease in oxygen supply to the heart muscle without causing muscle necrosis; angina pain is similar to the pain experienced with a myocardial infarction

Angiotensin—vasoconstrictor in the bloodstream that is produced by the kidney

Anomalies—contrasts from what is normally expected; congenital anomalies are generally due to faulty fetal development in the uterus

Anorexia—loss of appetite

Anovulation—temporary or permanent cessation of female ovulation

Anoxia—deficiency or absence of oxygen leading to tissue death

Antacids—substances used to neutralize stomach acid

Anterior—front

Antibacterial—substance used to destroy bacteria

Antibiotics—substances used to destroy pathogens

Antibodies—proteins formed within the body in response to an invading antigen

Anticholinergic—blocking of cholinergic responses through the parasympathetic nervous system (cholinergic effect is that of acetylcholine)

Anticholinesterase—blocks cholinesterase in the body

Anticoagulant—substance that prevents or delays blood from clotting

Anticonvulsive—substance that prevents, reduces the frequency of, or treats convulsions (seizures)

Antidepressants—medications used in the treatment of depression

Antidiarrheal—substance that prevents or treats diarrhea

Antiemetics—substances that prevent or treat nausea and vomiting

Antifungal—substance used to destroy fungus

Antigen—foreign substance in the body that stimulates the body to produce antibodies

Antihistamines—substances that counteract the effect of histamines, which are amino acids normally present in the body and released into the bloodstream in response to injury to the tissues; histamines are also released during allergic reactions when the body is in contact with a substance to which it is sensitive

Antihypertensive—medication used in the treatment of high blood pressure (hypertension)

Anti-inflammatory—substance used to treat or reduce inflammation

Antimicrobial—substance used in the treatment of microbes

Antineoplastic—substance used in the treatment of cancerous growths (neoplasm)

Antipyretic—substance used to decrease a fever

Antiseptic—substance used to disinfect a specific area; may refer to the skin, mucous membranes, or an inanimate object

Antispasmodics—substances that prevent or treat spasms

Antiviral—substance used in the treatment of a virus

Anus—external opening of the rectum

Aorta—normally the largest vessel in the body; artery that transports blood to the systemic circulatory system from the left ventricle

Aortic semilunar valve—valve connecting the left ventricle of the heart and the aorta

Apathy—absence of feelings or emotions

Aphasia—loss of ability to speak or understand written or spoken communication

Apnea—absence of respirations

Apneustic—respiratory center located in the pons of the brain

Appendix—small appendage located at the junction between the ileum of the small intestine and the opening into the large intestine

Apraxia—inability to respond correctly to commands or use objects correctly

Arachnoid—the middle meninx (membrane) that covers the brain and spinal cord

Areola—colored area of tissue around the nipple of the breast

Arrhythmia—abnormal rhythm of the beat of the heart

Arterial—pertains to artery

Arterial blood gases (ABGs)—test done to determine the amount of oxygen, carbon dioxide, and other gases present in the arterial blood

Arteriosclerosis—hardening of the arteries

Arteritis—inflammation of an artery of the body

Artery—blood vessel that carries blood away from the heart

Arthralgia—joint pain

Arthrodesis—surgical fusion of a joint causing immobilization of that joint

Arthroplasty—surgical repair or reconstruction of a joint

Articular cartilage—cartilage covering the joint ends of bones

Ascending colon—portion of the large intestine located between the distal ileum and the transverse colon

Ascites—accumulation of fluid within the peritoneal cavity

Aspiration—inhalation or drawing in of a foreign body into the lungs; also refers to removal of fluid from a certain site in the body, e.g. knee or spine

Asthma—disease characterized by reversible bronchospasm in the airway characterized by cough, dyspnea, wheezing, and increased mucous production

Asymmetry—unequal in size or shape compared to the corresponding body part on the opposite side of the body; also refers to irregular edges of a mole or rash

Asymptomatic—exhibiting no symptoms

Ataxia—lack of muscle coordination with voluntary or involuntary movement

Atelectasis—collapsed lung

Atherosclerosis—hardening of the arteries due to accumulation of fat and plaque within the lining of the arterial walls

Athetoid—specific category of cerebral palsy in which the motor cortex of the brain is damaged resulting in difficulty with smooth coordination and involuntary movement

Atrial fibrillation—irregular beating and contractions of the atria of the heart

Atria (atrium)—upper chambers of the heart

Atrophy—reduction in size of tissue or organ within the body

Auditory—in reference to hearing; eighth cranial nerve

Aura—sensation that is often perceived by an individual prior to the onset of an epileptic seizure or migraine headache; perceived by the individual as a sensation in hearing, smell, taste, or vision

Auscultate—process of listening to sounds within the body, generally with a stethoscope, as the organs within the body carry out their specific functions

Autoimmune—process by which antibodies within a person's body destroy normal cells within the body

Autologous—removed from the individuals themselves; generally refers to blood donation from oneself, e.g. prior to surgery; bone marrow from oneself

Autopsy—surgical examination of the body and tissues of the body after death; often done to determine the cause of death

Axillary—armpit

Axon—transfers neurological impulses away from the neuron, across the synapse, and on to the dendrite of the next neuron

Bacteremia—accumulation of bacteria in the blood

Bacteria—microorganisms present almost everywhere; divided into three classifications: rod-shaped (bacilli), spiral-shaped, and spherical. Spherical may appear in pairs (diplococci), chains (streptococci), or clusters (staphylococci)

Ball joint (ball and socket joint)—a joint where the ball-shaped end of one bone fits into the cup-shaped end of another bone

Basal ganglia—areas of gray matter located in the brain that assist in coordination of the muscles

Basophils—one of the three granular white blood cells (granular white blood cells are basophils, eosinophils, and neutrophils); make up 1 to 3% of the total number of white blood cells

B-cells—lymphocytes produced in the bone marrow and maturing in the spleen and lymph nodes; sensitive to only a specific antigen

Behavior modification—a method of controlling or encouraging change in a person's behavior with a reward system; positive behavior results in the granting of a reward or privilege, whereas negative behavior results in the loss of a reward or privilege

Beta blockers—medications that decrease blood pressure and heart rate; may also be used for the treatment of angina

Bilateral—refers to both sides, generally of the body

Bile—substance manufactured and secreted by the liver and stored in the gallbladder; the function of bile is to aid the body in digestion of fats

Bilirubin—product of hemoglobin breakdown; excreted by the liver; approximately 260 milligrams of bilirubin is produced daily, with the majority excreted through fecal material and the remainder (1%) excreted in urine

Bilirubinemia—accumulation of bilirubin in the blood

Binge—as in bulimia; constituted by the consumption of large amounts of food and calories

Biopsy—removal of a small piece of tissue for examination under a microscope; procedure used to diagnose specific diseases, especially cancer

Bisexual—sexual preference for a person of either sex

Bladder—muscular organ that stores urine until it is ready to be excreted from the body

Blast—an immaturely developed cell

Blepharitis—inflammation of the eyelid

Blood pressure—measurement of the pressure within the arteries of the body as it relates to the contraction (systole) and relaxation (diastole) of the heart

Bolus—large dosage of a substance or medication given in one administration; also refers to a mass of food that has been chewed and is ready to be swallowed

Bone marrow—tissue located in the bones of the body and refers either to yellow bone marrow (located in the medullary cavity) or red bone marrow, which is located in the spongy bone

Bouchard's nodes—nodes that appear in the middle joints of the fingers, which are characteristic of osteoarthritis

Brachycephalic—condition of a short head

Bradycardia—decreased heartbeat, generally less than 60 beats per minute

Bradykinesia—decreased or slowed movements

Brain stem—the portion of the brain that connects the brain with the spinal cord; the parts of the brain stem are the medulla, pons, and midbrain

Breech—refers to presentation or delivery of a fetus buttocks first

Bronchi—the two branches off the trachea; left and right bronchus

Bronchioles—the small branches off the bronchi within the lungs

Bronchitis—inflammation of the bronchial tubes

Bronchodilator—medication that dilates the bronchus

Bronchoscopy—visualization of the bronchus using a flexible instrument; this procedure is used to aid in diagnosis of disease and also permits biopsy

Bronchospasm—spasm or constriction of the bronchus causing a narrowing of the lumen of the bronchus; often occurs in asthma and decreases the exchange of oxygen and carbon dioxide

Brudzinski's sign—in a supine position when the neck is flexed, flexing of the hips automatically occurs; presence of this sign is a positive indicator of meningitis

Bruit—abnormal sound present when auscultating a vein or artery

Brushfield spots—spots present on the iris of the eye, generally white, light gray, or yellow in color; often present in individuals with Down syndrome

Burkitt's lymphoma—a type of lymphoma that commonly involves the lymph nodes, although it may involve other parts of the body; commonly associated with Epstein-Barr virus, which causes mononucleosis

Bursa (plural: **bursae**)—fluid-filled sac located at the joints of the body; purpose is to reduce the friction at the site of the joint

Cachexia—general wasting away of weight and body tissue often seen in chronic and debilitating illness

Calcium—mineral found in foods, such as dairy products and green leafy vegetables, which is necessary for the formation and strength of bones and teeth as well as the function of muscles and nerves; calcium is also stored in the bones of the body

Calcium channel blocker—medication that dilates vessels of the heart and reduces the oxygen requirements of the heart muscle; also used in the treatment of arrhythmias

Candida albicans—fungal infection found primarily in the mouth and digestive tract, characterized by white, painful lesions

Capillary—smallest of the blood vessels forming the junction of arteries and veins; also refers to the smallest of the lymphatic system vessels

Carbohydrate—important energy source found in many foods; substance made of hydrogen, oxygen, and carbon; primary food sources of carbohydrates are sugars (simple carbohydrates) and starches (complex carbohydrates)

Carbon dioxide (CO$_2$)—waste product of cellular metabolism; excreted from the body during the process of respiration

Carcinogens—substances that cause cancer or have the ability to cause or increase the risk of developing cancer

Carcinoma—cancerous tumor of the epithelium (lining of internal and external organs)

Cardiac—refers to the heart

Cardiac arrest—cessation of the beating of the heart

Cardiac arrhythmia—abnormal rhythm of the beat of the heart

Cardiac output—amount of blood that is pumped from the heart via the left ventricle per minute

Cardiogenic shock—shock that results due to severely compromised cardiac output

Cardiomegaly—enlargement of the heart

Cardiovascular—refers to the blood vessels of the heart

Caries—process of deterioration of the bones or teeth

Carotid—carotid arteries located in the neck that supply blood to the head

Carpal tunnel syndrome—pain, numbness, and loss of function of the thumb and first two or three fingers of the hand due to pressure or injury to the nerve in the wrist; often caused by frequent, repetitive movements

Cartilage—fibrous connective tissues that make up the nasal septum, external portion of the ear, eustachian tube, trachea, cushion between the vertebrae, and portions of the ribs

Cataract—visual impairment caused by an opacity (cloudiness) of the lens of the eye

Catecholamines—examples of catecholamines include epinephrine and norepinephrine; increase heart rate and act as vasoconstrictors

Catheter—tube inserted into an opening in the body to drain or inject fluid

Cecum—first part of the large intestine; situated between the ileum of the small intestine and the ascending colon

Celiac disease—disease that results in malabsorption of foods due to an allergy to glutens, which are proteins found in grains such as wheat

Central nervous system (CNS)—the voluntary and involuntary nerves of the brain and spinal column

Cerebellum—portion of the brain located directly under the cerebrum; responsible for coordination of balance and muscle tone

Cerebral—refers to the cerebrum, the largest portion of the brain

Cerebrospinal fluid (CSF)—fluid that surrounds the brain and spinal cord and protects from injury by acting as a cushion

Cerebrovascular—refers to the blood vessels of the brain

Cerebrum—largest portion of the brain; responsible for voluntary movement and thought processes

Cervical—the neck or cervix of the female reproductive organs

Cervix—opening to the vagina located at the base of the uterus

Cesarean section—surgical removal of a fetus through an incision in the lower abdomen

Chancre—skin lesion that is present during syphilis; generally appearing two to three weeks after exposure to *Treponema pallidum*

Chemotherapy—instillation of antineoplastic chemicals for the purpose of treating malignancies

Chest physiotherapy (chest percussion)—technique used to drain mucous from the lungs using manual vibration while the patient is in specific positions to enhance the effect of gravity on the mucous and secretions

Cholecystokinin (CCK)—hormone secreted by the small intestine that stimulates contraction of the gallbladder, then releases enzymes secreted by the pancreas

Cholesterol—substance found normally in many foods including animal fats and egg yolks

Cholinesterase—enzyme capable of breaking down acetylcholine

Chromosomal—pertaining to chromosomes, which contain the DNA in the cell nucleus that transmits genetic information; the normal cell contains 46 chromosomes (23 pair)

Chronic—long-term

Chronic obstructive pulmonary disease (COPD)—chronic lung disease that is the result of asthma, chronic bronchitis, and/or emphysema

Chyme—semisolid, partially digested food in the stomach and small intestine

Cilia—hairlike extensions found in the mucous membrane of the respiratory tract that aid in removing foreign bodies, e.g. dust or mucous, from the respiratory tract

Cirrhosis—chronic liver disease characterized by degeneration of liver cells and formation of scar tissue

Clinodactyl—abnormal outward deviation of one or more fingers

Coagulation—refers to the clotting of the blood

Coarctation—narrowing of the lumen of a vessel; frequently refers to the aorta

Cogwheel—rigidity of movement that is jerky and uneven when the extremity is moved or manipulated

Colectomy—surgical removal of a portion of the colon or all of the colon

Colon—the main portion of the large intestine extending from the ileum to the rectum

Colostomy—surgical creation of an opening between the colon and the abdomen as a method of excreting feces

Coma—stupor or unconsciousness from which a person cannot be aroused

Commode—portable toilet frequently seen in a hospital or long-term care facility; used for a patient who has difficulty ambulating to the bathroom

Complex carbohydrates—starches

Condoms—latex or rubber sheaths placed over the penis during sexual intercourse to aid in the prevention of pregnancy or sexually transmitted diseases

Condyloma—growth resembling a wart found on the genital area that is caused by the human papilloma virus

Confabulation—a person who has experienced memory loss may imagine or make up events to fill in the gaps of the loss of memory

Congenital—present from the time of birth

Congestive heart failure (CHF)—disease caused by inadequate pumping action of the heart resulting in fluid accumulation within the body

Conjunctivitis—inflammation of the mucous membrane lining the eyelid

Connective tissue—type of tissue within the body that supports and connects other tissues within the framework of the body; includes bones and cartilage

Constipation—difficulty having a bowel movement due to the feces being hard, dry, or large in diameter

Constriction—narrowing of a lumen or opening

Contagious—able to be transmitted either by direct or indirect contact; also known as communicable

Contraceptives—methods used to prevent a pregnancy from occurring

Contractility—able to contract or shorten in length

Contraction—any shortening of a muscle

Contracture—permanent shortening of a muscle often related to immobility

Convolution—surface that has many folds or coils

Convulsion—seizure; involuntary contraction and relaxation of muscles

COPD—chronic obstructive pulmonary disease

Coronary—heart

Corpus callosum—bundle of nerve fibers that connects the hemispheres of the cerebrum of the brain

Corpus uteri—the main body of the uterus

Cortex—outer covering or layer of an organ

Cortical—cortex or outer membrane of an organ

Corticosteroids—hormones secreted from the adrenal gland; also refers to a medication given to reduce inflammation

Cranial nerves—twelve pairs of nerves that originate in the brain and control various functions of the body

Cranium—the bones of the skull excluding the jaw bone and facial bones

Crepitus—grating sound heard with the movement of a joint

Crohn's disease—chronic inflammatory disease of the ileum

Cryptococcosis—fungal infection; most frequently involves the central nervous system

Cryptosporidiosis—disease caused by the organism *Cryptosporidium parvum*; characterized by diarrhea and abdominal cramps

C-section—*see* Cesarean section

Culture—growth of organisms obtained from a specimen in the body as a method of diagnosis of the causative pathogen of a disease; examples include sputum and wound drainage

Cushing's syndrome—overproduction and secretion of glucocorticoids from the adrenal glands

Cyanosis—blue discoloration of the skin due to decreased hemoglobin and oxygenation of the blood

Cystectomy—surgical removal of a fluid-filled sac or the urinary bladder

Cystic duct—gallbladder duct

Cystic fibrosis—disease affecting the respiratory tract and exocrine glands of the body; characterized by increased mucous production in the lungs and increased perspiration

Cystitis—inflammation of the urinary bladder

Cytology—study of the cell

Cytomegalovirus—virus that most frequently involves the salivary glands

Dander—small particles released from the hair or feathers of animals

Debilitating—causing extreme weakness

Decubitus ulcer—ulcer or sore on the skin that results from long periods of pressure to an area of skin and the decreased circulation that results; also known as bedsore

Defecation—bowel movement

Dehydration—reduced fluid level in the body resulting from extreme fluid loss from the body or severe reduction in the amount of fluid taken into the body

Delirium—extreme mental confusion or agitation

Delirium tremens—tremors, irritability, confusion, hallucinations, and possible seizures following the sudden cessation of alcohol

Delusion—false thought or belief that is not consistent with the actual external stimuli or with the truth

Dementia—diminished or deterioration of mental functioning; confusion

Dendrite—portion of the neuron that conducts an impulse toward the body of the cell

Descending colon—portion of the large intestine between the transverse colon and the sigmoid colon

Detoxification—destruction, removal, or reduction of toxic substances

Detoxify—process of detoxification by removing the toxic substance; in the case of drug or alcohol addiction, the process means complete withdrawal of the drug or alcohol

Diabetes—a condition in which there is either a complete lack of insulin, inadequate amounts of insulin, or the body's cells are not able to use the insulin efficiently

Dextrose—sugar

Diabetes insipidus—decreased production of vasopressin by the pituitary gland that results in excessive thirst and urination

Diabetes mellitus—disease in which the body is unable to break down and use carbohydrates for energy due to the lack of insulin or the inability of the body to use insulin adequately

Diabetologist—physician specializing in the care of patients with diabetes

Diaphoresis—extreme perspiration or sweating

Diaphragm—(a) primary muscle used for breathing, located at the base of the lungs; (b) a method of contraception that places a rubber cup over the cervix during sexual intercourse

Diarrhea—the passing of liquid or semisolid bowel movements (feces); diarrhea results due to the fact that the waste products pass through the intestinal tract so rapidly that fluid and nutrients are not reabsorbed into the body

Diastole—period of relaxation of the heartbeat that alternates with contraction, or systole, of the heart muscle

Diastolic—refers to the lower or bottom number of the blood pressure; the amount of pressure needed to keep the arteries open during relaxation of the ventricles of the heart

Diplegia—paralysis of extremities on both sides of the body with either extremity being affected similarly

Diplopia—double vision

Disseminated intravascular coagulation—accumulation of platelets in the small vessels in the body causing clots to form, while at the same time the platelets are depleted in other areas of the body and hemorrhaging occurs

Distal—farthest from the point of attachment

Distention—state of being swollen or distended

Diuresis—excreting large amounts of urine

Diuretic—medication or substance that increases urine output and decreases the fluid level of tissues in the body

Diverticulosis—presence of diverticulum (sacs or pouches) in the intestinal tract

Dopamine—important for the process of neurotransmission in the central nervous system (CNS); produced by the adrenal glands

Dressler's syndrome—syndrome occurring after a myocardial infarction (heart attack) characterized by fever, chest pain, pleuritis, and pericarditis

Duodenum—the first portion of the small intestine; approximately 10 to 12 inches in length

Dura mater—the outer meninx (membrane) that covers the brain and spinal cord

Dysarthria—difficulty with speech due to impairment of the nerves or muscles that control speech

Dysfunction—abnormal function

Dyskinesia—impairment of voluntary movement

Dyspareunia—pain occurring in the genital area during or after sexual intercourse

Dysphagia—difficulty with swallowing

Dyspnea—difficulty with breathing

Dysrhythmia—abnormality of the rhythm; refers to abnormally fast, slow, or irregular rhythm

Dysuria—painful urination

Eclampsia—complication of pregnancy that develops during the last portion of the pregnancy; characterized by hypertension, weight gain, headaches, and edema; severe cases may lead to seizures, coma, and possible death

Ectopic pregnancy—fertilized ovum that attaches frequently in the fallopian tubes or elsewhere outside of the endometrium of the uterus

Edema—accumulation of fluid in the tissues that results in swelling and weight gain

Ejaculation—forcible expulsion of semen from the penis

Electrolytes—compounds capable of transmitting an electrical current, e.g. sodium, potassium, and chloride

Embolism—substance or blood clot that travels through the vascular system of the body often causing obstruction by lodging in the lumen of a vessel

Emesis—vomiting

Emphysema—chronic lung disease; airways of the lungs become distended and lose their elasticity

Empyema—pus-filled cavity, generally located in the lung

Emulsify—breakdown of fats in the digestive system

Encephalitis—inflammation of the brain and the meninges

Encephalopathy—refers to any disease or disorder of the brain

Endarterectomy—surgical removal of plaque and fat buildup from the lumen of an artery

Endocrine—gland that secretes hormones directly into the bloodstream, such as adrenal, islets of Langerhans, ovaries, parathyroid, pineal, pituitary, testes, thymus, and thyroid

Endocrinologist—physician specializing in the area of endocrinology (study of the endocrine system)

Endometrial—of the mucous membrane that lines the interior of the uterus

Endoneurium—covering of the individual fibers of the nerve within the peripheral nerve

Enema—introduction of fluid into the rectum to stimulate a bowel movement; fluid may also be introduced for the purpose of treatments or testing (x-ray)

Engorgement—process by which blood vessels become filled with blood

Enteric—refers to the intestine

Enterostomal therapist—person with specific training to aid clients with the care of stomas

Enzyme—proteins that can change another substance chemically without themselves being changed or destroyed

Eosinophils—granular white blood cells; play an important part in the immune response of the body as well as during allergic reactions

Epidemiology—study of the cause of disease and disease transmission and methods to control disease

Epidermoid—the epidermis (skin)

Epididymitis—inflammation of the epididymis, which is a place of storage and maturation for sperm

Epithelium—covering of internal and external organs

Epstein-Barr virus—virus that causes mononucleosis

Equilibrium—state of being equal or balanced; refers to chemical or physical balance within the body

Erythrocytes—red blood cells; biconcave disc-shaped cells; function in the body to transport oxygen and carbon dioxide within the bloodstream; average of 5 million per cubic millimeter of blood

Esophageal reflux—backing up of stomach acid into the esophagus

Esophageal varices—dilation of the vessels of the esophagus; may result in inflammation and bleeding; condition often associated with cirrhosis of the liver

Esophagitis—inflammation of the esophagus

Esophagus—hollow muscular tube that connects the pharynx to the stomach; average of 10 to 12 inches in length; part of the gastrointestinal system

Estrogen—female sex hormone produced by the ovary

Exacerbated—the severity of the symptoms of a specific disease are increased

Excretion—eliminate or pass out of

Exocrine—gland that secretes directly to the surface of the skin or through ducts to the outside of the gland

Expectorants—medications or substances that promote the removal of fluids or phlegm from the respiratory tract

Expiration—the process of breathing out during respiration (breathing)

Exposure—process of having come in contact with an infectious person or an infectious agent; process of coming in contact with or being subjected to radiation

External—exterior or outside

Extremity—refers to the arms or legs of the body; limb

Extrinsic—outside

Fallopian tube—tube located between the ovary and the uterus; transports the ovum

Fasting—abstain from eating for a certain period of time

Fatal—resulting in death

Fatigue—feeling of tiredness or exhaustion

Fecal—refers to bowel movements or stools passed from the intestines

Feces—solid waste passed from the intestinal tract; stool or bowel movement

Fetid—foul smelling

Fetus—refers to an unborn child during the last two trimesters (6 months) in the uterus

Fiber—substances that remain after the digestion of foods in the digestive tract; bulk

Fibrinogen—protein in the blood that is necessary for clotting

Fibrocystic—abnormal growth of fibrous tissue

Fibrosis—fibrous tissue formation

Fibrous—similar to scar tissue

Fissure—formation of a groove or crack

Fistula—abnormal passageway from one organ to another or from an internal organ to the exterior of the body

Flaccid—limp; absence of muscle tone or movement

Flank—area of the back and side between the lower edge of the ribs to the upper area of the ilium

Flaring—spread outward

Flatus—gas in the intestinal tract

Flexion—bending

Fontanel—soft spot or open space between the skull bones in a fetus or infant

Forceps—instrument used to grasp or hold an object

Frontal lobe—anterior portion of the cerebrum of the brain

Fulminant hepatitis—sudden onset of symptoms with hepatitis that usually results in death

Fungus—plant organism, e.g. yeast and mold

Fusion—join or grow together

Gait—pattern of movement or ambulation

Gait belt—belt made of webbed fabric that is put around the waist of a person needing assistance with transfer or ambulation; added security by allowing the person who is assisting to have a firm hold on the belt

Gallbladder—organ located directly below the liver; function is to store and concentrate bile, which is manufactured by the liver

Gamma globulin—protein manufactured by the lymph system in response to toxins present in the system, e.g. bacteria or virus

Gastric—stomach

Gastrointestinal—refers to the system of the body that includes the mouth, esophagus, stomach, small intestine, and large intestine; function is to digest foods and remove the nutrients and fluids from them for use in the tissues of the body

Gastrostomy—opening from the abdomen to the stomach for the purpose of feeding

Gene—hereditary unit that makes up DNA

Genetic—heredity or reproduction

Genital—the reproductive organs of the male or female

Genitourinary—organs contained in the genital and urinary systems of the body

Gestational—occurring during the period of development of the fetus from conception to birth

Girth—measurement of the circumference of the abdomen

Gland—organ within the body that secretes a certain substance or hormone; endocrine and exocrine

Glomerulonephritis—inflammation of the glomeruli of the kidney

Glucagon—hormone secreted by the pancreas that has the capability of elevating the level of glucose in the blood; also available in a commercially manufactured form used to elevate the level of glucose in the blood during periods of hypoglycemia

Glucocorticoids—hormones secreted by the adrenal gland that affect the metabolism of carbohydrates and proteins in the body

Glucose—sugar manufactured in the body by the metabolism of carbohydrates; primary energy source for the body's cells

Glycogen—stored in the body and can be converted into glucose within the body during periods of hypoglycemia; glycogen is formed initially from carbohydrates

Gout—disease that causes inflammation of the joint(s) due to an accumulation of uric acid

Gram stain—procedure of staining a smear on a slide to determine the type of bacteria; gram-positive bacteria organisms stain dark purple in reaction to the crystal violet iodine solution and safranin O, gram-negative bacteria organisms stain pink or red

Granulocytes—the granular leukocytes (basophils, eosinophils, and neutrophils)

Gray matter—portions of the central nervous system made up primarily of the nerve cell bodies, which are gray in color

Groin—the area located at the junction of the abdomen and thighs

Gynecomastia—enlarged breasts in the male

Habilitation—process of improving the functional ability of a person with a disability

Hallucination—sensory perception that is not based on actual external stimuli; may relate to the sense of taste, smell, sight, sound, or touch

Heberden's nodes—nodules located on the joints of the fingers; present with osteoarthritis

Heimlich maneuver—technique used to remove an obstruction caused by a foreign body in the respiratory tract; technique consists of inward and upward abdominal thrusts, which cause pressure on the diaphragm

Hematemesis—presence of blood in emesis

Hematocrit—percentage by volume of the number of red blood cells in the blood

Hematuria—presence of blood in the urine

Hemianopia—loss of vision of half of the visual field of an eye or eyes

Hemiplegia—refers to paralysis of one half of the body

Hemisphere—refers to half of the cerebrum or cerebellum

Hemoccult®—test used to check for the presence of blood in feces

Hemochromatosis—metabolic disease in which the body stores an excess amount of iron

Hemoglobin—protein found in the red blood cells that contains iron; function is to enable the red blood cells to transport oxygen and carbon dioxide in the bloodstream

Hemiparesis—paralysis of one half of the body

Hemolytic—red blood cell destruction

Hemophilia—hereditary disorder in which there is an abnormality in the clotting mechanism of the blood and prolonged bleeding time

Hemoptysis—coughing up of blood from the respiratory tract

Hemorrhage—extreme bleeding or blood loss; may be internal or external

Hemorrhoids—enlargement of the vessels of the mucous membrane of the anus or rectum

Hepatic—refers to the liver

Hepatitis—inflammation of the liver; caused by viral, bacterial, or chemical agents

Hepatomegaly—refers to enlargement of the liver

Heredity—genetic characteristics or traits that are passed from parents to their offspring

Herpes simplex virus—virus that causes vesicles on the skin, generally in the facial area

Heterosexual—sexual preference or attraction for persons of the opposite sex

Hinge joints—joints that allow bones to swing back and forth like a door on a hinge; examples of hinge joints are the elbows and the knees

Histamine—protein substance that is normally present in the body and is released in response to injury or inflammation

Histiocyte—cell that carries on the process of phagocytosis

Homosexual—sexual preference or attraction for persons of the same sex

Hormonal receptor assay—test that helps in the determination of an estrogen- versus a progesterone-dependent tumor

Hormone—substance secreted by certain organs or tissues in the body that stimulate the activity of other tissues or glands in the body

Hospice—supportive care that is directed at meeting the social, spiritual, physical, psychological, and safety needs of a dying person and his or her family

Human immunodeficiency virus (HIV)—virus that causes acquired immune deficiency syndrome (AIDS)

Hydrocephalus—accumulation of cerebrospinal fluid within the cranium; the excess fluid may cause an enlargement of the skull in infants and causes extreme pressure on the brain; accumulation of fluid caused from overproduction of cerebrospinal fluid or inadequate drainage of the cerebrospinal fluid

Hyperaldosteronism—condition during which an abnormally large amount of aldosterone is manufactured and secreted by the adrenal glands

Hyperalimentation—introduction of solution into the body that is high enough in necessary nutrients to sustain life; may by introduced through either a parenteral route or enteral route

Hyperbaric—increased pressure and increased amounts of oxygen

Hyperextensible—more than normal extension of a joint, often causing injury

Hyperglycemia—increased amounts of glucose in the blood

Hypertension—high blood pressure

Hyperthyroidism—condition during which an abnormally large amount of thyroid hormones is manufactured and secreted by the thyroid

Hypertrophy—enlarged size of a tissue or organ

Hyperventilation—rapid rate of respirations that increases the amount of air in the lungs; often seen in stress or with lung diseases

Hypoalbuminemia—decreased amounts of albumin in the blood

Hypoglycemia—decreased amounts of glucose in the blood

Hypokalemia—decreased amounts of potassium in the blood

Hyponatremia—decreased amounts of sodium in the blood

Hypoparathyroidism—decreased secretion of hormones from the parathyroid gland

Hypopituitarism—decreased secretion of hormones from the pituitary gland

Hypotension—low blood pressure

Hypothermia—a body temperature that is abnormally low

Hypothyroidism—decreased secretion of hormones by the thyroid gland

Hypotonia—abnormal reduction in tone or strength of muscles

Hypotonic—decreased muscle tone

Hypoxemia—decreased amounts of oxygen in the bloodstream and, therefore, decreased amounts of oxygen available to the tissues of the body

Hypoxia—decreased oxygen intake

Hysterectomy—surgical removal of the uterus

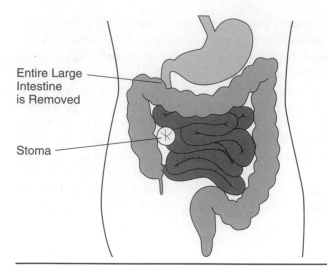

Entire Large Intestine is Removed

Stoma

Figure G-1 An ileostomy and stoma (large intestine removed) (From Hegner, *Nursing Assistant: A Nursing Process Approach, 7th edition*, copyright © 1995, Delmar Publishers)

Idiopathic—disease that has no specifically known cause

Ileostomy—opening from the ileum to the abdominal wall for the purpose of excreting waste products (See Figure G-1)

Ileum—distal portion of the small intestine; small intestine is divided into three parts: the duodenum, jejunum, and ileum; varies in total length from 8 to 15 feet

Imaging—imaging oneself in a different setting, often used as a method of pain relief

Immobility—inability or a decrease in the ability to be mobile (movement)

Immune—resistant to disease either by natural defenses in the body (antibodies) or through the use of a vaccine

Immune system—system of the body that has the primary function of detecting pathogens in the body and removing or destroying the foreign pathogen; also known as the lymph system

Immunity—the body's resistance to a disease or injury from a pathogen; most frequently refers to contagious diseases

Immunoglobin—protein that is able to function as an antibody

Immunologic—condition of being immune

Immunosuppressives—medications that suppress the body's formation of antibodies in response to an antigen

Immunotherapy—therapy that builds up the body's natural immune system by injecting small amounts of antibodies, which have been produced by a donor, into the person's system

Impotence—incapability of the male to achieve an erection during sexual arousal

Inanimate—refers to an object that is not alive

Incontinent—inability to control urination or defecation; may be due to muscle damage, neurological damage, or confusion

Incubation—the length of time it takes from exposure to a disease to develop the symptoms of the disease

Infectious—ability to transmit a disease

Inferior—below another part

Infertility—inability to become pregnant (female) or to cause a pregnancy (male)

Inflammation—localized response to injury; symptoms may include redness, swelling, pain, or increased local temperature

Influenza—acute viral respiratory infection characterized by fever, cough, chills, headache, and sore throat

Insidious—refers to a gradual onset of symptoms

Insomnia—inability to fall asleep or stay asleep once sleep is achieved

Inspiration—process of drawing oxygen-rich air into the lungs

Insulin—hormone produced by the beta cells of the islets of Langerhans of the pancreas, which is necessary for the metabolism of glucose for energy by the cells of the body; also a commercially prepared substance that can be injected into the body in the absence or diminished production of insulin by the body

Intake and output (I and O)—record that is kept of all fluids taken into the body and all the fluids that leave the body

Integumentary—system of the body that includes the skin, hair, and nails

Interstitially—relating to the spaces between the cells and tissues of the body

Intima—lining of the blood vessels

Intoxication—intake of large amounts of alcohol that alter a person's ability to function and reason clearly

Intracranial—refers to the area within the cranium

Intravenous (IV)—the area within the veins of the body or the introduction of fluids into the veins of the body

Intravesical—inside the bladder

Intrinsic—within the body

Intubation—insertion of a hollow tube through the nose or mouth into the trachea for the purpose of delivering oxygen to a patient in an emergency

Iron—mineral found in meats, legumes, and fortified grains that is necessary for the production of hemoglobin; hemoglobin is the protein portion of the red blood cell that transports oxygen

Ischemia—diminished blood supply to a portion of the body

Jaundice—yellow discoloration of the skin, mucous membranes, and eyes due to an accumulation of bilirubin in the blood

Jejunum—the middle portion of the small intestine; the small intestine is divided into three parts: the duodenum, jejunum, and ileum; the jejunum is approximately 8 feet in length

Jobst stockings—highly elasticized stocking that is worn to increase venous blood return and lymphatic vessel return from the extremities

Joint—the place where two bones meet

Joint aspiration—removal of fluid from the space around a joint

Joint capsule—fibrous tissue that surrounds the joint

Kaposi's sarcoma—type of cancer that frequently involves the skin; may involve other sites of the body as well; frequently found in patients with AIDS

Karyotype—arrangement of the chromosomes according to order of size

Keratitis—inflammation of the cornea of the eye

Kernicterus—buildup of bilirubin in the brain and spinal cord of an infant

Kernig's sign—inability to straighten the leg while in a sitting position without extreme pain to the hamstring area; frequent symptom of meningitis

Ketoacidosis—accumulation of ketone bodies in the bloodstream that causes a decreased pH level in the body (acidosis)

Ketone—end product of the metabolism of fat in the body

Kyphosis—curvature of the spine in the thoracic region; also known as hunchback

Lability—instability; generally refers to the state of emotional well-being

Lanugo—fine hair that covers the body; generally seen in newborn infants and especially premature infants

Larynx—voice box, located at the base of the throat region

Lassitude—extreme fatigue

Laxatives—medications or substances given to promote a bowel movement by increasing peristalsis or by absorbing fluid from the surrounding tissues to loosen the consistency of the feces

Lesion—infection or injury to the skin

Lethargy—sluggishness; extreme fatigue or exhaustion

Leukemia—malignant disease characterized by uncontrolled growth of immature white blood cells

Leukocytes—white blood cells; divided into two groups: granular (basophils, eosinophils, neutrophils) and nongranular (lymphocytes, monocytes)

Leukocytosis—increased number of leukocytes in the blood

Leukopenia—decreased number of white blood cells

Libido—sexual desires

Ligament—connective tissue that connects bones to one another

Lipoproteins—proteins that are bound to lipids (fats) in the bloodstream

Liver—organ of the body located in the upper right quadrant of the abdomen

Lobe—specific portion of an organ

Lobectomy—surgical removal of the lobe of an organ; frequently refers to the lung or brain

Lumen—diameter of the interior of a vessel or duct

Lumpectomy—surgical removal of a lump

Lupus erythematosus—disease of the skin and connective tissues of the body

Luteinizing hormone—hormone secreted by the anterior pituitary gland that regulates ovulation and the endometrium in response to pregnancy

Lymphadenopathy—refers to disease of the lymph nodes; generally accompanied by enlargement of the lymph nodes

Lymphedema—swelling of an extremity due to obstruction of the lymph vessels

Lymph nodes—tissue located along the lymph vessels that is an important part of the lymph system (immune system); lymph nodes filter pathogens from the bloodstream and produce monocytes and lymphocytes

Lymphoblast—immature lymphocyte

Lymphocyte—one of the two nongranular leukocytes; responsible for providing immunity for the body against diseases

Lymphocytosis—increased number of lymphocytes

Lymphomas—tumors of the lymph tissues

Lymph system—system of the body that has the primary function of detecting pathogens in the body and removing or destroying the foreign pathogen; also known as the immune system

Malabsorption—inadequate or altered absorption of vitamins, minerals, and other nutrients from the digestive tract

Malaise—feeling of fatigue and vague discomfort

Malalignment—displaced alignment; refers frequently to the bones or teeth

Malignancy—cancerous

Malnutrition—poor nutrition resulting in inadequate intake of vitamins, minerals, and other nutrients necessary for proper health and maintenance of the body

Malodorous—refers to foul or unpleasant odor

Mammography—x-ray of the breast tissue; used in the diagnosis of breast cancer and other diseases affecting the breast

Manifests—makes itself known; usually refers to the appearance of symptoms

Mast cells—cells present in the connective tissues that are responsible for manufacturing and storing histamine; stimulated as part of the inflammatory response of the body

Mastectomy—surgical removal of the breast

Maternal—refers to the mother

Mechanical ventilation—providing oxygenation of the lungs through artificial methods with the use of an endotracheal tube (intubation) and the use of an ambu bag or mechanical ventilator (respirator)

Mediastinum—the area between the lungs in the chest

Medulla—lowest section of the brain stem

Membrane—external or internal covering of an organ

Meninges—membranes covering the brain and spinal cord (dura mater, arachnoid, and pia mater); *singular*, meninx

Meningitis—inflammation of the meninges of the brain and spinal cord

Menopause—cessation of the menstrual cycle in the female; generally occurring between the ages of 45 and 55

Menses—menstruation

Menstruation—monthly discharge of blood and tissues from the lining of the uterus in a female who is not pregnant; generally a cycle of 28 days

Metabolic—refers to metabolism

Metabolic alkalosis—condition caused by a loss of acids and an increase in the pH and bicarbonate levels in the blood

Metabolized—combined chemical and physical changes occur within the body

Metastasized—spread from one point to another point within the body; generally refers to the spread of cancer within the body

Midbrain—uppermost section of the brain stem

Milliliter (ml)—unit of liquid measurement; 1/1000 of a liter

Miscarriage—spontaneous expulsion of the fetus from the uterus prior to viability of the fetus

Mitochondria—energy source within the cell

Mitral valve (bicuspid)—valve located in the heart between the left atrium and the left ventricle

Mobility—the capability of movement or of being mobile

Monocytes—nongranular white blood cells (lymphocytes are the other nongranular white blood cells)

Monogamy—sexual relationships with one person exclusively; generally refers to married couples remaining faithful to one another

Mononucleosis—disease affecting the lymph system; often referred to as "kissing disease"

Monoplegia—paralysis of a single limb

Monotone—voice lacking character

Mortality—refers to the state of being subject to death

Motor neuron—controls the motor movements of the muscles and organs of the body from stimulation received from the central nervous system

Mucous—fluid secreted by the mucous membranes of the body

Mucous membrane—membrane that lines organs or systems that are open to the air and secrete mucous

Mucous plug—hardened mucous secretions that block a portion of the airway within the lung

Multiple sclerosis (MS)—disease of the nervous system caused by destruction of the myelin sheath

Muscular dystrophy—disease characterized by muscle weakness and degeneration of the muscle tissue

Myalgia—muscle pain

Myasthenia gravis—disease of the muscular system caused by a lack of acetylcholine

Mycobacterium—families of organisms that cause leprosy and tuberculosis

Mycoplasma—organism lacking a cell wall; frequently causes infections of the genitourinary or respiratory systems

Mycosis fungoides—malignant cancerous growth located on the skin of the body and scalp that has the potential of becoming ulcerated and infected

Myelin sheath—fatlike covering around the nerve fibers

Myocardial—heart muscle

Myocardial infarction (MI)—heart muscle death due to complete or partial obstruction of the coronary arteries that supply the specific regions of the heart muscle with blood; also known as heart attack

Nasal—nose

Nasal flaring—increase in the size of the nostrils generally due to respiratory distress in children

Nasogastric tubes (NG)—tubes that are passed through the nose and into the stomach; option of using the tubes to drain stomach contents or instillation of fluids into the stomach

Nasopharyngeal—nose and throat

Necrosis—tissue death

Neoplasm—new growth or formation of abnormal tissue often crowding out healthy tissue

Neoplastic—refers to the tissue growth of a neoplasm

Nerve fiber—term for neuron, which is the nerve cell

Neurofibrillary tangles—nerve fibers twisted in tangles that are located in the neuron of the cell; present in Alzheimer's disease

Neurological—refers to the nervous system

Neuromuscular—refers to a combination of the muscles and the nerves

Neuromuscular junction—place at which nerves and muscles meet or connect

Neuropathy—refers to a disease of the nerves

Neurotransmitters—substances that enable an impulse to travel from the axon of a neuron, across the synapse, and to the dendrite of another neuron

Neutropenia—decrease in the total number of neutrophils

Neutrophils—one of the three granular white blood cells or leukocytes (granular leukocytes include basophils, eosinophils, and neutrophils)

Nicotine—poisonous substance found in tobacco

Nitrogen—element occurring in the form of a gas in the atmosphere

Nocturia—increased frequency of urination during the night

Nocturnal—refers to night time

Nodule—refers to a node or a swelling of a specific location on the body

Nonsteroidal anti-inflammatory drugs (NSAID)—medications that decrease inflammation, relieve pain, and reduce fever

Norepinephrine—hormone produced by the adrenal gland that acts as a vasoconstrictor

Noxious—poisonous or harmful

Nuchal—refers to the neck

Nulliparity—condition referring to a female who has not produced a viable (living or capable of living) offspring

Obesity—the state of being overweight; generally refers to those people who are a minimum of 20 to 30% over their recommended weight

Obstruction—blockage

Occipital lobe—lobe of the cerebrum located directly above the cerebellum in the posterior of the brain

Olfactory—the first of the twelve cranial nerves; responsible for the sense of smell

Oophorectomy—surgical removal of the ovary

Oophoropexy—repair of an ovary that is not in the correct position

Ophthalmologist—specialist (physician) whose main focus is diagnosing and treating diseases and disorders of the eye

Opisthotonos—spasm involving the entire body in which the back is arched backward; seen as a symptom of meningitis, tetanus, and poisoning

Opportunistic illness—illness or infection that occurs during a time when the immune system is depressed or defective

Orally—taken by mouth

Orchiectomy—surgical removal of the testicle

Orthopnea—difficulty breathing unless in an upright position

Orthostatic hypotension—results when a person moves from a recumbent to a standing position; also known as postural hypotension

Orthotics—appliances used in the treatment or rehabilitation of neuromuscular illness or disorders

Osteoplasty—surgical repair of a bone

Osteoporosis—refers to loss of bone tissue and skeletal mass

Osteotomy—refers to surgically cutting into a bone

Otitis media—inflammation of the middle ear

Ova and parasites—test done on feces to check for the presence of parasites

Ovarian—relating to the female reproductive glands that store the ovum and produce estrogen and progesterone

Overhydration—fluid overload in the body

Ovum—female reproductive cell or egg

Oximeter—noninvasive machine used to determine the amount of oxygen in the blood

Oxygen (O$_2$)—gas present in the atmosphere that is necessary for the respiratory process of humans and other animals

Pacemaker—instrument capable of delivering an electrical current to the heart to stimulate contraction of the heart muscle

Palliative—treatment offered for purposes of comfort rather than purposes of cure

Pallor—pale; absence of color

Palpate—to examine or feel with the fingers or hand

Palpitations—unusually strong, bounding pulse of the heart that is often felt or noticed by the patient

Pancreas—organ located in the upper left quadrant of the abdomen that secretes insulin and digestive enzymes

Pancreatitis—inflammation of the pancreas

Pannus—tissue covering a surface of the body

Papillary—nipple of the breast

Paracentesis—removal of fluid from a cavity through a surgically made puncture site

Paralysis—loss of feeling or movement to a certain portion of the body

Paranoia—mental disturbance characterized by delusions of persecution or illusions of grandeur

Paraplegia—paralysis involving both legs of the body and may involve the entire lower portion of the body

Parasite—organism that is only able to live when it gains nourishment from another living organism (host)

Parathyroid—gland located adjacent to the thyroid gland in the neck that secretes parathyroid hormone

Parenteral—route for nourishment or medication that does not include the alimentary canal, e.g. intravenous, intramuscular, and subcutaneous

Paresthesia—refers to a feeling of numbness or tingling

Parietal lobe—sections of the cerebrum located at the side

Parkinson's disease—disease of the nervous system characterized by weakness, muscle rigidity, and tremor

Parotid glands—salivary glands in the mouth

Paroxysmal—sudden exacerbation of symptoms of a short duration

Paternal—refers to the father

Pathogen—disease-producing substance

Pectoral—chest

Pelvic inflammatory disease (PID)—infection involving the internal female reproductive organs

Pelvis—region located below the abdomen

Penis—male sex organ used for the purpose of urination and sexual intercourse

Pepsin—enzyme secreted by the stomach that is responsible for the breakdown of proteins

Perforation—creation of a hole or opening

Pericardial fluid—fluid in the sac (cavity) surrounding the heart

Pericarditis—inflammation of the sac around the heart

Perinatal—refers to the time directly before, during, and after birth

Perineal—external floor of the pelvis

Perineurium—tissue that divides fibers of nerves within the peripheral nerve

Peripheral—refers to a part of the body away from the midline

Peristalsis—muscular contractions of the gastrointestinal tract

Peritoneal—refers to peritoneum

Peritoneal fluid—fluid located in the peritoneum that cushions the organs from one another and prevents friction between the organs

Peritoneum—tissue that lines the organ of the abdomen and the interior abdominal wall

Peritonitis—inflammation of the peritoneum (membrane that lines the abdominal cavity)

Peyer's patches—lymph nodes located in the ileum of the small intestine

Phagocytosis—white blood cells that surround and destroy pathogens in the body

Pharynx—throat

Pheochromocytoma—tumor located in the adrenal medulla that secretes epinephrine and norepinephrine

Philadelphia chromosome—abnormality in chromosome 9 or 22; commonly found in patients with chronic myelocytic leukemia

Phlebotomy—withdrawal of blood from a vein

Phlegm—mucous from the respiratory tract

Photophobia—increased sensitivity to light

Pia mater—innermost meninx (membrane) covering the brain and spinal cord

Pineal body (pineal gland)—gland in the brain stem that secretes melatonin, which controls the secretion of melanin in the skin

Pituitary gland—gland located in the brain that secretes hormones responsible for controlling the other glands of the body

Placenta previa—placental attachment near the opening of the uterus (cervix) rather than the normal position higher on the uterine wall

Plantar—refers to the sole of the foot

Plaque—abnormal accumulation of a substance; generally refers to the lumen of the blood vessel or to the teeth

Plasma—liquid portion of the blood

Plasmapheresis—separating the plasma from the cells in a specimen of blood by means of centrifuge; the red blood cells are then reinjected into the original donor or another person

Platelet—disklike structure in the blood that is important for the clotting of blood; also known as thrombocyte

Pleura—membrane that encloses the lung

Pleural—refers to the pleura of the lung

Pleural effusion—fluid accumulation in the cavity surrounding the lung

Pleural fluid—the fluid that accumulates with pleural effusion

Pleurisy—inflammation of the pleura of the lung

Pneumococcal—caused by pneumococci

Pneumocystis carinii pneumonia—type of pneumonia caused by the *Pneumocystis carinii* organism; commonly seen with AIDS

Pneumonectomy—surgical removal of the lung

Pneumonia—inflammation or infection of the lungs

Pneumotoxic—produced by pneumococci

Polycythemia—increased number of red blood cells in the blood

Polycythemia vera—chronic disease in which the RBCs and hemoglobin are increased

Polydipsia—extreme thirst; common sign of diabetes mellitus

Polyps—growths originating in a mucous membrane

Polypectomy—surgical removal of a polyp

Polyphagia—increased appetite and consumption of food; common symptom of diabetes

Polyposis—condition of having many polyps

Polyunsaturated—fats that become liquid at room temperature

Polyuria—extreme amounts of urine produced and discharged from the urethra; a common symptom of diabetes

Pons—portion of the brain anterior to the cerebellum and between the medulla and the midbrain

Portal—refers to the vessel that carries blood to and through the liver

Posterior—back side or back part

Postmenopausal—after cessation of the menstrual cycle (menopause)

Postnatal—refers to the period after birth

Postural drainage—procedure in which the patient is positioned in alternating positions to facilitate drainage and expectoration of secretions in the lung through the use of gravity

Potassium—mineral found in bananas, potatoes, yellow vegetables, citrus fruits, and milk; necessary for the regulation of fluid balance in the body as well as muscle and nerve function

Predisposition—presence of conditions that could increase the tendency toward developing a disease or illness

Prenatal—refers to the period before birth

Proctitis—inflammation of the anus, rectum, and surrounding tissues

Progesterone—hormone secreted by the ovary

Progestin—class of hormones that includes the hormone progesterone

Prognosis—projected outcome of a disease or illness

Proliferation—ability for rapid multiplication or reproduction

Prone—positioned on the abdomen

Prostatectomy—surgical removal of the prostate gland

Prostate gland—male gland that surrounds the urethra and secretes the liquid portion of semen

Prostatitis—inflammation of the prostate gland

Prosthesis—artificial limb or body part; frequently refers to breast prosthesis or artificial limb

Protein—substance found in meats, vegetables, and dairy products; necessary for growth, energy, and muscle strength

Proteinuria—increased amounts of protein or albumin in the urine

Prothrombin—part of the clotting factor that is converted to thrombin through interaction with thrombokinase

Protozoa—single-celled organisms found in water and soil; capable of causing disease

Pruritus—itchiness of the skin

Ptosis—drooping of a body part; frequently refers to the eyelid

Puberty—time when a person becomes able to reproduce; generally occurs during adolescence

Pulmonary—refers to the lung

Pulmonary artery—artery that carries blood to the lungs from the right ventricle of the heart

Pulmonary embolism—obstruction of a portion of the arterial circulation of the lungs due to a blood clot that travels from another part of the body and lodges in the arterial circulation

Pulmonary semilunar valve—valve located between the right ventricle of the heart and the pulmonary artery

Pulmonary vein—vein that carries blood from the lungs to the left atrium of the heart

Purge—emptying of the gastrointestinal tract by manually forcing oneself to vomit or through the use of laxatives

Pyelonephritis—inflammation of the kidney(s)

Quadrant—a specific region of the abdomen that has been divided into four separate portions by one horizontal and one vertical line through the umbilicus (See Figure G-2)

Quadriplegia—paralysis of all four limbs of the body; generally includes the trunk of the body

Radiation—therapy for the treatment of malignancies and certain other disorders through the use of specified amounts of radiation directed at the specific location of the body to be treated

Rales—abnormal respiratory sound that occurs as a result of air moving within lungs that have an increased amount of secretions present within them

Range of motion (ROM)—exercises during which each of the joints of the body is put through its entire range of movements; generally done when a patient is immobile to prevent the formation of contractures, decubitus ulcers, and other complications that may occur as a result of immobility

Rectal—refers to the rectum (distal 5 inches of the large intestine)

Rectum—distal 5 inches of the large intestine; responsible for storing feces until they are ready to be expelled from the body

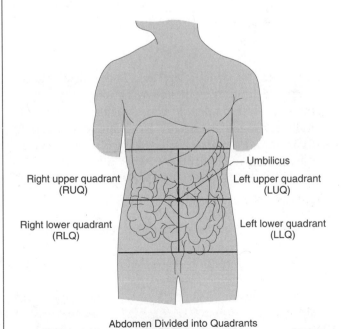

Right upper quadrant (RUQ)

Left upper quadrant (LUQ)

— Umbilicus

Right lower quadrant (RLQ)

Left lower quadrant (LLQ)

Abdomen Divided into Quadrants

Figure G-2 The abdominal quadrants (From Smith et al., *Medical Terminology: A Programmed Text*, 7th edition, copyright © 1995, Delmar Publishers)

Red blood cells (RBCs)—biconcave cells present in the blood; combine with hemoglobin to transport oxygen and carbon dioxide throughout the body; normal accumulation of 5,000,000 per cubic millimeter in the human body; also known as erythrocytes

Reed-Sternberg cells—cells present in the connective tissue with Hodgkin's disease

Remission—period of diminished or absent symptoms of a disease or illness

Renal—refers to the kidney

Renal failure—failure of the kidney to function

Resection—partial surgical removal of an organ or other part of the body

Respiration—process of breathing in (inspiration) and out (expiration) that brings oxygen into the body (inspiration) and releases the waste product of carbon dioxide (expiration)

Respiratory arrest—respirations cease

Respiratory failure—increase in carbon dioxide levels in the blood and decreased levels of oxygen in the blood due to poor air exchange within the lungs

Retention—holding something in the body that usually is excreted from the body; often refers to fluid within the cells of the body

Retina—portion at the posterior of the eye that receives the visual image from the lens

Retinopathy—refers to disease of the retina

Retraction—pulling back

Retrovirus—special group of viruses

Rickettsia—microorganism belonging to the Rickettsia family

Rigidity—stiffness

Rubella—infectious disease of short duration caused by a virus characterized by rash and fever; also known as German measles

Sacral—the five vertebrae located at the distal end of the spinal column directly above the coccyx

Salicylate—salt of salicylic acid, which, in the form of acetylsalicylic acid, is used as an analgesic (aspirin)

Saliva—liquid secreted by the salivary glands to aid in the digestion of food

Salivary gland—glands located in the oral cavity that secrete saliva

Satiated—being full or satisfied

Saturated fat—fats from animal sources that are solid at room temperature

Scleritis—inflammation of the sclera (fibrous tissue that covers the "white of the eye")

Sclerosis—formation of scar tissue from normal, healthy tissue

Seborrhea—increased secretions from the sebaceous (oil-producing) glands of the body; frequently refers to the sebaceous glands of the scalp; commonly called dandruff

Secondary sex characteristics—physical characteristics that develop at the time of puberty and were not present at birth; examples include development of breasts and pubic hair in females and development of facial hair and increased body hair in males

Sedentary—life style that includes very little physical labor, exertion, or exercise; inactive

Seizure—episode affecting the nervous system that is characterized by symptoms ranging from alteration in consciousness to severe tremors involving the entire body, which can be accompanied by a temporary loss of consciousness

Semen—thick, white fluid that is discharged from the urethra of the penis of the male during sexual arousal and climax

Semi-Fowler's position—position of sitting up in bed with the back supported

Sensitivity—determining which treatment would be most effective in treating the microorganism that has been cultured

Sensory nerves—nerves that transmit sensory impulses to the brain

Septum—division between two cavities or spaces within the body; frequently refers to the septum of the heart or the nasal septum

Serotonin—chemical that acts as a vasoconstrictor

Serum—portion of the blood remaining after the clotting factors have been removed or separated

Sexually transmitted disease (STD)—disease that is transmitted as a result of sexual activity with an infected person

Shock—condition in which the heart and circulatory system fail to provide adequate oxygenated blood to all the organs and tissues of the body

Sickle cell anemia—disease in which the red blood cells are elongated rather than biconcave and increase the thickness or viscosity of the blood

Sigmoid colon—portion of the large intestine between the transverse colon and the rectum

Simian crease—crease present on the palm of the hand; a common symptom of Down syndrome

Sinus—hollow space or cavity

Sinusitis—inflammation of the sinus cavity

Sitz baths—baths that soak the buttocks and hips; frequently used after the vaginal delivery of an infant or after rectal surgery

Skull—the bones that form the head

Sodium—mineral found in salt, cured meats, salted foods, and processed foods that is necessary for the maintenance of fluid balance within the body

Somatostatin—hormone that inhibits the secretion of the human growth hormone from the anterior pituitary gland

Spasm—uncontrolled movement caused by contraction of the muscles

Spasticity—increased muscular tone that makes movement or stretching of the muscles difficult

Specific gravity—weight of a material using water as a control or comparison

Sperm—male reproductive cells that are released in the semen during sexual arousal and climax

Spermicide—material or solution that destroys sperm

Sphincter—muscular opening between two parts of the body that, when contracted, prevents passage of material from one part to the next and also prevents reflux back into the original part of the body

Spider angiomata—burst capillaries located on the skin; frequently seen in patients with cirrhosis and other forms of liver disease

Spinal ganglion—root of the spinal nerve that is made up of cell bodies

Spleen—organ located in the upper left quadrant of the abdomen that is necessary for the filtering, storage, and formation of blood and blood cells

Splenectomy—surgical removal of the spleen

Splenomegaly—enlargement of the spleen

Spongy bone—lightweight bone located at the ends of the bone; the area resembles a sponge in appearance; this formation adds strength to the ends of the bone without adding extra weight

Spontaneous—voluntary occurrence

Spur—hard, bonelike growth located on the bone at the joint; common in arthritis

Sputum—material that is coughed up from within the respiratory tract

Stature—height when in an upright position

Stem cells—cells capable of reproducing cells for specific tissues in the body

Sternal retraction—retraction of the sternum during periods of extreme respiratory difficulty in children

Sternum—breastbone

Stillbirth—fetus that is dead at birth

Stoma—artificial opening created between two cavities in the body or between a cavity and the outside (surface) of the body

Stomatitis—inflammation of the mouth

Stool—solid waste material excreted from the bowels; bowel movement

Stricture—narrowing of an opening or lumen of a passageway in the body due to formation of scar tissue; strictures may also be congenital

Stroke—nerve and brain damage resulting from diminished blood flow or cessation of blood flow to a specific portion of the brain

Subarachnoid—located below the arachnoid (middle membrane or meninx that covers the brain and spinal cord)

Subcutaneous—below the skin

Substantia nigra—area of cells within the brain that produce dopamine

Sulfonylureas—medications that stimulate insulin production by the pancreas and increase the body cells' sensitivity to the insulin; used for the control of diabetes mellitus

Superior vena cava—one of the two main vessels that return blood from the body to the right atrium of the heart

Suppositories—cone-shaped, semisolid substances that may be inserted into the rectum, vagina, or urethra for the purpose of administering treatment or medication

Suprapubic—located above the pubic region

Symptomatic—presence of symptoms

Synapse—junction between the axon of one neuron and the dendrite of another neuron in the nervous system pathway; nerve impulse travels across this junction to continue the impulse along the nervous system pathway

Syncope—fainting; loss of consciousness

Synovectomy—surgical removal of synovial membrane

Synovial fluid—fluid that is secreted by the synovial membrane; located in bursae and cavities of joints; functions to protect and lubricate joints

Synovial membrane—lining of the synovial (joint) capsule

Synovitis—inflammation of the synovial membrane

Synovium—synovial membrane

Syrup of Ipecac—medication used to induce vomiting in certain cases of poisoning

Systemic—refers to the entire body

Systole—refers to the period of contraction of the ventricles of the heart

Systolic—refers to the first or top number in blood pressure; maximum blood pressure during contraction of the ventricles of the heart

Tachycardia—rapid heart rate; generally refers to a pulse greater than 100 to 110 beats per minute

Tachypnea—rapid respiratory rate; generally refers to a respiratory rate greater than 40 breaths per minute

T-cells—lymphocytes that are manufactured in the bone marrow and travel to the thymus gland of the body to mature; part of the immune system of the body; able to recognize antigens in the body and either destroy the antigens themselves or signal phagocytes to destroy the foreign substance

TED hose—elastic stockings used to aid in venous return of blood to the heart and decrease or prevent edema

Telemetry—transmission of heart rhythm to a distant screen through the use of electronics while the patient wears a small, portable monitor

Temporal lobe—lobe of the brain necessary for hearing and smelling

Tenacity—sticky or adhering

Tendon—fibrous tissue that connects muscles to bones

Tenesmus—spasms of the anal sphincter or urinary sphincter that gives the feeling of needing to empty the bowel or bladder; may cause pain with defecation or urination

Tenting—loss of elasticity of the skin caused by dehydration; causes skin to return slowly to its normal position when pinched

Terminal—pertaining to the end of life; often refers to a disease or illness that is expected to hasten death or be the direct cause of death

Testicles—male reproductive glands located in the scrotum directly adjacent to the penis

Testosterone—male hormone that is responsible for secondary sex characteristics production in men; produced in the testes

Thalamotomy—surgical removal or destruction of all or part of the thalamus

Thalamus—the portion of the brain that receives sensory input

Thoracic—chest or thorax

Thrombocytes—disklike structures in the blood that are important for the clotting of blood

Thrombocytopenia—decrease in the number of platelets in the blood, which could predispose the patient to abnormal bleeding

Thrombocytosis—increase in the number of platelets in the blood

Thromboembolism—blood clot that has moved from its site of origin

Thrombophlebitis—inflammation of a blood vessel due to the formation of a clot

Thrombosis—blood clot formation within the blood vessels

Thymectomy—surgical removal of the thymus gland

Thymoma—tumor of the thymus gland

Thymus gland—gland located in the mediastinum; part of the lymph system; responsible for the maturation of T-cells (lymphocytes) that have been produced in the bone marrow

Thyroid—gland in the neck region that regulates metabolism in the body

Topical—a specific area of the body; often refers to medication or ointments applied to the skin

Total parenteral nutrition (TPN)—total nutritional requirements provided through intravenous method; used for patients who are unable to take nutrition by mouth

Toxemia—toxic substances present in the blood that cause generalized symptoms due to their disbursement throughout the body

Toxicity—refers to a state of overwhelming poisonous substances in the body

Toxic megacolon—extreme dilation of the colon that predisposes the colon to rupturing

Toxin—poisonous substance

Toxoplasmosis—infection caused from the *Toxoplasma gondii* organism that can cause infections of the lungs, liver, immune system, and central nervous system

Trachea—airway that connects the larynx to the bronchial tubes

Tracheotomy—surgical creation of an opening between the trachea and the surface of the anterior neck

Transcutaneous electrical nerve stimulation (TENS)—transmission of an electrical stimulus over the body to the area of pain that interferes with pain sensation and transmission

Transient ischemic attack (TIA)—"mini-stroke"; caused by the temporary lack of blood supply to a specific portion of the brain

Transverse colon—portion of the large intestine located between the ascending and the descending colons

Tricuspid valve—valve located between the right atrium and right ventricle of the heart

Triplegia—paralysis involving the lower limbs of the body and one of the upper limbs

Tuberculosis—respiratory disease caused by the organism *Mycobacterium tuberculosis*; this disease may also infect the central nervous system, gastrointestinal system, skeletal system, immune system, integumentary system, or genitourinary system

Turgor—the normal elasticity and characteristics of the skin

Ulceration—lesion on the skin or mucous membrane

Ulcerative colitis—condition of inflammation of the colon resulting in formation of ulcers in the mucous membrane of the colon

Ultrasound—sound-wave visualization of organs and tissues of the body as the sound waves "bounce off" the various tissues and organs of the body and are recorded

Umbilical cord—network of blood vessels that connects the placenta to the fetus

Umbilical hernia—herniation in the area of the umbilicus (navel or "belly button")

Unilateral—one side of the body

Universal precautions—practice of maintaining a barrier between yourself and the potential contact with any blood or body fluids; essential to assume that any and all blood or body fluids are contaminated and have the capability of causing disease and illness

Urea—presence of by-products of protein metabolism (carbonic acid) in the urine, blood, or lymph; carbonic acid is one of the main substances that make up urine

Ureter—narrow tube that carries urine from the kidney to the bladder

Urethra—tube from which urine passes from the bladder to the outside of the body

Uricemia—accumulation of uric acid in the blood

Urinal—container males use to urinate into

Urination—process of eliminating urine from the body

Uterus—female organ that holds the developing fetus during pregnancy

Vaccinations—small amounts of an infectious agent given to a person to build up that person's immunity to the infectious agent

Vaccine—liquid suspension that includes an infectious agent used to build up immunity or resistance to that specific agent

Vagal nerve—tenth cranial nerve; responsible for swallowing and speaking as well as functioning of the aorta, stomach, and esophagus

Vaginal—relating to the external opening to the cervix and uterus; birth canal

Valvular—related to structures in the body that allow blood or other fluids in the body to flow in a single direction

Vascular—refers to the blood vessels of the body

Vasoconstriction—constriction of the vessels of the body or a specific area of the body

Vasodilation—refers to dilation of the vessels of the body

Vasodilator—medication or substance that causes dilation of the vessels of the body

Vein—blood vessel that returns blood to the heart

Ventricle—refers to a cavity within the body; generally refers to either the ventricles within the brain or the ventricles in the lower chambers of the heart

Vertigo—dizziness

Villi—fingerlike projections in the small intestine that absorb nutrients and fluids from food

Viruses—organisms that rely on other cells (hosts) for the nutrients necessary to sustain themselves

Vital signs—the measurements of temperature, pulse, respirations, and blood pressure; *see* Appendix D

Vitamin A—vitamin present in green leafy vegetables, carrots, dairy products, and fish that is necessary for healthy gums, hair, nails, teeth, and function of the eyes

Vitamin B$_{12}$—vitamin present in meats, eggs, and shellfish that is necessary for the function of the nervous system

Vitamin D—vitamin present in fortified dairy products, fish, and egg yolks that is necessary for the body's absorption of calcium

Vomit—expulsion of material from the stomach to the mouth

Vulva—external female reproductive parts or genitalia

Wheezing—whistling sound heard during the process of respirations due to constriction of the respiratory tract

White blood cells (WBCs)—responsible for fighting infection within the body; divided into granular white blood cells (basophils, eosinophils, and neutrophils) and nongranular white blood cells (lymphocytes and monocytes); also known as leukocytes

White matter—portions of the central nervous system made up primarily of the axons that are white in color

Bibliography

ABCs of viral hepatitis. (February 1991). *Health News.* Toronto, Ontario, Canada: University of Toronto.

Ahlskog, J. & Wilkinson, J. (February 1990). New concepts in the treatment of Parkinson's disease. *American Family Physician.* pp. 574–584.

Algra, B. (1992). *The facts about HIV and AIDS.* Health and Drug Education Series. Bakersfield, CA: Algra Corporation.

Algra, B. (1992). *How the AIDS virus is transmitted.* Health and Drug Education Series. Bakersfield, CA: Algra Corporation.

Altman, L. (November 9, 1990). High blood pressure: An overtreated condition? *The New York Times.*

Alzheimer's Association: Someone To Stand By You. (N.D.). *The dementias: Hope through research.*

Alzheimer's Association: Someone To Stand By You. (Summer 1993). Newsletter. Volume 13, No. 2, pp. 1, 4–6.

Alzheimer's Association: Someone To Stand By You. (1991). *Care for advanced Alzheimer's disease.*

Alzheimer's Association: Someone To Stand By You. (1991). *Directions in Alzheimer's disease research.*

Alzheimer's Association: Someone To Stand By You. (1991). *If you have Alzheimer's disease: What you should know, what you can do.*

Alzheimer's Association: Someone To Stand By You. (1990). *Alzheimer's disease: An overview.*

Alzheimer's Association: Someone To Stand By You. (1990). *Caregiving at home.*

Alzheimer's Association: Someone To Stand By You. (1990). *Communicating with the Alzheimer patient.*

Alzheimer's Association: Someone To Stand By You. (1990). *Especially for the Alzheimer caregiver.*

Alzheimer's Association: Someone To Stand By You. (1990). *If you think someone you know has Alzheimer's disease.*

Alzheimer's Association: Someone To Stand By You. (1989). *Information on Alzheimer's association.*

Alzheimer's Disease Education and Referral Center. (N.D.). *Alzheimer's disease fact sheet.*

American Cancer Society. (1990). *How to do breast self-examination.*

American Cancer Society. (1984). *How to examine your breasts.*

American Cancer Society. (1980). *Facts on colorectal cancer.*

American Cancer Society. (1978). *Facts on bladder cancer.*

American Cancer Society. (1978). *Facts on uterine cancer.*

American Cancer Society. (1977). *Cancer facts for men.*

American Cancer Society. (1973). *Stay healthy! Learn about uterine cancer.*

American Council for Healthful Living. (1990). *Common sexually transmitted diseases.*

American Council on Science and Health. (April 1988). *Answers about AIDS, 6th ed.,* pp. 38–40.

American Diabetes Association. (1993). *Nutrition and insulin-dependent diabetes.*

American Diabetes Association. (1989). *Exchange lists for meal planning.*

American Diabetes Association. (1989). *What is insulin-dependent diabetes?*

American Diabetes Association. (1989). *What is non-insulin-dependent diabetes?*

American Heart Association. (1985). *The American heart association diet: An eating plan for healthy Americans.*

American Heart Association. (1989). *Cholesterol and your heart.*

American Heart Association. (1989). *Heart attack.*

American Heart Association. (1989). *Heart attack and stroke: Signals and action.*

American Heart Association. (1988). *Fact sheet on heart attack, stroke, and risk factors.*

American Heart Association. (1985). *What you should know about PTCA.*

American Heart Association. (1979). *Your heart and how it works.*

American Heart Association. (1973). *The heart and blood vessels.*

American Liver Foundation. (N.D.). *Viral hepatitis: Everybody's problem?* pp. 1–3

American Lung Association. (1992). *Childhood asthma: A matter of control.*

American Lung Association. (1992). *Facts about . . . Home control of allergies and asthma.*

American Lung Association. (1991). *Facts in brief about lung disease.*

American Lung Association. (1990). *Facts about . . . Emphysema.*

American Lung Association. (July 1979). *Lung cancer.*

American Lung Association. (1977). *What everyone should know about asthma.*

American National Red Cross. (November 1988). *Children, parents, and AIDS.*

439

American National Red Cross. (November 1988). *Men, sex, and AIDS.*

American National Red Cross. (November 1988). *Teenagers and AIDS.*

American National Red Cross. (November 1988). *Your job and AIDS: Are there risks?*

American Parkinson Disease Association, Inc. (N.D.). *Basic information about Parkinson's disease.*

American Social Health Association. (1990). *Some questions and answers about chlamydia.*

American Social Health Association. (1986). *Some questions and answers about HIV infections and AIDS.*

American Social Health Association. (1983). *Some questions and answers about herpes.*

American Social Health Association. (1983). *Women and VD.*

Anorexia Nervosa and Related Eating Disorders, Inc. (1992). *Eating and exercise disorders.*

Arbetter, S. (March 1989). Eating disorders: Emotional food fights. *Current Health 2.*

Arthritis Foundation. (1993). *Rheumatoid arthritis.*

Arthritis Foundation. (1990). *Basic facts: Answers to your questions.*

Arthritis Foundation. (1990). *Osteoarthritis.*

Arthritis Foundation. (1988). *Arthritis: A serious look at the facts.*

Arthritis Foundation. (1987). *Arthritis: Medical information series: Rheumatoid arthritis.*

Association for Retarded Citizens. (March 1991). *Down syndrome.*

Barnett, C. & Funnell, M. (1987). *Life with diabetes: Diabetes defined.* Ann Arbor, MI: Michigan Diabetes Research Center, University of Michigan, pp. 15–17.

Beaser, R., Weir, G., & Hill, J. (January/February 1991). Diabetes research update. *Diabetes in the News 10.*

Berger, T., Obuch, M. L., & Goldschmidt, R. H. (June 1990). Dermatologic manifestations of HIV infections. *American Family Physician* 41, no. 6, 1,737–1,738.

Black, P. (June 21, 1993). Demystifying multiple sclerosis. *Business Week Magazine,* p. 166.

Blakeslee, S. (November 12, 1991). Fetal cell transplants show early promise in Parkinson patients. *The New York Times.*

BM Publications. (1989). *Home Emergency Guide.*

Brody, J. (Wednesday, November 23, 1983). A disease afflicting the mind. *The New York Times.*

Browder, S. (November 3, 1992). Mammograms. *Woman's Day Magazine.*

Busse, W. W. (May/June 1990). *What is asthma?* Advance Plus: Asthma and Allergy Foundation of America.

California Medical Association. (March 1991). Acquired immunodeficiency syndrome (AIDS): An overview. *Health Tips.*

California Medical Association. (March 1991). AIDS transmission: The risk of acquiring AIDS. *Health Tips.*

California Medical Association. (March 1991). Children and AIDS. *Health Tips.*

California Medical Association. (March 1991). Women and AIDS. *Health Tips.*

California Medical Association. (June 1989). Muscular dystrophies. *Health Tip Index* 362.

Cancer prevention: Foods, lifestyles, and medical care to keep you healthy. By the Editors of *Prevention Magazine Health Books.*

Center for Digestive Disorders. (March 1980). *Ulcerative colitis.*

Centers for Disease Control. (N.D.). HIV/AIDS prevention: Facts about HIV/AIDS and Race/Ethnicity.

Centers for Disease Control. (N.D.). How you won't get AIDS.

Centers for Disease Control. (1993). HIV/AIDS prevention: Facts about adolescents and HIV/AIDS.

Centers for Disease Control. (1993). HIV/AIDS prevention: Facts about the scope of the HIV/AIDS epidemic in the United States.

Centers for Disease Control. (1993). HIV/AIDS prevention: Facts about women and HIV/AIDS.

Centers for Disease Control. (1993). HIV infection and AIDS: Are you at risk?

Centers for Disease Control. (1991). Voluntary HIV counseling and testing: Facts, issues, and answers.

Centers for Disease Control. (1986). *Chronic disease reports: Deaths from lung cancer—United States.*

Channing L. Bete Co., Inc. (1972). *What everyone should know about arthritis, America's most crippling disease.*

Christman, C. & Bennett, J. (January 1987). Diabetes: New names, new test, new diet. *Nursing 87,* pp. 34–41.

Clayman, C. (editor). (1989). Pneumonia. *American Medical Association Encyclopedia of Medicine.* New York: Random House.

Clode, T. (March 1993). Chlamydia: The silent disease that has everyone talking. *Human Sexuality Supplement to Current Health 2.*

College of Pharmacy, S.D.S.U. (1977). *Bronchial asthma.*

Cote, L. & Sprinzeles, L. (N.D.). *The Parkinson patient at home.* Parkinson's Disease Foundation.

Crohn's and Colitis Foundation. (N.D.). *IBD and the emotions: Is There a Connection?*

Crohn's and Colitis Foundation. (1993). *Questions and answers about complications.*

Crohn's and Colitis Foundation. (1993). *Questions and answers about Crohn's disease and ulcerative colitis.*

Dahl, L. (January 1993). Cerebral palsy. *The Pacesetter.* p. 11.

Daum, M. (N.D.). *Nutrition and inflammatory bowel disease.* Crohn's and Colitis Foundation.

Dennison, R. (April 1986). Cardiopulmonary assessment: How to do it. *Nursing 86.*

Department of Health, Education, and Welfare. (1976). *Sexually transmitted diseases.*

Department of Health and Human Services. (N.D.). *Condoms and sexually transmitted diseases . . . especially AIDS.*

Department of Health and Human Services. (May 1992). *Questions and answers about breast lumps.*

Department of Health and Human Services. (August 1992). *Sexually transmitted diseases.*

Department of Health and Human Services. (September 1992). *Noninsulin-dependent diabetes.*

Department of Health and Human Services. (November 1992). *Breast exams: What you should know.*

Department of Health and Human Services. (1992). *Preventing HIV and AIDS: What you can do.*

Department of Health and Human Services. (January 1990). *Diabetes overview.* National Institute of Diabetes and Digestive Kidney Diseases.

Department of Health and Human Services. (January 1990). *Smart advice for women 40 and over: Have a mammogram.*

Department of Health and Human Services. (March 1990). *Questions and answers about breast lumps.*

Department of Health and Human Services. (April 1990). *Insulin-dependent diabetes.*

Department of Health and Human Services. (October 1990). *Diabetes in adults.*

Department of Health and Human Services. (1990). *Surgeon General's report on acquired immune deficiency syndrome.* C. Everett Koop.

Department of Health and Human Services. (January 1989). *The diabetes dictionary.*

Department of Health and Human Services. (September 1987). *Diet, nutrition, and cancer prevention: The good news.*

Department of Health and Human Services. (1986). *Coping with AIDS: Psychological and social considerations in helping people with HTLV-III infection.*

Department of Health and Human Services. (1986). *Surgeon General's report on acquired immune deficiency syndrome.* C. Everett Koop.

Department of Health and Human Services. (October 1984). *Breast cancer: Understanding treatment options.*

Department of Health and Human Services and National Cancer Institute. (January 1985). *Research report: Hodgkin's disease and the non-Hodgkin's lymphomas.*

Diabetes mellitus. (1990). *Mosby's Medical, Nursing, and Allied Health Dictionary, 3rd edition.* St. Louis: pp. 361–362.

Diabetes Update. (October 1990). *Nursing 90,* pp. 49–51.

Dorros, S. & Dorros, D. (N.D.). *Patient perspectives on Parkinson's.* National Parkinson Foundation.

Drug to treat spasticity available under treatment IND. (June 1990). *FDA Consumer.*

Eaton Laboratories. (N.D.). *Coming back.*

Eggland, E. (January 1987). Teaching the ABCs of COPD. *Nursing 87,* pp. 60–64.

Eli Lilly and Company. (1990). *Glucagon emergency kit.*

Facts about Down syndrome for women over 35. *Obstetrics and Gynecology.*

Faulk, D. (N.D.). *Sensible nutrition helps in managing ileitis, colitis.* Center for Digestive Disorders.

Fisons Corporation. (1992). *Asthma: What every parent should know.*

Freese, A. (1979). *Stroke: New approaches to prevention and treatment.* Public Affairs Pamphlet No. 576.

Gable, C. (December 12, 1990). Pneumoccal vaccine: Efficacy and associated cost savings. *Journal of the American Medical Association* 264.

Garrett, J. (1988). The AIDS patient: Helping him and his parents cope. *Nursing 88,* pp. 50–52.

Glanze, W. D., Anderson, K. N., & Anderson, L. E. (eds.). (1990). Computed tomography (CT). In *Mosby's Medical, Nursing, and Allied Health Dictionary.*

Guiteras, P. (March 1991). What you should know about . . . The alphabet of hepatitis. *Executive Health Report.*

Hahn, K. (September 1987). Left vs. right: What a difference the side makes in stroke. *Nursing 87,* pp. 44–47.

Hahn, K. (April 1987). Slow-teaching the COPD patient. *Nursing 87,* pp. 34–41.

Hernandez, P. (October 31, 1982). The secret food obsession that afflicts one in five young women: Bulimia. *San Francisco Examiner and Chronicle.*

High blood pressure: The silent killer. (January 1993). Condensed report from the Fifth Report of the Joint National Committee on the Detection, Evaluation, and Treatment of High Blood Pressure, National Institutes of Health, National Heart, Lung, and Blood Institute. *Be Stroke Smart Newsletter* published by the National Stroke Association.

Holland, L. (N.D.). *The ABCs of hepatitis.*

How to handle hypertension. (September 1989). *The Johns Hopkins Medical Letter.*

Hughes, B. (May 1987). Diabetes management. *Nursing 87,* pp. 63–64.

Hypertension: How effective are nondrug therapies? (February 1990). *Consumers Reports Health Letter* 2.

Institute For Advanced Studies in Immunology and Aging. (1993). *A town forum on Alzheimer's disease: Exploring the progress and the future of medical research.*

Irwin, M. (1986). *AIDS: Fears and facts.*

James, J. (1985). *The herpes perplex.* Do It Now Foundation.

Jess, L. (March 1992). Chronic bronchitis and emphysema: Airing the differences. *Nursing 92*, pp. 34–41.

Juvenile Diabetes Foundation. (December 1990). *Information about insulin.*

Karlasberg, E. (December 1992). I have an eating disorder. *TEEN Magazine*, pp. 96–98.

Kazilimani, E. (Winter 1990). The precautions of prenatal testing. *Priorities.*

Kee, J. L. (1983). *Laboratory and diagnostic tests with nursing implications.* Prentice-Hall Company.

Keesey, J. C. (N.D.). *A practical guide to: Myasthenia gravis.*

Klein, D. M. (July 1988). Angina. *Nursing 88.*

Know the warning signs of stroke. (1991). Syntex Laboratories Inc.

Konradi, D. & Stockert, P. (June 1989). A close-up look at leukemia. *Nursing 89.*

Kushner, I. (N.D.). *Understanding Arthritis.* Chapter 11: Rheumatoid Arthritis, pp. 126–133.

Levy, D. & Pollard, T. (December 1988). Failure of the heart. *Emergency Magazine.*

Lieberman, A. N., Gopinathan, G., Neophytides, A., & Goldstein, M. (N.D.). *Parkinson's disease handbook: A guide for patients and their families.* American Parkinson Disease Association Inc.

Lifson, A. (March 4, 1988). Do alternate modes for transmission of human immunodeficiency virus exist? *Journal of the American Medical Association* 259, no. 9, pp. 1,353–1,356.

Light For the Way Inc. (1984). *An introduction to your child who has Down syndrome.*

Link, M. (April 1993). Living with leukemia. *Current Health 2.*

Lippincott Manual of Nursing Practice, 2nd edition. (1978). J. B. Lippincott Company.

Lippincott Manual of Nursing Practice, 5th edition. (1991). J.B. Lippincott Company.

Lombard, J. (N.D.). *Handy, helpful hints . . . For independent living after stroke.* National Easter Seal Society.

Lumpectomy vs. mastectomy. (October 1990). *Consumer Reports Health Letters.*

March of Dimes Birth Defects Foundation. (1993). Public Health Education Information Sheet. *Down syndrome.*

March of Dimes Birth Defects Foundation. (1992). *Genital herpes.*

March of Dimes Birth Defects Foundation. (October 1984). *Sexually transmitted diseases.*

Marion Laboratories Inc. (1973). *TIAs . . . The early warning system of impending stroke: A physician learning system.*

Marx, J. (January 1993). Viral hepatitis: Unscrambling the alphabet. *Nursing 93*, pp. 34–41.

McGriff, S. (May 1989). *Learning to live with neuromuscular disease: A message for parents.*

Memmier, R., Cohen, B., & Wood, D. (1992). *The human body in health and diseases, 7th edition.* J. B. Lippincott Company.

Merck and Co. Inc. (December 4–6, 1992). What every man should know about his prostate. *USA Weekend*, pp. 10–11.

Merki, M. (1993). *AIDS and society.* Teacher's Annotated Edition. Macmillan/McGraw-Hill School Publishing Company.

Merck Sharp and Dohme. (N.D.). *The Parkinson's patient: What you and your family should know.*

Miller, B. & Keane, C. (1972). *Encyclopedia and dictionary of medicine and nursing.* W. B. Saunders Company.

Miracle, V. (January 1988). Understanding the different types of MI. *Nursing 88.*

Muscular Dystrophy Association. (May 1990). *Facts about muscular dystrophy.*

National Cancer Institute. (1990). *Cancer of the prostate: Research report.*

National Cancer Institute. (November 1989). *What you need to know about lung cancer.*

National Cancer Institute. (1989). *Cancer of the lung: Research report.*

National Cancer Institute. (January 1988). *What you need to know about breast cancer.*

National Cancer Institute. (March 1988). *Cancer of the colon and rectum: Research report.*

National Digestive Diseases Information Clearinghouse. (October 1989). *Ulcerative colitis.*

National Down Syndrome Congress. (N.D.). *Facts about Down syndrome.*

National Down Syndrome Congress. (1988). *Down syndrome.*

National Easter Seal Society for Crippled Children and Adults. (1979). *Understanding stroke.*

National Eye Institute. (November 1990). *Diabetic retinopathy.*

National Heart, Lung, and Blood Institute. (1987). *Facts about coronary artery bypass surgery.*

National Institute of Aging. (1992). *Progress report on Alzheimer's disease.*

National Institute of Allergy and Infectious Diseases. (June 1992). *Chlamydial Infection.*

National Institute of Allergy and Infectious Diseases. (June 1992). *Genital herpes.*

National Institute of Allergy and Infectious Diseases. (June 1992). *Hepatitis.*

National Institute of Allergy and Infectious Diseases. (June 1992). *HIV infection and AIDS.*

National Institute of Allergy and Infectious Diseases. (June 1992). *Syphilis.*

National Institute of Allergy and Infectious Diseases. (April 1991). *Allergic diseases.*

National Institute of Child Health and Human Development. (1984). *Facts about Down syndrome,* pp. 1–3.

National Institutes of Health: National Institute of Mental Health. (January 1993). *Eating disorders.*

National Institute of Neurological Disorders and Stroke. (June 1983). *Parkinson's disease: Hope through research.* NIH Pub. No. 83-139.

National Institute on Drug Abuse. (March 1991). Treating Eating Disorders. *Employee Assistance.*

National Jewish Center for Immunology and Respiratory Medicine. (1985). *Understanding asthma.*

National Jewish Center for Immunology and Respiratory Medicine. (1985). *Understanding immunology.*

National Multiple Sclerosis Society. (1988). *What is multiple sclerosis?*

National Myasthenia Gravis Foundation. (N.D.). *Mestinon.*

National Parkinson Foundation. (N.D.). *The Parkinson handbook: A guide for Parkinson patients and their families.*

National Stroke Association. (1993). *Stroke: Reducing your risk.*

Newman, J. (March 1992). HBV: Overshadowed by AIDS. *Emergency,* p. 62.

Nutrition notes. (March 1990). *Diabetes Forecast*

Parkinson's Disease Foundation. (N.D.). *Exercises for the Parkinson patient with hints for daily living.*

Parkinson's Disease Foundation. (1992). *Progress, promise, and hope!*

Parkinson's disease: New hope on the horizon. (September 1990). *The University of Texas Lifetime Health Letter 2,* No. 9.

Parys, E. (Feburary 1987). Assessing the failing state of the heart. *Nursing 87,* pp. 42–49.

Patlak, M. (July/August 1989). The puzzling picture of multiple sclerosis. *FDA Consumer.*

Peppers, M. (March 1992). Viral vaccines. *Emergency,* pp. 23–25.

Petty, T. & Nett, L. (July 1991). *Save your breath, America.*

Pharmaceutical Manufacturers Association. (1993). *New medicines in development for older Americans.*

Pharmacia Laboratories. (1978). *Ulcerative colitis and Crohn's disease.*

Phillips, E. (July 20, 1993). Just tired or are you really sick? *Woman's Day Magazine,* pp. 31, 39.

Pneumococcal vaccine. (March 1991). *Medical Update 14.*

Professional Guide to Diseases, 3rd edition. (1989). Springhouse Corporation.

Prostate cancer: What it is and how it is treated. (1993). Zeneca Pharmaceuticals.

Quinless, F. (October 1990). Myocardial infarction. *Nursing 90.*

Rees, A. M. & Willey, C. (eds). (N.D.). *Personal Health Reporter.*

Reinke, L. F. & Hoffman, L. A. (October 1992). How to teach asthma co-management. *American Journal of Nursing.*

Romanik, K. (1992). *Around the clock with COPD.* American Lung Association.

Sachar, D. (December 1985). *Inflammatory bowel disease.* National Digestive Diseases Education and Information Clearinghouse.

Samonds, R. J. & Cammermeyer, M. (September 1985). The patient with multiple sclerosis. *Nursing 85.*

Scardino, P. T. (November 1989). Early detection of prostate cancer. *Urologic Clinics of North America 16,* no. 4.

Schroeder, S., et al. (editors). (1992). *Current medical diagnosis and treatment 1991.* Norwalk, CT: Appleton and Lange.

Schumacher, H. (1988). *Primer on the rheumatic diseases.* American Arthritis Foundation.

Sioux Valley Hospital, Sioux Falls, SD. (N.D.). *Eating disorder program criteria for hospitalization.*

Sioux Valley Hospital, Sioux Falls, SD. (1988). *Eating disorders study guide: Anorexia nervosa and bulimia nervosa.*

South Dakota Department of Health. (N.D.). *Sexually transmitted diseases and you!!*

South Dakota Department of Health. (April 1993). *HIV/AIDS surveillance report.*

Spence, W.R. (1991). AIDS: What you don't know can kill you.

Steiner-Grossman, P., ed. (1993). *Questions and answers about surgery in Crohn's disease.* Crohn's and Colitis Foundation.

Stroke (cerebrovascular accident). *Home Health Handbook.* Group 7, Card 66.

Susan G. Komen Breast Cancer Foundation. (1992). *Caring for your breasts.*

Taber's Cyclopedic Medical Dictionary. (1993). Edited by Clayton L. Thomas. F.A. Davis Company.

Taylor, L. & Taylor, L. (1989). *Fundamentals of nursing.* Lippincott Company.

Thibodeau, G. & Parker-Anthony, C. (1988). *Structure and function of the body.* Times Mirror/Mosby College Publishing.

Thompson, McFarland, Hirsch, Tucker, & Bowers. (1986). *Clinical Nursing.* C. V. Mosby Company.

Trottier, D. J. & Kochar, M. S. (November 1992). Hypertension and high cholesterol: A dangerous synergy. *American Journal of Nursing.*

United States Department of Health and Human Services. (N.D.). *Alzheimer's disease: Fact sheet.*

United States Department of Health and Human Services. (March 1990). *What you need to know about asthma.*

United States Department of Health and Human Services. (October 1981). *How to cope with arthritis.*

Upjohn Company. (1976). *You and diabetes.*

Weinhouse, B. (July 21, 1992). The asthma explosion. *Family Circle Magazine,* pp. 55–58.

Weiss, J. (N.D.). *A practical approach to the emotions of asthma.* American Lung Association.

West, D., et al. (June 1990). Vaccination of infants and children against hepatitis B. *Pediatric Clinics of North America 37,* no. 3.

What every man should know about his prostate. (N.D.). Merck Pharmaceuticals.

Wilson, J., et al. (editors). (1991). *Pneumocystis carinii pneumonia.* In *Harrison's Principles of Internal Medicine, 12th edition.* New York: McGraw-Hill, pp. 799–800.

Wong, D. & Whaley, L. (1990). *Clinical manual of pediatric nursing.* C. V. Mosby Company.

Zamula, E. (1990). *Childhood asthma.* Department of Health and Human Services.

Index